current procedural terminology

cpt® 2009
Changes
An insider's view

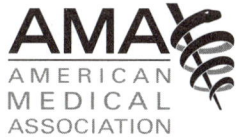
AMERICAN MEDICAL ASSOCIATION

American Medical Association
Executive Vice President, Chief Executive Officer: Michael D. Maves, MD, MBA
Chief Operating Officer: Bernard L. Hengesbaugh
Senior Vice President, Publishing and Business Services: Robert A. Musacchio, PhD
Vice President and General Manager, Publishing: Frank J. Krause
Publisher, Physician Practice Solutions: Jay T. Ahlman
Vice President, Business Operations: Vanessa Hayden
Director, CPT Product Development: Dan Reyes
Director, Production and Manufacturing: Jean Roberts
Director, Business Marketing and Communication: Pam Palmersheim
Manager, Marketing and Strategic Planning: Erin Kalitowski
Director of Sales, Business Products: J. D. Kinney
Director of Coding Editorial and Regulatory Services: Marie Mindeman
Senior Coding Specialists: Mary O'Heron, Desiree Rozell, Lianne Stancik, and DeHandro Hayden
Coding Specialists: Peggy Thompson and Ada Walker
RBRVS Data and Methods Manager: Todd Klemp
Developmental Editor: Elizabeth Kennedy
Production Manager: Rosalyn Carlton
Senior Print Production Specialist: Ronnie Summers
Marketing Manager: Leigh Adams

© 2008 American Medical Association
All rights reserved.
Printed in the United States of America.

Current Procedural Terminology (CPT®) copyright 1966, 1970, 1973, 1977, 1981, 1983–2008, American Medical Association. All rights reserved.

CPT is a registered trademark of the American Medical Association.

www.ama-assn.org

No part of this publication may be reproduced, stored in a retrieval system, transmitted in any form, or by any means, electronic, mechanical, photocopying, recording, or otherwise, without prior written permission of the publisher.

For information regarding the reprinting or licensing of *CPT® Changes 2009: An Insider's View*, please contact:

CPT Intellectual Property Services
American Medical Association
515 N. State St.
Chicago, IL 60654
312 464-5022

Additional copies of this book may be ordered by calling: 800 621-8335 or from the secure AMA Web site at www.amabookstore.com. Refer to product number OP512909.

This book is intended for information purposes only. It is not intended to constitute legal advice. If legal advice is desired or needed, a licensed attorney should be consulted.

ISBN: 978-1-60359-059-4
AC34:08-P-004:11/08

Contents

Foreword vii

Using This Book ix
    The Symbols ix
    The Rationale ix
    Reading the Clinical Examples x
    The Tabular Review of the Changes x
    CPT Codebook Text and Guidelines x

Introduction 1

Evaluation and Management 5
    Evaluation and Management (E/M) Services Guidelines 7
    Hospital Inpatient Services 7
    Critical Care Services 8
    Prolonged Services 10
    Case Management Services 12
    Preventive Medicine Services 12
    Newborn Care Services 14
    Inpatient Neonatal Intensive Care Services and
    Pediatric and Neonatal Critical Care Services 17
    Initial and Continuing Intensive Care Services 23

Anesthesia 25
    Head 27
    Thorax (Chest Wall and Shoulder Girdle) 29
    Other Procedures 35

Surgery 37
    General 39
    Integumentary System 39
    Musculoskeletal System 44
    Respiratory System 58
    Cardiovascular System 59
    Digestive System 72
    Urinary System 89
    Male Genital System 91
    Female Genital System 93

    Nervous System 94

    Eye and Ocular Adnexa. 110

    Operating Microscope 113

Radiology 115

    Diagnostic Radiology (Diagnostic Imaging) 117

    Diagnostic Ultrasound 117

    Radiologic Guidance 118

    Breast, Mammography 119

    Bone/Joint Studies 119

    Radiation Oncology 120

    Nuclear Medicine 123

Pathology and Laboratory 125

    Organ or Disease-Oriented Panels 127

    Evocative/Suppression Testing 128

    Chemistry 129

    Hematology and Coagulation 133

    Immunology 134

    Microbiology 134

    In Vivo (eg, Transcutaneous) Laboratory Procedures 136

Medicine 137

    Immune Globulins 139

    Immunization Administration for Vaccines/Toxoids 139

    Vaccines, Toxoids 139

    Biofeedback 142

    Dialysis 142

    Gastroenterology 159

    Ophthalmology 160

    Special Otorhinolaryngologic Services 160

    Audiologic Function Tests 160

    Cardiovascular 161

    Pulmonary 195

    Allergy and Clinical Immunology 195

    Endocrinology 196

Neurology and Neuromuscular Procedures	197
Health and Behavior Assessment/Intervention	200

Category II Codes **207**
    Composite Codes 209
    Structural Measures 252

Category III Codes **255**
    Remote Real-Time Interactive Videoconferenced Critical Care Services 266

Appendices **277**
    Appendix A 279
    Appendix H 280

Tabular Review of the Changes **285**

Foreword

The American Medical Association is pleased to offer *CPT® Changes 2009: An Insider's View*. Since this book was first published in 2000, it has served as the definitive text on additions, revisions, and deletions to the CPT code set.

In developing this book, it was our intention to provide CPT users with a glimpse of the logic, rationale, and proposed function of CPT changes that resulted from the decisions of the CPT Editorial Panel and the yearly update process. American Medical Association (AMA) staff members have the unique perspective of being both participants in the CPT editorial process and users of the CPT code set. *CPT Changes* is intended to bridge understanding between clinical decisions made at the CPT Editorial Panel regarding appropriate service or procedure descriptions, with functional interpretations of coding guidelines, code intent, and code combinations necessary for users of the CPT code set. A new edition of this book, like the codebook, is published annually.

To assist CPT users in applying new and revised CPT codes, this book includes clinical examples that describe the typical patient who might receive the procedure and detailed descriptions of the procedure. Both of these are required as a part of the CPT code change proposal process and are used by the CPT Editorial Panel in crafting language, guidelines, and parenthetical notes associated with the new or revised codes. In addition, many of the clinical examples and descriptions of the procedures are used in the AMA/Specialty Society RVS Update process for conducting surveys on physician work and in developing work relative value recommendations to the Centers for Medicare and Medicaid Services (CMS) as part of the Medicare Physician Fee Schedule (MPFS).

We are confident that the information contained in *CPT Changes* each year will prove to be a valuable resource to CPT users not only as they apply changes for the year of publication but also as a resource for frequent reference as they continue their education in CPT coding. The AMA makes every effort to be a voice of clarity and consistency in an otherwise confusing system of health care claims and payment, and *CPT Changes 2009: An Insider's View* demonstrates our continued commitment to assist users of the CPT code set.

Using This Book

This book is designed to serve as a reference guide to understanding the changes contained in *Current Procedural Terminology (CPT®) 2009* and is not intended to replace the CPT codebook. Every effort is made to ensure accuracy; however, if differences exist, you should always defer to the information contained in the CPT codebook for 2009.

The Symbols

This book uses the same coding conventions that appear in the CPT nomenclature.

- ● Indicates that a new procedure number was added to the CPT nomenclature

- ▲ Indicates that a code revision has resulted in a substantially altered procedure descriptor

- ✚ Indicates a CPT add-on code

- ⊘ Indicates a code that is exempt from the use of modifier 51 but is not designated as a CPT add-on procedure/service

- ►◄ Indicate revised guidelines, cross-references, and/or explanatory text

- ⊙ Indicates a code that typically includes moderate sedation

- ⁄ Indicates a code for a vaccine that is pending FDA approval

- ○ Indicates a reinstated or recycled code

Whenever possible, complete segments of text from the CPT codebook are provided; however, in some cases, the text has been abbreviated.

The Rationale

After each change or series of changes is a rationale. The rationale is intended to provide a brief explanation as to why changes occurred but may not answer every question that may arise as a result of the changes.

Reading the Clinical Examples

The clinical examples and their procedural descriptions included in this text with many of the codes give practical situations for which the new and/or revised codes in the *CPT 2009* codebook would be appropriately reported. It is important to note that these examples do not suggest limiting the use of a code but only represent the typical patient and service or procedure. They do not describe the universe of patients for whom the service or procedure would be appropriate. In addition, third-party payer reporting policies may differ.

The Tabular Review of the Changes

The table beginning on page 275 allows you to see all of the code changes at a glance. By reviewing the table you can easily determine the level to which your particular field of interest has been affected by the changes in *CPT 2009*.

CPT Codebook Text and Guidelines

In *CPT Changes 2009*, guideline and revised CPT codebook text appears in brown indented type. Any revised text, guidelines, and/or headings are indicated with the ►◄ symbols. This convention in *CPT Changes 2009* differs slightly from the CPT codebook. Within the codebook, symbols are placed at the beginning and end of a paragraph that contains a revision or revisions. *CPT Changes 2009* offers readers a more detailed view of the changes to the codes and guidelines. In this book, the revision symbols (►◄) are placed around each specific change.

Introduction

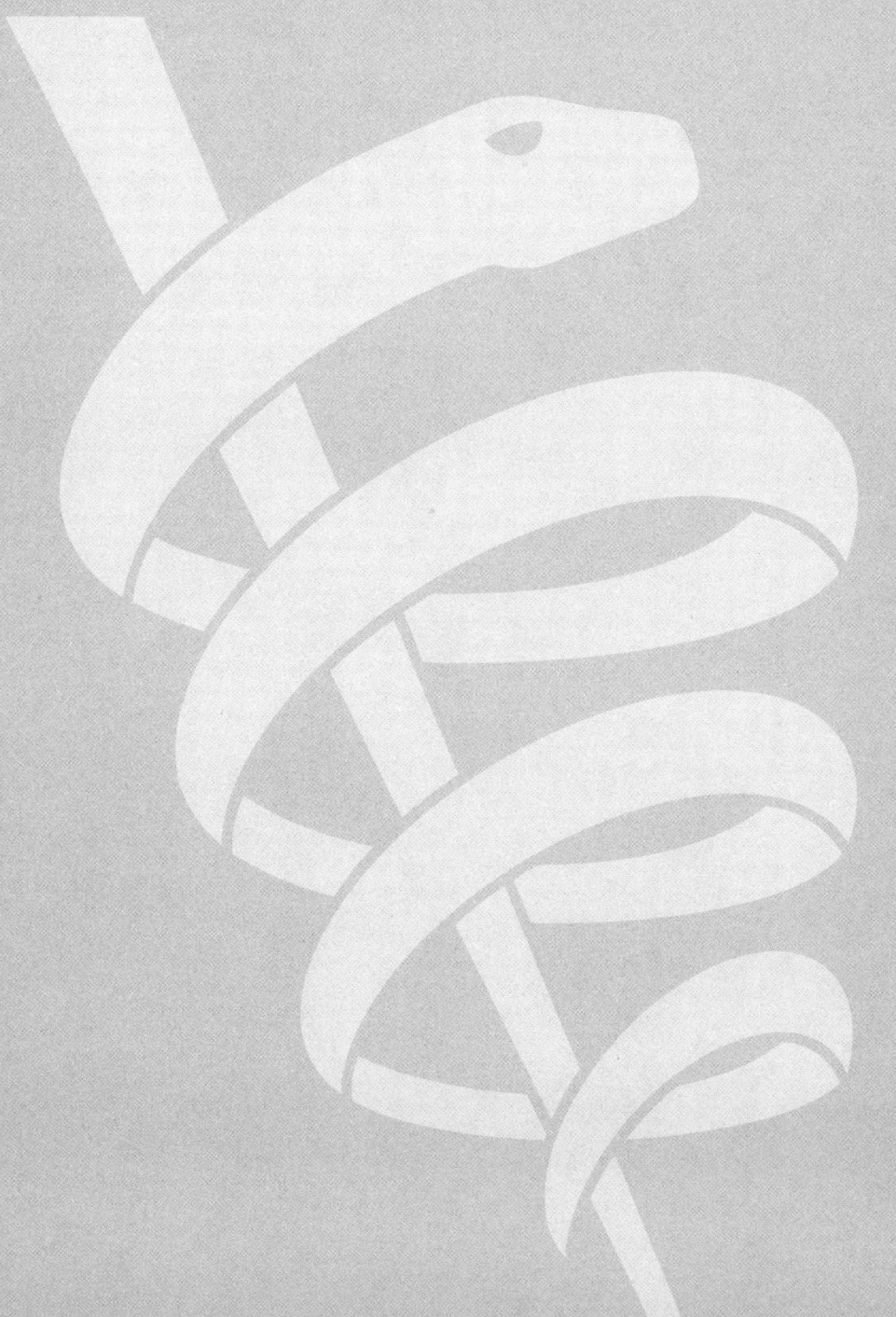

Introduction

Current Procedural Terminology (CPT®), Fourth . . .

Inclusion of a descriptor and its associated . . .

The CPT code set is published annually in the late summer or early fall as both electronic data files and books. The release of CPT data files on the Internet typically precedes the book by several weeks. In any case, January 1 is the effective date for use of the update of the CPT code set. The interval between the release of the update and the effective date is considered the implementation period and is intended to allow physicians and other providers, payers, and vendors to incorporate CPT changes into their systems. The exceptions to this schedule of release and effective dates are CPT Category III and vaccine product codes, which are released twice a year on January 1 or July 1 with effective dates for use six months later, and CPT Category II codes. ▶Changes to the CPT code set are meant to be applied prospectively from the effective date.◀

The main body of the material is listed in six sections . . .

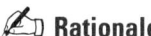 **Rationale**

The Introduction to the CPT codebook has been revised to define the initial date on which application of guidelines are intended to become effective and to also discourage retroactive application of revisions to the text of the CPT codebook.

Evaluation and Management

The revisions of the Evaluation and Management Services section include extensive revisions of all of Pediatric Evaluation and Management services, with renumbering of all of the codes to a new subsection. These revisions include the Pediatric Patient Transport, Inpatient Neonatal and Pediatric Critical Care Services and Newborn Care Services sections. Renumbering of the codes in these sections also results in numerous revisions of the Critical Care Services guidelines.

Evaluation and Management

Evaluation and Management (E/M) Services Guidelines

Definitions of Commonly Used Terms

Certain key words and phrases are used throughout the E/M section. The following definitions are intended to reduce the potential for differing interpretations and to increase the consistency of reporting by physicians in differing specialties. ▶E/M services may also be reported by other qualified health care professionals who are authorized to perform such services within the scope of their practice.◀

🖉 Rationale

The Definitions of Commonly Used Terms included in the Evaluation and Management service guidelines have been revised to include "other qualified health care professionals."

Hospital Inpatient Services

Subsequent Hospital Care

HOSPITAL DISCHARGE SERVICES

99238 **Hospital discharge day management;** 30 minutes or less

99239 more than 30 minutes

(For discharge services provided to newborns admitted and discharged on the same date, use ▶99463◀)

🖉 Rationale

In support of the extensive editorial revisions in the Neonatal and Pediatric Critical Care section, the Pediatric Critical Care Patient Transport, and the Neonatal Critical Care services subsections, the cross-reference following 99239 has been revised to instruct the user to report 99463 for discharge services provided to normal newborns admitted and discharged on the same date.

99288 **Physician direction of** emergency medical systems (EMS) emergency care, advanced life support

▶(99289 has been deleted. To report, use 99466)◀

▶(99290 has been deleted. To report, use 99467)◀

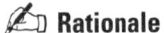 **Rationale**

In tandem with the extensive editorial revisions in the Neonatal and Pediatric Critical Care section, the Pediatric Critical Care Patient Transport section has been deleted, renumbered, and relocated. Two new cross-references have been included to instruct the user to report codes 99466 and 99467 for pediatric critical care services.

Critical Care Services

Critical care is the direct delivery . . .

Providing medical care to a critically . . .

Inpatient critical care services provided to infants 29 days through ▶71◀ months of age are reported with pediatric critical care codes ▶99471-99476◀. The pediatric critical care codes are reported as long as the infant/young child qualifies for critical care services during the hospital stay through ▶71◀ months of age. Inpatient critical care services provided to neonates (28 days of age or less) are reported with the neonatal critical care codes ▶99468◀ and ▶99469◀. The neonatal critical care codes are reported as long as the neonate qualifies for critical care services during the hospital stay through the 28th postnatal day. The reporting of the pediatric and neonatal critical care services is not based on time or the type of unit (eg, pediatric or neonatal critical care unit) and it is not dependent upon the type of provider delivering the care. To report critical care services provided in the outpatient setting (eg, emergency department or office) for neonates and pediatric patients up through ▶71◀ months of age, see the critical care codes 99291, 99292. If the same physician provides critical care services for a neonatal or pediatric patient in both the outpatient and inpatient settings on the same day, report only the appropriate neonatal or pediatric critical care code ▶99468-99472◀ for all critical care services provided on that day. ▶Also report 99291-99292 for neonatal or pediatric critical care services provided by the physician providing critical care at one facility but transferring the patient to another facility. Critical care services provided by a second physician of a different specialty not reporting a per-day neonatal or pediatric critical care code can be reported with codes 99291, 99292.◀ For additional instructions on reporting these services, see the Neonatal and Pediatric Critical Care section and codes ▶99468-99476.◀

Services for a patient who is not critically ill but happens to be in a critical care unit are reported using other appropriate E/M codes.

Critical care and other E/M services . . .

The following services are included in . . .

Codes 99291, 99292 should be reported for the physician's attendance during the transport of critically ill or critically injured patients over 24 months of age to or from a facility or hospital. For physician transport services of critically ill or critically injured pediatric patients 24 months of age or less, see ▶99466, 99467.◀

The critical care codes 99291 and 99292 are used to report the total duration of time spent by a physician providing critical care services to a critically ill or critically injured patient, even if the time spent by the physician on that date is not continuous. For any given period of time spent providing critical care services, the physician must devote his or her full attention to the patient and, therefore, cannot provide services to any other patient during the same period of time.

Time spent with the individual patient should be recorded in the patient's record. The time that can be reported as critical care is the time spent engaged in work directly related to the individual patient's care whether that time was spent at the immediate bedside or elsewhere on the floor or unit. For example, time spent on the unit or at the nursing station on the floor reviewing test results or imaging studies, discussing the critically ill patient's care with other medical staff, or documenting critical care services in the medical record would be reported as critical care, even though it does not occur at the bedside. Also, when the patient is unable or lacks capacity to participate in discussions, time spent on the floor or unit with family members or surrogate decision makers obtaining a medical history, reviewing the patient's condition or prognosis, or discussing treatment or limitation(s) of treatment may be reported as critical care, provided that the conversation bears directly on the management of the patient.

Time spent in activities that occur outside of the unit or off the floor (eg, telephone calls whether taken at home, in the office, or elsewhere in the hospital) may not be reported as critical care since the physician is not immediately available to the patient. Time spent in activities that do not directly contribute to the treatment of the patient may not be reported as critical care, even if they are performed in the critical care unit (eg, participation in administrative meetings or telephone calls to discuss other patients). Time spent performing separately reportable procedures or services should not be included in the time reported as critical care time. ▶No physician may report remote real-time interactive videoconferenced critical care services (0188T, 0189T) for the period in which any physician reports 99291-99292.◀

Code 99291 is used to report . . .

Code 99292 is used to report . . .

 ## Rationale

Revisions to the Critical Care Services section are the result of further clarifications of the Neonatal and Pediatric Critical Care code revisions, which were revised for the CPT® 2009 codebook. With the implementation of these codes for reporting the Pediatric Critical Care Services, this section remained in its current location. The introductory guidelines were further revised to reflect the addition of the pediatric critical care codes by revising the upper age limit to 71 months. Other revisions to the guidelines direct the user to the renumbered pediatric transport codes. Revisions to this section also clarify the use of these codes for the physician in the transferring facility who will not be reporting a full day code with codes 99468, 99469, 99471, and 99472. Instructions have also been added to preclude any physician reporting remote real-time interactive videoconferenced critical care services (0188T, 0189T) during the period in which another physician reports 99291-99292 or a full day neonatal or pediatric critical care code (99293, 99294, 99295 or 99296).

▶(99293 has been deleted. To report, use 99471)◀

▶(99294 has been deleted. To report, use 99472)◀

▶(99295 has been deleted. To report, use 99468)◀

▶(99296 has been deleted. To report, use 99469)◀

Rationale

In tandem with the extensive editorial revisions in the Neonatal and Pediatric Critical Care section, the Inpatient Neonatal and Pediatric Critical Care and Intensive Services subsection has been deleted, renumbered, and relocated. Four new cross-references have been included to instruct the user to report codes 99468, 99469, 99471, and 99472 for inpatient neonatal and pediatric critical care and intensive services.

▶(99298 has been deleted. To report, use 99478)◀

▶(99299 has been deleted. To report, use 99479)◀

▶(99300 has been deleted. To report, use 99480)◀

Rationale

In tandem with the extensive editorial revisions in the Neonatal and Pediatric Critical Care section, the Continuing Intensive Care Services subsection has been deleted, renumbered, and relocated. Three new cross-references have been included to instruct the user to report codes 99478, 99479, and 99480 for continuing intensive care services.

Prolonged Services

Prolonged Physician Service With Direct (Face-to-Face) Patient Contact

Codes 99354-99357 are used when a physician provides prolonged service involving direct (face-to-face) patient contact that is beyond the usual service in either the inpatient or outpatient setting.
▶This service is reported in addition to the designated evaluation and management services at any level and any other physician services provided at the same session as evaluation and management services.◀ Appropriate codes should be selected for supplies provided or procedures performed in the care of the patient during this period.

Codes 99354-▶99355◀ are used to report the total duration of face-to-face time spent by a physician on a given date providing prolonged service, even if the time spent by the physician on that date is not continuous. ▶Codes 99356-99357 are used to report the total duration of unit time spent by a physician on a given date providing prolonged service to a patient, even if the time spent by the physician on that date is not continuous.◀

Code 99354 or 99356 is used to report the first hour of prolonged service on a given date, depending on the place of service.

▶Either code should be used only once per date, even if the time spent by the physician is not continuous on that date. Prolonged service of less than 30 minutes total duration on a given date is not separately reported, because the work involved is included in the total work of the evaluation and management codes.◀

Code 99355 or 99357 is used . . .

▶The use of the time-based add-on codes requires that the primary evaluation and management service have a typical or specified time published in the CPT codebook.◀

The following examples illustrate the correct . . .

Total Duration of Prolonged Services	Code(s)
Less than 30 minutes (less than 1/2 hour)	Not reported separately
30-74 minutes (1/2 hr. – 1 hr. 14 min.)	99354 X 1
75-104 (1 hr. 15 min. – 1 hr. 44 min.)	99354 X 1 AND 99355 X 1
▶105 or more (1 hr. 45 min. or more)◀	99354 X 1 AND 99355 X 2 ▶or more for each additional 30 minutes◀

+▲ 99354   Prolonged physician service in the office or other outpatient setting requiring direct (face-to-face) patient contact beyond the usual service; first hour (List separately in addition to code for office or other outpatient **Evaluation and Management Service**)

(Use 99354 in conjunction with 99201-99215, 99241-99245, ▶99324-99337, 99341-99350, 90809, 90815)◀

+▲ 99355   each additional 30 minutes (List separately in addition to code for prolonged physician service)

(Use 99355 in conjunction with 99354)

+▲ 99356   Prolonged physician service in the inpatient setting, requiring unit/floor time beyond the usual service; first hour (List separately in addition to code for inpatient Evaluation and Management service)

(Use 99356 in conjunction with 99221-99233, 99251-99255, ▶99304-99310, 90822, 90829◀)

+▲ 99357   each additional 30 minutes (List separately in addition to code for prolonged physician service)

(Use 99357 in conjunction with 99356)

🖉 Rationale

The guidelines for the face-to-face outpatient and inpatient prolonged evaluation and management services, reported with codes 99354-99357, have been revised to indicate that these are intended to be reported with evaluation and management services in addition to any other physician services reported at the same session. The guidelines for the outpatient services have been revised to indicate that only the outpatient services are intended to report the total duration of face-to-face time with the patient, while the inpatient codes are intended to report the total duration of the time spent (continuous or non-continuous) by the physician on the unit.

Directions have also been added to instruct that if a time-based add-on code is reported, it can only be used with evaluation and management services codes with typical or specified times included in their descriptors. An abbreviated table of time examples has been revised for clarity. The referenced codes in the parenthetical instructions following codes 99354 and 99356 have been revised to reflect appropriate services (psychotherapy with medical evaluation and management) and sites of services (inpatient nursing facility services) for these categories.

These services should not be reported in addition to the team conference services (99366-99368), telephone (99441-99443), or other non-face-to-face services.

Physician Standby Services

99360 **Physician standby service,** requiring prolonged . . .

(99360 may be reported in addition to ▶99460, 99465◀ as appropriate)

(Do not report 99360 in conjunction with ▶99464◀)

 Rationale
In support of the extensive editorial revisions in the Neonatal and Pediatric Critical Care section, the cross-references following code 99360 have been revised to instruct the user to report code 99360 in conjunction with codes 99460 and 99465 for physician standby services. As indicated in the exclusionary parenthetical note, code 99360 should not be reported with code 99464.

Case Management Services

Anticoagulant Management

Anticoagulant services are intended to describe . . .

When reporting these services, the work of anticoagulant . . .

These services are outpatient services only. When anticoagulation therapy is initiated or continued in the inpatient or observation setting, a new period begins after discharge and is reported with 99364. Do not report 99363-99364 with 99217-99239, 99291, ▶99292◀, 99304-99318, ▶99471-99480◀, or other code(s) for physician review, interpretation, and patient management of home INR (International Normalized Ration) prothrombin testing for a patient with mechanical heart valve(s).

 Rationale
In support of the extensive editorial revisions in the Neonatal and Pediatric Critical Care section, the Anticoagulant Management subsection guidelines have been revised to delete code 99300 and include code 99292. As indicated in the exclusionary parenthetical note, codes 99471-99480 should not be reported with codes 99363 and 99364.

Preventive Medicine Services

▶Vaccine/toxoid products, immunization administrations,◀ ancillary studies involving laboratory, radiology, other procedures, or screening tests ▶(eg, vision, hearing, developmental)◀ identified with a specific CPT code are reported separately. For immunization administration ▶and vaccine risk/benefit counseling,◀ see 90465-90474. ▶For vaccine/toxoid products, see 90476-90749.◀

NEW PATIENT

▲ **99381** **Initial comprehensive preventive medicine** evaluation and management of an individual including an age and gender appropriate history, examination, counseling/anticipatory guidance/risk factor reduction interventions, and the ordering of laboratory/diagnostic procedures, new patient; infant (age younger than 1 year)

▲ **99382** early childhood (age 1 through 4 years)

▲ **99383** late childhood (age 5 through 11 years)

▲ **99384** adolescent (age 12 through 17 years)

▲ **99385** 18-39 years

▲ **99386** 40-64 years

▲ **99387** 65 years and older

ESTABLISHED PATIENT

▲ **99391** **Periodic comprehensive preventive medicine** reevaluation and management of an individual including an age and gender appropriate history, examination, counseling/anticipatory guidance/ risk factor reduction interventions, and the ordering of laboratory/diagnostic procedures, established patient; infant (age younger than 1 year)

▲ **99392** early childhood (age 1 through 4 years)

▲ **99393** late childhood (age 5 through 11 years)

▲ **99394** adolescent (age 12 through 17 years)

▲ **99395** 18-39 years

▲ **99396** 40-64 years

▲ **99397** 65 years and older

Rationale

The last paragraph of the introductory language for the Preventive Medicine Services section has been revised to distinguish between the two groups of codes required to report immunizations (ie, vaccine/toxoid product and immunization administrations), which are to be separately reported when performed in conjunction with a preventive medicine service. Also, for clarification, examples of the types of screening tests that may be separately reported in addition to a preventive medicine service have been added to include vision, hearing, and developmental tests. The term *toxoid* was added to the reference listing the vaccine product codes 90476-90749.

Codes 99381 and 99391 were revised to exclude reference to immunization services. These services are separately reportable, as indicated in the introductory language that directs the use of codes 90465-90474 for immunization administration and vaccine risk/benefit counseling and codes 90476-90749 for reporting vaccine/toxoid products.

Counseling Risk Factor Reduction and Behavior Change Intervention

NEW OR ESTABLISHED PATIENT

These codes are used to report . . .

Preventive medicine counseling and risk factor . . .

Behavior change interventions are for persons . . .

For counseling groups of patients with . . .

▶Health and Behavior Assessment/Intervention services (96150-96155) should not be reported on the same day.◀

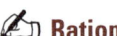 Rationale

The Counseling Risk Factor Reduction and Behavior Change Intervention guidelines have been revised to indicate that the entire series of codes for Health and Behavior Assessment/Intervention services (96150-96155) consists of similar services and should not be separately reported with codes 99401-99412.

99429   **Unlisted preventive** medicine services

▶(99431 has been deleted. To report, use 99460)◀

▶(99432 has been deleted. To report, use 99461)◀

▶(99433 has been deleted. To report, use 99462)◀

▶(99435 has been deleted. To report, use 99463)◀

▶(99436 has been deleted. To report, use 99464)◀

▶(99440 has been deleted. To report, use 99465)◀

Rationale

To support the extensive editorial revisions of the Neonatal and Pediatric Critical Care section, the **Newborn Care Services** subsection has been deleted, renumbered, and relocated to codes 99460, 99461, 99462, 99463, 99464 and 99465.

▶Newborn Care Services◀

▶The following codes are used to report the services provided to newborns (birth through the first 28 days) in several different settings. Use of the normal newborn codes is limited to the initial care of the newborn in the first days after birth prior to home discharge.

Evaluation and Management (E/M) services for the newborn include maternal and/or fetal and newborn history, newborn physical examination(s), ordering of diagnostic tests and treatments, meetings with the family, and documentation in the medical record.◀

▶When delivery room attendance services (99464) or delivery room resuscitation services (99465) are required, report these in addition to normal newborn services E/M codes.

For E/M services provided to newborns who are other than normal, see codes for hospital inpatient services (99221-99233) and neonatal intensive and critical care services (99466-99469, 99477-99480). When normal newborn services are provided by the same physician on the same date that the newborn later becomes ill and receives additional intensive or critical care services, report the appropriate E/M code with modifier 25 for these services in addition to the normal newborn code.

Procedures (eg, 54150, newborn circumcision) are not included with the normal newborn codes, and when performed, should be reported in addition to the newborn services.

When newborns are seen in follow-up after the date of discharge in the office or outpatient setting, see 99201-99215, 99381, 99391 as appropriate.◀

●**99460**　Initial hospital or birthing center care, per day, for evaluation and management of normal newborn infant

●**99461**　Initial care, per day, for evaluation and management of normal newborn infant seen in other than hospital or birthing center

●**99462**　Subsequent hospital care, per day, for evaluation and management of normal newborn

●**99463**　Initial hospital or birthing center care, per day, for evaluation and management of normal newborn infant admitted and discharged on the same date

▶(For newborn hospital discharge services provided on a date subsequent to the admission date, see 99238, 99239)◀

Rationale

Extensive revisions have been made to the Newborn Care Services codes and guidelines for the CPT 2009 codebook. The revisions provide further clarification of the intent of the newly revised Newborn Care Services subsection. The newborn care services section is now divided into two sections: (1) newborn care services, which includes codes 99460-99463, and (2) a new subsection that was added to include Delivery/Birthing Room Attendance and Neonatal Resuscitation Services and codes 99464 and 99465.

Codes 99431-99435, the introductory guidelines, and the associated cross-references have been deleted, relocated, and renumbered to codes 99460-99463 in the new Newborn Care Services section. The guidelines have been revised with greater detail in instruction for reporting the newborn care service codes. For purposes of reporting newborn care services, the use of the normal newborn codes is limited to the initial care of the newborn in the first days after birth prior to home discharge. The newborn services include the maternal and/or fetal and newborn history, newborn physical examination(s), ordering of diagnostic tests and treatments, meeting with family members, and documentation of the services. The delivery room attendance services (99464) or delivery room resuscitation services (99465) may also be appropriately reported when performed, in addition to the normal newborn services E/M codes.

The guidelines have also been revised instructing the appropriate reporting of separate evaluation and management services when the normal newborn services are provided by the same physician on the same date that the newborn later becomes ill and receives additional intensive or critical care services. When reporting an evaluation and management service code in addition to the normal newborn code, modifier 25 should be appended to the appropriate evaluation and management service code. As indicated in the new instruction, it is also appropriate to separately report code 54150 for newborn circumcision when performed, as this service is not considered an inclusive component of the normal newborn codes.

▶Delivery/Birthing Room Attendance and Resuscitation Services◀

●99464 Attendance at delivery (when requested by the delivering physician) and initial stabilization of newborn

▶(99464 may be reported in conjunction with 99460, 99468, 99477)◀

▶(Do not report 99464 in conjunction with 99465)◀

●99465 Delivery/birthing room resuscitation, provision of positive pressure ventilation and/or chest compressions in the presence of acute inadequate ventilation and/or cardiac output

▶(Do not report 99465 in conjunction with 99460, 99468, 99477)◀

▶(Do not report 99465 in conjunction with 99464)◀

▶(Procedures that are performed as a necessary part of the resuscitation [eg, intubation, vascular lines] are reported separately in addition to 99465. In order to report these procedures, they must be performed as a necessary component of the resuscitation and not as a convenience before admission to the neonatal intensive care unit)◀

Rationale

Codes 99436 and 99440 have been deleted and renumbered to codes 99464 and 99465 in a new subsection titled Delivery/Birthing Room Attendance and Resuscitation Services. This new placement in the hierarchy is also intended to provide further clarity for understanding and reporting these codes. Code 99465 was editorially revised to delete "newborn" and include "delivery/birthing room" in the code descriptor for consistency purposes within the subsection.

Cross-references have also been included following these codes to instruct appropriate coding. An instructional parenthetical note was included to instruct that when procedures are performed as a necessary part of the resuscitation (eg, intubation, vascular lines) these services are separately reported in addition to code 99465. Resuscitation services that are performed immediately prior to admission to the neonatal intensive care unit are not separately reported and are included in the neonatal intensive care per diem services.

▶Inpatient Neonatal Intensive Care Services and Pediatric and Neonatal Critical Care Services◀

▶Pediatric Critical Care Patient Transport◀

▶The following codes (99466, 99467) are used to report the physical attendance and direct face-to-face care by a physician during the interfacility transport of a critically ill or critically injured pediatric patient 24 months of age or less. For the purpose of reporting codes 99466 and 99467, face-to-face care begins when the physician assumes primary responsibility of the pediatric patient at the referring hospital/facility, and ends when the receiving hospital/facility accepts responsibility for the pediatric patient's care. Only the time the physician spends in direct face-to-face contact with the patient during the transport should be reported. Pediatric patient transport services involving less than 30 minutes of face-to-face physician care should not be reported using codes 99466, 99467. Procedure(s) or service(s) performed by other members of the transporting team may not be reported by the supervising physician.

For the definition of the critically ill or critically injured pediatric patient and the list of services included in critical care, see the **Neonatal and Pediatric Critical Care Services** section. Any services performed, which are not listed may be reported separately.

The direction of emergency care to transporting staff by a physician located in a hospital or other facility by two-way communication is not considered direct face-to-face care and should not be reported with 99466, 99467. Physician-directed emergency care through outside voice communication to transporting staff personnel is reported with 99288.

Emergency department services (99281-99285), initial hospital care (99221-99223), critical care (99291, 99292), initial date neonatal intensive (99477), or critical care (99468) are only reported after the patient has been admitted to the emergency department, the inpatient floor, or the critical care unit of the receiving facility. If inpatient critical care services are reported in the referring facility prior to transfer to the receiving hospital, use the critical care codes (99291, 99292).

Code 99466 is used to report the first 30 to 74 minutes of direct face-to-face time with the transport pediatric patient and should be reported only once on a given date. Code 99467 is used to report each additional 30 minutes provided on a given date. Face-to-face services of less than 30 minutes should not be reported with these codes.◀

●99466 **Critical care** services delivered by a physician, face-to-face, during an interfacility transport of critically ill or critically injured pediatric patient, 24 months of age or less; first 30-74 minutes of hands-on care during transport

+●99467 each additional 30 minutes (List separately in addition to code for primary service)

▶(Use 99467 in conjunction with 99466)◀

▶(Critical care of less than 30 minutes total duration should be reported with the appropriate E/M code)◀

🖎 Rationale

The Pediatric Critical Care Patient Transport subsection, guidelines, and codes 99289 and 99290 have been relocated and renumbered. Codes 99289 and 99290 have been renumbered to 99466 and 99467, respectively. This section has been included in the newly revised Inpatient Neonatal Intensive Care Services and Pediatric and Neonatal Critical Care Services section. These revisions support the expansion of the Neonatal and Pediatric Critical Care Services section. Codes 99466 and 99467 have been editorially renumbered and remain time-based codes, and are intended to identify the physical attendance and direct face-to-face care by a physician during the interfacility transport of a critically ill or critically injured patient. These codes are intended to be reported only once on a given date. Face-to-face care begins when the physician assumes primary responsibility for the patient at the referring hospital/facility and ends when the receiving hospital/facility accepts responsibility for the patient's care. Only the time the physician spends in direct face-to-face contact with the patient during the transport should be reported. It is not appropriate to report codes 99466 and 99467 for critical care transport services requiring less than 30 minutes.

A physician providing direct emergency care through outside voice communication to transporting staff personnel should continue to use code 99288. Procedure(s) or service(s) performed by other members of the transporting team may not be reported by the supervising physician. The following Neonatal and Pediatric Critical Care Services section contains a complete listing of services that are included in the critical care services and not separately reported.

▶Inpatient Neonatal and Pediatric Critical Care◀

▶The same definitions for critical care services apply for the adult, child, and neonate.

Codes 99468, 99469 are used to report services provided by a physician directing the inpatient care of a critically ill neonate or infant 28 days of age or less. They represent care starting with the date of admission (99468) and subsequent day(s) (99469) that the neonate remains critical. These codes may be reported only by a single physician and only once per day, per patient.

The initial day neonatal critical care code (99468) can be used in addition to 99464 or 99465 as appropriate, when the physician is present for the delivery (99464) or resuscitation (99465) is required. Other procedures performed as a necessary part of the resuscitation (eg, endotracheal intubation [31500]) are also reported separately when performed as part of the pre-admission delivery room care. In order to report these procedures separately, they must be performed as a necessary component of the resuscitation and not simply as a convenience before admission to the neonatal intensive care unit.

Codes 99471-99476 are used to report services provided by a physician directing the inpatient care of a critically ill infant or young child from 29 days of postnatal age through 5 years of age. They represent care starting with the date of admission (99471, 99475) and subsequent day(s) (99472, 99476) the infant or child remains critical. These codes may be reported only by a single physician and only once per day, per patient in a given setting. Service for the critically ill or critically injured child older than 5 years of age would be reported with critical care codes (99291, 99292).

The pediatric and neonatal critical care codes include those procedures listed for the critical care codes (99291, 99292). In addition, the following procedures are also included (and not separately reported) in the pediatric and neonatal critical care service codes (99468-99472, 99475, 99476), the intensive care services codes (99477-99480), and the pediatric critical care patient transport codes (99466, 99467):◀

▶Invasive or non-invasive electronic monitoring of vital signs

Vascular access procedures

Peripheral vessel catheterization (36000)

Other arterial catheters (36140, 36620)

Umbilical venous catheters (36510)

Central vessel catheterization (36555)

Vascular access procedures (36400, 36405, 36406)

Vascular punctures oral (36420, 36600)

Umbilical arterial catheters (36660)

Airway and ventilation management

Endotracheal intubation (31500)

Ventilatory management (94002-94004)

Bedside pulmonary function testing (94375)

Surfactant administration (94610)

Continuous positive airway pressure (CPAP) (94660)

Monitoring or interpretation of blood gases or oxygen saturation (94760-94762)

Transfusion of blood components (36430, 36440)

Oral or nasogastric tube placement (43752)

Suprapubic bladder aspiration (51100)

Bladder catheterization (51701, 51702)

Lumbar puncture (62270)

Any services performed which are not listed above may be reported separately.

When a neonate or infant is not critically ill, but requires intensive observation, frequent interventions, and other intensive care services, the Continuing Intensive Care Services codes (99477-99480) should be used to report these services.

To report critical care services provided in the outpatient setting (eg, emergency department or office) for neonates and pediatric patients of any age, see the Critical Care codes 99291, 99292. If the same physician provides critical care services for a neonatal or pediatric patient in both the outpatient and inpatient settings on the same day, report only the appropriate Neonatal or Pediatric Critical Care codes 99468-99476 for all critical care services provided on that day. Critical care services provided by a second physician of a different specialty not reporting a per-day neonatal or pediatric critical care code can be reported with 99291, 99292.

When critical care services are provided to neonates or pediatric patients less than 5 years of age at two separate institutions by a physician from a different group on the same date of service, the physician from the referring institution should report their critical care services with the critical care◄

▶codes (99291, 99292) and the receiving institution should report the appropriate global admission code (99468, 99471, 99475, 99476) for the same date of service.

Critical care services to a pediatric patient 6 years of age or older are reported with the critical care codes 99291, 99292.

Critical care services to a neonate or pediatric patient provided in an outpatient environment are reported with the critical care codes 99291, 99292.

Critical care services provided by a second physician of a different specialty not reporting a 24-hour global code can be reported with the critical care codes 99291, 99292.

No physician may report remote real-time videoconferenced critical care (0188T, 0189T) when neonatal or pediatric intensive or critical care services (99468-99476) are reported.◀

- **99468** **Initial inpatient neonatal critical care,** per day, for the evaluation and management of a critically ill neonate, 28 days of age or less

- **99469** **Subsequent inpatient neonatal critical care,** per day, for the evaluation and management of a critically ill neonate, 28 days of age or less

- **99471** **Initial inpatient pediatric critical care,** per day, for the evaluation and management of a critically ill infant or young child, 29 days through 24 months of age

- **99472** **Subsequent inpatient pediatric critical care,** per day, for the evaluation and management of a critically ill infant or young child, 29 days through 24 months of age

- **99475** **Initial inpatient pediatric critical care,** per day, for the evaluation and management of a critically ill infant or young child, 2 through 5 years of age

- **99476** **Subsequent inpatient pediatric critical care,** per day, for the evaluation and management of a critically ill infant or young child, 2 through 5 years of age

Rationale

The Neonatal and Pediatric Critical Care Services sections have undergone comprehensive revisions to reflect the typical and current neonatal care services practices. Previously these sections for newborn and pediatric care services were scattered throughout the Evaluation and Management (E/M) Services section of the CPT codebook. The CPT 2009 codebook revisions include expansion of the Inpatient Neonatal and Pediatric Critical Care section with condensation of the Neonatal (99468, 99469) and Pediatric (99471, 99472) Critical Care codes and guidelines into one location. These revisions provide an aggregation of the instructions in a single location, with greater detail in the instruction on the use of the codes and the relationships of the codes to other neonatal and pediatric sections and codes. Descriptions of the typical service for each of the critical care and intensive care codes in this section also no longer follow the code descriptor but are included in the guidelines.

The inpatient neonatal critical care codes 99295 and 99296 have been deleted and renumbered to codes 99468 and 99469, respectively. These codes are intended to identify the initial and subsequent neonatal critical care services codes describing the initial day and each subsequent hospital day evaluation and management service provided to a critically ill neonate, 28 days of age or less.

The inpatient pediatric critical care codes 99293 and 99294 have been deleted and renumbered to codes 99471 and 99472, respectively. These codes are intended to identify the initial and subsequent pediatric critical care services codes and describe the initial day and each subsequent hospital day evaluation and management service provided to a critically ill infant, 28 days of age (postnatal) to 2 years of age. The care for these patients is typically managed in pediatric intensive care units (PICU) by pediatric critical care specialists, neonatologists, and pediatric surgeons. These codes are only applicable to patients until their second birthday. This age limit in the code descriptor reflects a significant number of PICU patients in this population and provides a reporting mechanism for continuity of global reporting for neonates who have passed 28 days of postnatal age receiving the same pattern of care, frequency of visits, and intensity of services as the neonates.

Two new codes, 99475 and 99476, and related cross-references have been established to report the initial and subsequent inpatient pediatric critical care services that describe the initial day and each subsequent hospital day evaluation and management provided to a critically ill infant or young child, 25 months through 71 months of age. These codes will describe the care management of children beyond 2 years of age who meet the accepted definition of critically ill or injured with single or multiple organ failure where the physician's presence is required to reassess the patient frequently and supervise the health care team over a 24-hour period, making complex, integrated decisions. Optimally, these codes include repetitive evaluation of the patient's status by the physician, therapy adjustment, review of laboratory results, monitoring and imaging data, and physician supervision of the health care team. These evaluations occur in encounters of variable length and intensity throughout the day and cannot reasonably be "counted" or documented at each patient contact, often representing a dozen or more per day. It is for this reason that these codes are "per diem" codes, reported per calendar day.

Optimal ongoing patient management will require frequent visits and ongoing supervision of the health care team by the physician in order to make and perform applications.

The most typical physiologic abnormalities in children beyond the age of 2 years are respiratory failure or respiratory distress with impending respiratory failure. Other indications for intensive care management of the critically ill pediatric patient are for postoperative care, trauma, head injury, and transplant, requiring care in the PICU for respiratory or cardiorespiratory support. Other diseases requiring intensive care management include sepsis or systemic inflammatory response syndrome (SIRS) with impending multi-organ system dysfunction or failure.

The inpatient pediatric critical care model typically consists of an in-house team managing many patients who are cared for in a large unit, with an in-house critical care physician present for 16-24 hours and intermittent frequent bedside and unit time visits throughout the calendar day. The codes do not, however, require 24 hour in-house presence by the reporting physician. The physician supervises the care team and evaluates the patient on multiple occasions throughout the first and subsequent days of care, speaks with the parents and referring physician, and evaluates imaging and laboratory data.

The pediatric intensive care codes include obtaining access through the central circulation via placement of a femoral, internal jugular, or subclavian catheter and the sometimes challenging establishment of vascular access, including peripheral, arterial, as well as central venous lines in sites that may be difficult to gain access to or are no longer available due to scarring from prior line placement in patients with chronic disease. The initial and subsequent services by the admitting physician often require performance of a series of repetitive procedures, including intubation, vascular access, interpretation of blood gas results, family interviews, records review, discussions with prior or primary care physicians, review of initial laboratory data, and initiation of the appropriate course of treatment. Appropriate multi-system organ management requires frequent and multiple laboratory testing and evaluation during the initial hours following admission, with subsequent changes made in ventilator settings, IV fluid rates and composition, initiation, and manipulation of vasoactive or inotropic drugs, antibiotics, and other therapeutic maneuvers. Endotracheal intubation to secure the airway and vascular access to provide vasoactive infusions, correction of acid-base balance, and provision of other medications may be necessary to stabilize and prevent further decompensation of patients who are compromised with multiple complications. All of the services that are inherent in critical care continue to be listed in the guidelines, but have been editorially revised as a visual listing to highlight the grouping of these services, which should not be separately reported.

An exclusionary statement has been added to preclude any physician reporting remote real-time interactive videoconferenced critical care services (0188T, 0189T) during the period in which another physician reports (99468, 99469, 99471, 99472, 99475, 99476).

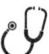
Clinical Example (99475)

A 4-year-old child is admitted to the pediatric intensive care unit (PICU) from the emergency room with impending respiratory failure due to asthma that has failed management in the emergency department. Treatment included continuous bronchodilator therapy and complex pharmacologic support. Blood gases define respiratory failure, and the child is sent to the PICU for close cardiovascular, respiratory, and blood gas monitoring and possible mechanical ventilation.

Description of Procedure (99475)
The physician completes the child's history with the child's family and undertakes a complete physical examination of the child. Lines are placed, laboratory work and blood gases are ordered, imaging is ordered, and the child is sedated and paralyzed, intubated, and placed on the ventilator due to deteriorating respiratory and mental status. Ventilator settings are varied based upon the initial blood gas results. The child's initial orders are written and treatment is initiated at the bedside.

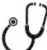
Clinical Example (99476)

A 3-year-old child is receiving continued care, including cardiovascular support and monitoring in the pediatric intensive care unit, after admission for fever, neutropenia, and circulatory shock following a diagnosis of bacteremia and sepsis during chemotherapy for acute lymphocytic leukemia.

Description of Procedure (99476)

The physician completes an interval exam, makes changes with the management of the patient, and discusses the changes in management with the bedside care team. The child is re-examined, and laboratory, imaging, and monitoring values are interpreted and changes in therapy ordered multiple times during the day.

▶Initial and Continuing Intensive Care Services◀

▶Code 99477 represents the initial day of inpatient care for the child who is not critically ill but requires intensive observation, frequent interventions, and other intensive care services. Codes 99478-99480 are used to report subsequent day services provided by a physician directing the continuing intensive care of the low birth weight (LBW 1500-2500 grams) present body weight infant, very low birth weight (VLBW less than 1500 grams) present body weight infant, or normal (2501-5000 grams) present body weight newborn who does not meet the definition of critically ill but continues to require intensive observation, frequent interventions, and other intensive care services. These services are for infants and neonates who are not critically ill but continue to require intensive cardiac and respiratory monitoring, continuous and/or frequent vital sign monitoring, heat maintenance, enteral and/or parenteral nutritional adjustments, laboratory and oxygen monitoring, and constant observation by the health care team under direct physician supervision. Codes 99477-99480 may be reported by only one physician and only once per day, per patient. These codes include the same procedures that are outlined in the **Pediatric Critical Care Services** section, and these services should not be separately reported.

For the subsequent care of the sick neonate less than 28 days of age but more than 5000 grams who does not require intensive or critical care services, use codes 99231-99233.◀

99477   **Initial hospital care,** per day, for the evaluation and management of the neonate, 28 days of age or less, who requires intensive observation, frequent interventions, and other intensive care services

(For the initiation of inpatient care of the normal newborn, use ▶99460◀)

(For the initiation of care of the critically ill neonate, use ▶99468◀)

(For initiation of inpatient hospital care of the ▶ill◀ neonate not requiring intensive observation, frequent interventions, and other intensive care services, see 99221-99223)

●**99478**   **Subsequent intensive care,** per day, for the evaluation and management of the recovering very low birth weight infant (present body weight less than 1500 grams)

●**99479**   **Subsequent intensive care,** per day, for the evaluation and management of the recovering low birth weight infant (present body weight of 1500-2500 grams)

●**99480**   **Subsequent intensive care,** per day, for the evaluation and management of the recovering infant (present body weight of 2501-5000 grams)

Rationale

The Initial and Continuing Intensive Care Service subsection and codes 99298, 99299, and 99300 have been relocated to follow the new Inpatient Neonatal and Pediatric Critical Care section. The introductory guidelines have been revised to reflect current pediatric and neonatal intensive care services. Code 99477 was established in 2008 to report the initial intensive care for a critically ill neonate 28 days of age or younger who requires intensive observation, frequent interventions, and other intensive care services and has been included in this section for 2009. Previously, code 99477 was listed under Other Evaluation and Management Services. Codes 99478, 99479, and 99480 are intended to identify the subsequent intensive care services for the evaluation and management of the recovering low birth weight infants ranging from present body weight less than 1500 grams to 5000 grams.

The introductory guidelines were further revised to instruct that the subsequent hospital care codes 99231-99233 should be reported when subsequent care of the sick neonate who is less than 28 days of age but weighs more than 5000 grams and does not require intensive care or critical care services.

Anesthesia

The revisions of the Anesthesia section are minimal, focusing on clarification of the intent of the populations described by the anesthesia services for coronary artery bypass graft procedures.

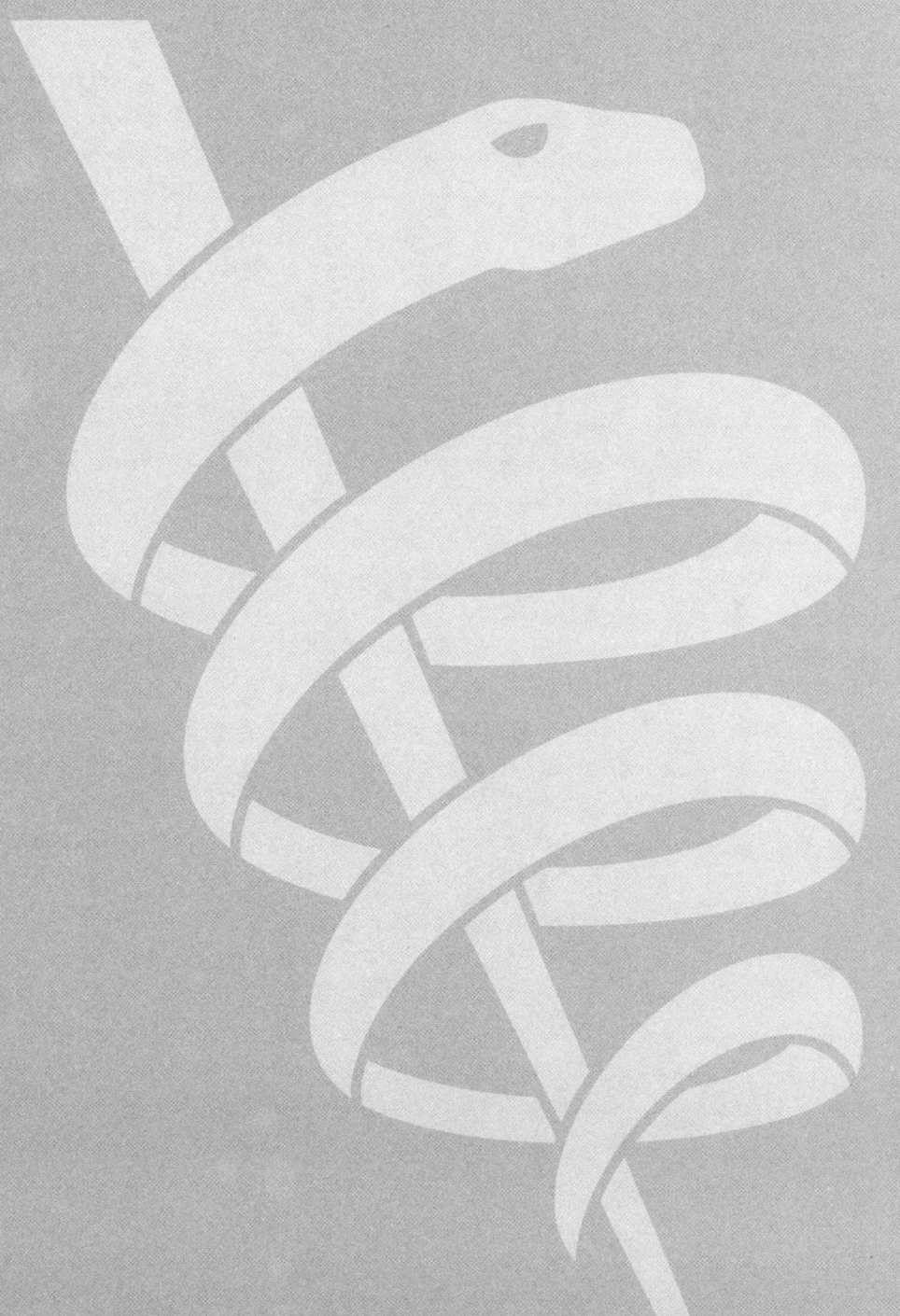

Anesthesia

Head

00210 Anesthesia for intracranial procedures; not otherwise specified

●**00211** craniotomy or craniectomy for evacuation of hematoma

00222 electrocoagulation of intracranial nerve

Rationale

Code 00211 was established to report anesthesia services for intracranial procedures (ie, craniotomy, craniectomy). This code differs in use from code 00210 that is used to report unspecified anesthesia services for surgical intracranial procedures. Code 00211 describes anesthesia for procedures that require either a craniotomy or a craniectomy for evacuation of a hematoma. The effort in providing anesthesia for these procedures includes (1) the urgent/emergent nature of providing anesthesia services for intracranial hematomas, (2) the typical worsening neurologic symptoms of the patient, (3) typical patient issues with coagulation or concomitant trauma, and (4) typical involvement of one or more systemic complications such as neurogenic pulmonary edema or cardiac involvement including dysrhythmias and ischemia.

Clinical Example (00211)

A 63-year-old man presents with headache, nausea, left-sided weakness, and mental status changes after a recent fall. His past medical history is notable for hypertension. Medications include an antihypertensive medication and aspirin. Current clotting studies are normal. Initial computed tomographic (CT) scan shows a large hematoma on the right with midline shift. A craniotomy is scheduled for urgent evacuation of the hematoma.

Description of Procedure (00211)

In the preanesthesia holding area, secure intravenous access with a large-bore catheter is established and the patient may receive light sedation if needed. Access for central venous pressure (CVP) may be selected either for certainty of intravenous access or in anticipation of the need to monitor intravascular volume or utilize vasoactive infusions and possibly diuretics. Arterial cannulation (art line) for direct and continuous monitoring of blood pressure is used for most procedures to allow careful monitoring and control of blood pressure. When either a CVP or an art line is placed, placement is separately reported. Interpretation of the information obtained from these monitors is included in the anesthetic work.

The patient is transferred to the operating room and appropriate monitoring devices are applied. The Joint Commission (formly The Joint Commission on Accreditation of Healthcare Organizations [JCAHO])–mandated "time out" is performed, confirming the correct patient, correct site, and correct surgery. The anesthesiologist confirms the preoperative antibiotic order with the surgeon and administers the prescribed medication before incision. After preoxygenation with oxygen, anesthesia is carefully induced in such a way as to minimize alteration in intracranial pressure while rapidly securing the airway to avoid opportunity for aspiration of gastric contents. Once adequate neuromuscular blockade is confirmed with a nerve blockade monitor, the anesthesiologist performs direct laryngoscopy and intubates the trachea, with careful titration of anesthetic agents to avoid any vasomotor perturbation. Proper tracheal placement is confirmed via capnography and the endotracheal tube is secured. An esophageal stethoscope with a temperature probe is placed. The anesthesiologist confirms the drug and dose of the prophylactic antibiotic with the surgeon and administers this prior to skin incision.

The patient is carefully positioned for the surgical procedure, often in a slightly head-up position and possibly in the lateral position to allow appropriate surgical access. A head holder involving the placement of pins through the scalp and into the skull may be used; its placement is intensely stimulating and therefore requires careful titration of anesthesia to attenuate changes in intracranial pressure. The operating room table is most often turned, with the anesthesiologist positioned at the patient's side or feet rather than at the head of the table. After the table is positioned to facilitate the surgical procedures, bilateral breath sounds are auscultated again, proper functioning of the monitors and vascular access is confirmed, and pressure points are padded. A warm air heating blanket is positioned on the patient unless the patient is febrile or there is a deliberate desire to cool the patient during the surgery.

Narcotics and muscle relaxants are intermittently administered as necessary and anesthetic level is titrated with an inhaled anesthetic agent. During the procedure, the anesthesiologist adjusts the ventilator to ensure adequate ventilation as determined by capnography, without compromising cerebral blood flow. The surgeon may request hyperventilation to a specific arterial partial pressure of carbon dioxide to decompress the brain. Similarly, the anesthesiologist and surgeon may specify a narrow range of blood pressure measurements to target during the procedure to ensure adequate cerebral perfusion pressure (CPP) without adversely increasing cerebral blood flow, intracranial pressure (ICP), and the risk of additional bleeding. The anesthesiologist carefully monitors the patient's oxygenation status with pulse oximetry and may obtain serial arterial blood samples as indicated to assess ventilation ($PaCO_2$) and pH. Coordinating with the surgeon, a variety of medications may be administered including anticonvulsants, osmotic diuretics, calcium antagonists, and corticosteroids in an attempt to regulate ICP. It may also be necessary to employ carefully titrated vasoactive medication in an attempt to maintain CPP at an appropriate level.

These procedures can result in significant blood loss, especially if the patient was using anticoagulants or platelet-inhibiting medications prior to surgery. In those circumstances, the anesthesiologist carefully monitors the volume of lost blood, the central venous pressure, and urine output. When appropriate, and after communication and agreement with the surgeon, blood component therapy is initiated after verifying that the blood products are appropriately matched and intended for the patient.

Arterial blood gas samples may be obtained to determine blood gas findings, particularly $PaCO_2$, hemoglobin, and certain electrolytes. Coagulation studies may be obtained when the patient has a preexisting coagulopathy or develops excessive intraoperative bleeding. The results of these tests are interpreted and therapeutic decisions are made to guide fluid, blood, and electrolyte therapy.

At the conclusion of the procedure, the anesthetic agents are discontinued and residual neuromuscular blockade is reversed pharmacologically. The anesthesiologist evaluates the patient's respiratory effort, oxygenation, level of consciousness, and the reversal of neuromuscular agents. If the patient meets acceptable criteria, the anesthesiologist extubates the patient's trachea. Patients undergoing these procedures are at risk for changes in ICP and possible pulmonary aspiration during tracheal extubation, so caution and careful assessment are necessary. If the patient is unstable or neurologically impaired, tracheal extubation may not be appropriate. Under this circumstance, a portable monitor and ventilation circuit are connected to the patient for transport and the patient is taken to the postanesthesia care unit (PACU) or intensive care unit (ICU) while ventilated en route by the anesthesiologist.

When the surgeon determines that a CT scan should be performed immediately postoperatively, the anesthesiologist transports the patient to the scanner and then to the ICU or PACU. During these transports and scanning, the anesthesiologist maintains the same level of monitoring and life support functions as are required in the operating room. Careful monitoring of the patient's vital signs is continuously performed during transport, and hemodynamic infusions are maintained and manipulated if necessary. If continued airway and ventilatory control is chosen rather than immediate extubation, sedation is usually continued to avoid coughing and straining, which may promote a recurrence of intracranial bleeding or increase in ICP. It is considered optimal to design an anesthetic plan that, although maintaining a significantly deep level of anesthesia during the procedure, allows a return to baseline consciousness and alertness as quickly possible to allow early assessment of the patient's neurological function after the trespass of surgery.

Thorax (Chest Wall and Shoulder Girdle)

Intrathoracic

00560	Anesthesia for procedures on heart, pericardial sac, and great vessels of chest; without pump oxygenator	
00561	with pump oxygenator, younger than one year of age	
▲ 00562	with pump oxygenator, ►age 1 year or older, for all non-coronary bypass procedures (eg, valve procedures) or for re-operation for coronary bypass more than 1 month after original operation◄	
▲ 00566	Anesthesia for direct coronary artery bypass grafting►;◄ without pump oxygenator	
●00567	with pump oxygenator	

Rationale

Code 00567 was established to report anesthesia services for on-pump coronary artery bypass grafting. Codes 00562 and 00566 have been revised to accommodate addition of code 00567 and to provide further differentiation in the descriptors from code 00562. Previously, code 00562 was used to identify all pump oxygenator procedures when the number of cardiac surgery codes were more limited. Over the years, however, an increasing number of the services described by code 00562 were more complex cardiac cases performed with a pump oxygenator. As a result, code 00567 has been added to include surgical anesthesia services involving coronary artery bypass (CABG) with pump oxygenator. This allows code 00562 to be used to report anesthesia services for more complex surgical procedures including valvular repairs and redo procedures. Code 00562 has been revised to better clarify that code 00561 is used to report anesthesia services for procedures on the heart, pericardial sac, and great vessels of the chest with pump oxygenator when the patient is under 1 year of age. Code 00562 is used to describe anesthesia services for these procedures when the patient is 1 year of age or older. In addition, code 00562 has been further revised to clearly capture the anesthesia work associated with CABG and valvular reoperations such as the one described by code 33533, Reoperation, coronary artery bypass procedure or valve procedures, more than one month after original operation (List separately in addition to code for primary procedure).

To accommodate the addition of code 00567, code 00566 was editorially revised to include the addition of a semicolon.

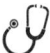

Clinical Example (00562)

The typical patient is a 66-year-old man who presents for an aortic valve replacement for critical aortic stenosis.

Description of Procedure (00562)

In the preanesthesia holding area, the patient is identified; secure intravenous access with a large-bore catheter is established; and intravenous sedation is carefully titrated as needed. An intravenous large-bore catheter is placed and infusion begins. Further medication is administered as needed. The patient is brought into the operating room and monitors are placed for five-lead electrocardiogram, pulse oximetry, and blood pressure. The Joint Commission-mandated "time out" is performed, confirming the correct patient, correct site, and correct surgery. The anesthesiologist confirms the preoperative antibiotic order with the surgeon and administers the prescribed medication before incision. Monitors are placed and vital signs obtained. If invasive lines (arterial, central venous pressure, or pulmonary artery catheter) have previously been placed (separately reported), the transducers are zeroed, calibrated, and connected to the operating room cardiac monitor. Blood samples are drawn for blood gas analysis as well as point-of-care blood coagulation analysis (eg, activated clotting time [ACT]; a thromboelastogram [TEG] is used as needed). The vasoactive infusions are readied to be infused into the central line but not started until their need is determined by the anesthesiologist. Anesthesia charting is performed. Baseline and subsequent hemodynamic parameters are documented.

A baseline arterial blood gas is drawn prior to induction. Manual ventilation with oxygen is provided. The anesthesiologist determines the medications for induction of anesthesia. Careful titration of medication is essential to maintain hemodynamic stability throughout induction and intubation. A warming blanket is placed for use after cardiopulmonary bypass (CPB).

The patient is carefully positioned for the surgical procedure. After preoxygenation with oxygen, general anesthesia is administered and the patient is paralyzed with muscle relaxants, with close attention paid to the patient's hemodynamic status. An immediate intervention is often necessary for a patient with coronary artery disease. This intervention may include rapid titration of hemodynamic medication infusions during the induction process, or resuscitation in the case of severe cardiovascular response to the induction of general anesthesia. Once adequate neuromuscular blockade is confirmed with a nerve blockade monitor, the patient's trachea is intubated; breath sounds are confirmed and hemodynamic parameters are reassessed after intubation. Ventilation is adjusted according to the blood gas results. Other tasks performed include padding of all pressure points and placement of an orogastric tube, esophageal stethoscope with temperature probe, neuromuscular monitor, noninvasive level of consciousness monitor, and a cerebral oximeter as indicated. Intermittent blood gas and blood coagulation analysis are measured throughout the surgery.

The anesthetic is maintained with the intravenous and inhalation agents as deemed appropriate by the anesthesiologist to optimize coronary perfusion, cardiac output, and hemodynamic stability while carefully considering the pathophysiology associated with the patient's valvular disease. Episodes of hemodynamic instability commonly occur at multiple times prior to CPB. Arrhythmias are treated as needed. Careful efforts to maintain hemodynamic, glucose, and acid-base stability and to prevent myocardial ischemia may require the use of vasodilators, vasopressors, insulin, and/or inotropes. Episodes of hemodynamic instability are common due to sudden changes in intravascular volume, aortic artery clamping, contractile dysfunction, ischemia, and physical manipulation of the heart and great vessels. Therefore, continuous monitoring for sudden hemodynamic alterations including hypotension, hypertension, tachycardia, bradycardia, dysrhythmias, myocardial ischemia, and ventricular dysfunction is required. Anticoagulating doses of heparin (or an alternative anticoagulant such as a direct thrombin inhibitor) are administered.

Once surgery has begun, ventilation is momentarily stopped during sternotomy. Baseline check of coagulation is performed (ACT or TEG). After the surgeon adequately dissects the great vessels, heparin is administered intravenously and a repeat clotting time is measured. The aorta and right atrium or vena cavae are cannulated when the ACT indicates adequate anticoagulation for cardiopulmonary bypass. Ventilation is discontinued with the establishment of CPB.

During bypass:
During CPB the anesthesiologist maintains the anesthetized state and muscular paralysis of the patient, while continuously monitoring, interpreting, and documenting blood pressure, kidney perfusion, brain wave activity, and brain

oxygenation. Adjustments are made to the anesthetic depth and acid-base status, and to correct any deviations from adequate tissue perfusion, particularly to the brain, kidney, spinal cord, and heart, while not permitting an undesirable blood pressure that could contribute to increased bronchial-coronary collateral blood flow and thereby disrupt the CABG surgical field. The anesthesiologist also works to avoid increased shearing forces on the occluded aorta, which might potentiate ischemia and/or bleeding. Acid-base status, electrolytes, blood glucose, anticoagulation status, anesthesia, and neuromuscular relaxation status are all closely monitored. This part of the procedure requires continual assessment and treatment of the patient.

Preparations are made to separate the patient from bypass after the completion of cardiac intervention. The length of bypass time generally indicates the severity of the insult to the heart and complexity of the procedure (eg, valve repairs, failed repairs, combination valve and coronary bypass, or intramyocardial coronaries), and serves as an indicator of difficulty in separation from CPB, as well as the instability of the patient following bypass. The adequacy of repair is carefully observed to predict the need for exogenous circulatory support to separate from bypass. Near the anticipated end of bypass and after adequate rewarming, ventilation is restarted, de-airing maneuvers are initiated, and cardiac rhythm is assessed. The anesthesiologist establishes the pacemaker settings and temporary epicardial pacing is initiated. In addition, inotropic cardiac support and afterload reduction allow safe separation from CPB. Antibiotics are re-dosed according to institution standards.

Post CPB:
Once cardiac and pulmonary parameters are stabilized, reversal of anticoagulation is confirmed with an ACT and TEG as needed, and blood products may be checked and administered as indicated. Blood gases and laboratory values are intermittently checked and treatment of acid-base, electrolyte, and metabolic abnormalities ensues. Cardiac function, brain activity, and tissue perfusion continue to be monitored, as the anesthetic is adjusted on the basis of the hemodynamic response.

At the conclusion of surgery, transport monitors and infusion pumps are checked for proper function and then connected to the patient for transport to the intensive care unit (ICU). The patient is carefully placed on the ICU/transport bed with all monitors and infusions. Manual ventilation is begun and the patient is transported to the ICU, with treatment continuing along the way as necessary to ensure stable respiratory and hemodynamic parameters. On arrival in the ICU, hemodynamic and respiratory monitor connections are transferred to the unit's systems. Ventilation is transferred to a bedside ventilator and parameters are adjusted to satisfactory patient outcomes as determined by oximetry, respirator indices, end-tidal CO_2 monitoring, examination, and arterial blood gas monitoring.

A written record of vital signs, drugs and fluids administered, procedures performed, and a narrative of important intraoperative events is maintained throughout the anesthetic period.

Clinical Example (00567)

The typical patient is a 62-year-old man undergoing direct CABG with pump oxygenator for ischemic heart disease. He has diabetes requiring insulin or oral agents.

Description of Procedure (00567)

In the preanesthesia holding area, the patient is identified, intravenous access with a large-bore catheter is established, and intravenous sedation is carefully titrated as needed. An intravenous large bore catheter is placed and the intravenous infusion begins. Further medication is administered as needed. The patient is transferred to the operating room and appropriate monitoring devices are applied. The Joint Commission-mandated "time out" is performed, confirming the correct patient, correct site, and correct surgery. The anesthesiologist confirms the preoperative antibiotic order with the surgeon and administers the prescribed medication before incision. Monitors are placed and vital signs obtained. If invasive lines (arterial, CVP, or pulmonary artery catheter) have previously been placed (separately reported), the transducers are zeroed, calibrated, and connected to the operating room cardiac monitor. Blood samples are drawn for blood gas analysis, as well as point-of-care blood coagulation analysis (eg, ACT; a TEG is used as needed). The vasoactive infusions are readied to be infused into the central line but not started until their need is determined by the anesthesiologist. Anesthesia charting is performed. Baseline and subsequent hemodynamic parameters are documented.

The patient is carefully positioned for the surgical procedure. After preoxygenation with oxygen, general anesthesia is administered and the patient is paralyzed with muscle relaxants, with close attention paid to the patient's hemodynamic status, as immediate intervention is often necessary for a patient with coronary artery disease. This intervention may include rapid titration of hemodynamic medication infusions during the induction process, or resuscitation in the case of severe cardiovascular response to the induction of general anesthesia. Once adequate neuromuscular blockade is confirmed with a nerve blockade monitor, the patient is intubated, breath sounds are confirmed, and hemodynamic parameters are reassessed after intubation. Ventilation is adjusted as indicated by the blood gas results. Other tasks performed include padding of pressure points and placement of an orogastric tube, esophageal stethoscope with temperature probe, neuromuscular monitor, noninvasive level of consciousness monitor, and a cerebral oximeter as indicated. Intermittent blood gas and blood coagulation analysis are measured throughout the surgery.

The anesthesia is maintained with the intravenous and inhalation agents as deemed appropriate by the anesthesiologist. Careful efforts to maintain hemodynamic, glucose, and acid-base stability and to prevent myocardial ischemia may require the use of vasodilators, vasopressors, insulin, and/or inotropes. Episodes of hemodynamic instability are common due to sudden changes in intravascular volume, aortic artery clamping, contractile dysfunction, ischemia, and physical manipulation of the heart and great vessels. Continuous monitoring for sudden hemodynamic alterations including hypotension, hypertension, tachycardia, bradycardia, dysrhythmias, myocardial ischemia, and ventricular dysfunction is therefore required. Anticoagulating doses of heparin (or an alternative anticoagulant such as a direct thrombin inhibitor) are administered.

It is desirable to monitor neurological function to ensure adequate perfusion during the procedure. The anesthesiologist administers drugs to facilitate organ protection as well as maintain adequate perfusion to the brain, kidney, spinal cord, and heart. Intermittent blood gas analysis, compressed electroencephalographic activity, cerebral oximetry, muscle relaxation, glucose, acid-base status, and coagulation status are interpreted to guide treatment throughout the surgery. Opioids, benzodiazepines, and muscle relaxants are intermittently administered as necessary.

During bypass:
During CPB the anesthesiologist maintains the anesthetized state and muscular paralysis of the patient, while continuously monitoring, interpreting, and documenting blood pressure, kidney perfusion, brain wave activity, and brain oxygenation. Adjustments are made to the anesthetic depth and acid-base status, and to correct any deviations from adequate tissue perfusion, particularly to the brain, kidney, spinal cord, and heart, while not permitting an undesirable blood pressure that could contribute to increased bronchial-coronary collateral blood flow and thereby disrupt the CABG surgical field. The anesthesiologist also works to avoid increased shearing forces on the occluded aorta, which might potentiate ischemia and/or bleeding. Acid-base status, electrolytes, blood glucose, anticoagulation status, anesthesia, and neuromuscular relaxation status are all closely monitored. This part of the procedure requires continual assessment and treatment of the patient.

During bypass, preparations are made to separate the patient from bypass. The length of bypass time generally indicates the severity of the insult to the heart and complexity of the procedure (eg, intramyocardial coronaries), and serves as an indicator of difficulty in separation from CPB, as well as the instability of the patient following bypass. The adequacy of repair is carefully observed to predict the need for exogenous circulatory support separate from bypass. Near the anticipated end of bypass and after adequate rewarming, ventilation is restarted, de-airing maneuvers are initiated, and cardiac rhythm is assessed. When indicated, the anesthesiologist establishes the pacemaker settings and begins temporary epicardial pacing. In addition, the anesthesiologist initiates inotropic cardiac support and afterload reduction, to allow safe separation from CPB. Antibiotics are redosed according to institution standards.

Post CPB:
Once cardiac and pulmonary parameters are stabilized, reversal of anticoagulation is confirmed with an ACT and TEG as needed, and blood products may be checked and administered as indicated. Blood gases and laboratory values are intermittently checked and treatment of acid-base, electrolyte, and metabolic abnormalities ensues. Cardiac function, brain activity, and tissue perfusion continue to be monitored, as the anesthetic is adjusted on the basis of the hemodynamic response.

At the conclusion of surgery, transport monitors and infusion pumps are checked for proper function and then connected to the patient for transport to the ICU. The patient is carefully placed on the ICU/transport bed with all monitors and infusions. Manual ventilation is begun and the patient is transported to the ICU, with treatment continuing along the way as necessary to ensure stable respiratory and hemodynamic parameters. On arrival in the ICU, hemodynamic and respiratory monitor connections are transferred to the unit's systems. Ventilation is transferred to a bedside ventilator and parameters are adjusted to satisfactory patient outcomes as determined by oximetry, respirator indices, end-tidal CO_2 monitoring, examination, and arterial blood gas monitoring.

Other Procedures

01991 Anesthesia for diagnostic or therapeutic nerve blocks and injections (when block or injection is performed by a different provider); other than the prone position

01992 prone position

(Do not report 01991 or 01992 in conjunction with 99143-99150)

(When regional intravenous administration of local anesthetic agent or other medication in the upper or lower extremity is used as the anesthetic for a surgical procedure, report the appropriate anesthesia code. To report a Bier block for pain management, use 64999. For intra-arterial or intravenous injections, see 90773, 90774)

(For intra-arterial or intravenous therapy for pain management, see ▶96373, 96374◀)

✎ Rationale

In tandem with the deletion and renumbering of the infusion services procedures, the cross-reference following code 01992 has been revised to instruct users to report code 96373 or 96374 for intra-arterial or intravenous therapy for pain management.

Surgery

Changes to this section include many revisions of the Integumentary System codes and the Skin Replacement guidelines to clarify the intent of spatial references within the code descriptors. Other important revisions resulting from the addition of codes include clarification of the hemorrhoid destruction, prostate resection codes and the nerve injection and keratoplasty codes.

New codes have been added in the Musculoskeletal section for the spine and pelvis, with revisions of codes in the hip, shoulder, and femur. Other new codes have been added for non-coronary bypass graft procedures, tongue base reductions, pancreatic duct cannulation, esophageal repair, laparoscopic hernia repairs, and stereotactic cranial and spinal radiosurgery.

Surgery

General

10021 Fine needle aspiration; without imaging guidance

10022 with imaging guidance

(For percutaneous needle biopsy other than fine needle aspiration, see 20206 for muscle, 32400 for pleura, 32405 for lung or mediastinum, 42400 for salivary gland, 47000, 47001 for liver, 48102 for pancreas, 49180 for abdominal or retroperitoneal mass, 60100 for thyroid, ▶62267 for nucleus pulposus, intervertebral disc, or paravertebral tissue,◀ 62269 for spinal cord)

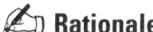 **Rationale**

To support the addition of code 62267 to report percutaneous aspiration within the nucleus pulposus, intervertebral disc, or paravertebral tissue for diagnostic purposes, the cross-reference following code 10022 was revised to refer users to 62267 when reporting interdiscal percutaneous diagnostic aspiration.

Integumentary System

Skin, Subcutaneous and Accessory Structures

EXCISION—DEBRIDEMENT

11000 Debridement of extensive eczematous or infected skin; up to 10% of body surface

+▲11001 each additional 10% of the body surface, or part thereof (List separately in addition to code for primary procedure)

REMOVAL OF SKIN TAGS

11200 Removal of skin tags, multiple fibrocutaneous tags, any area; up to and including 15 lesions

+▲11201 each additional 10 lesions, or part thereof (List separately in addition to code for primary procedure)

Introduction

11920 Tattooing, intradermal introduction of insoluble opaque pigments to correct color defects of skin, including micropigmentation; 6.0 sq cm or less

11921 6.1 to 20.0 sq cm

+▲11922 each additional 20.0 sq cm, or part thereof (List separately in addition to code for primary procedure)

✏️ Rationale

Codes 11001, 11201, and 11922 have been editorially revised with the addition of "or part thereof" to clarify that the existing phrase "each additional 10% of the body surface," "each additional 10 lesions," or "each additional 20.0 sq cm" is intended to include repair of any additional percentage within the stated measurement. These revisions were made to address confusion regarding reporting for repairs over the initial measurement, whether by percentage, number of lesions, or area measurement, and to provide consistency with other add-on integumentary codes that include measurement as a reporting mechanism.

Repair (Closure)

REPAIR—INTERMEDIATE

Sum of lengths of repairs for each group of anatomic sites.

▲ 12031 Repair, intermediate, wounds of scalp, axillae, trunk and/or extremities (excluding hands and feet); 2.5 cm or less

▲ 12032 2.6 cm to 7.5 cm

▲ 12034 7.6 cm to 12.5 cm

▲ 12035 12.6 cm to 20.0 cm

▲ 12036 20.1 cm to 30.0 cm

▲ 12037 over 30.0 cm

▲ 12041 Repair, intermediate, wounds of neck, hands, feet and/or external genitalia; 2.5 cm or less

▲ 12042 2.6 cm to 7.5 cm

▲ 12044 7.6 cm to 12.5 cm

▲ 12045 12.6 cm to 20.0 cm

▲ 12046 20.1 cm to 30.0 cm

▲ 12047 over 30.0 cm

▲ 12051 Repair, intermediate, wounds of face, ears, eyelids, nose, lips and/or mucous membranes; 2.5 cm or less

▲ 12052 2.6 cm to 5.0 cm

▲ 12053 5.1 cm to 7.5 cm

▲ 12054 7.6 cm to 12.5 cm

▲ 12055 12.6 cm to 20.0 cm

▲ 12056 20.1 cm to 30.0 cm

▲ 12057 over 30.0 cm

Rationale

The intermediate repair codes 12031-12057 have been revised for consistency in terminology to describe intermediate wound repair. Unlike the simple (12001-12021) and complex (13100-13160) wound repair codes, whose descriptor language was congruent with the existing guidelines and headings in the CPT® coding system, the reference to "layer closure" and absence of "intermediate repair" language in codes 12031-12057 caused confusion in interpretation. The revision in terminology now adds congruency both between the wound repair code sets and with the wound repair guidelines.

SKIN REPLACEMENT SURGERY AND SKIN SUBSTITUTES

Identify by size and location of . . .

When a primary procedure such as . . .

Use codes 15002-15005 for initial wound recipient site preparation.

▶Use codes 15100-15261 for autologous skin grafts. For autologous tissue-cultured epidermal grafts, use codes 15150-15157. For harvesting of autologous keratinocytes and dermal tissue for tissue-cultured skin grafts, use code 15040. Procedures are coded by recipient site. Use codes 15170-15176 for acellular dermal replacement.◀

Repair of donor site requiring skin . . .

Codes 15002-15005 describe burn and wound . . .

These codes are not intended to be reported for simple graft application alone or application stabilized with dressings (eg, by simple gauze wrap). The skin substitute/graft is anchored using the surgeon's choice of fixation. When services are performed in the office, the supply of the skin substitute/graft should be reported separately. Routine dressing supplies are not reported separately. ▶When square centimeters are indicated, this refers to 1 sq cm up to the stated amount. Add-on codes begin with the next sq cm (eg, 130 sq cm would be coded using a code for the first 100 sq cm and an add-on code for the next 30 sq cm). Use modifier 58 for staged application procedure(s).◀

(For microvascular flaps, see 15756-15758)

Surgical Preparation
(15000, 15001 have been deleted. To report, see 15002-15005)

15002   Surgical preparation or creation of recipient site by excision of open wounds, burn eschar, or scar (including subcutaneous tissues), or incisional release of scar contracture, trunk, arms, legs; first 100 sq cm or 1% of body area of infants and children

+▲ **15003**   each additional 100 sq cm, or part thereof, or each additional 1% of body area of infants and children (List separately in addition to code for primary procedure)

15004   Surgical preparation or creation of recipient site by excision of open wounds, burn eschar, or scar (including subcutaneous tissues), or incisional release of scar contracture, face, scalp, eyelids, mouth, neck, ears, orbits, genitalia, hands, feet and/or multiple digits; first 100 sq cm or 1% of body area of infants and children

+▲ 15005 each additional 100 sq cm, or part thereof, or each additional 1% of body area of infants and children (List separately in addition to code for primary procedure)

Grafts

Acellular Dermal Replacement

15200 Full thickness graft, free, including direct closure of donor site, trunk; 20 sq cm or less

+▲ 15201 each additional 20 sq cm, or part thereof (List separately in addition to code for primary procedure)

15220 Full thickness graft, free, including direct closure of donor site, scalp, arms, and/or legs; 20 sq cm or less

+▲ 15221 each additional 20 sq cm, or part thereof (List separately in addition to code for primary procedure)

15240 Full thickness graft, free, including direct closure of donor site, forehead, cheeks, chin, mouth, neck, axillae, genitalia, hands, and/or feet; 20 sq cm or less

+▲ 15241 each additional 20 sq cm, or part thereof (List separately in addition to code for primary procedure)

15260 Full thickness graft, free, including direct closure of donor site, nose, ears, eyelids, and/or lips; 20 sq cm or less

+▲ 15261 each additional 20 sq cm, or part thereof (List separately in addition to code for primary procedure)

Allograft/Tissue Cultured Allogeneic Skin Substitute

15340 Tissue cultured allogeneic skin substitute; first 25 sq cm or less

+▲ 15341 each additional 25 sq cm, or part thereof (List separately in addition to code for primary procedure)

Rationale

The guidelines for the Skin Replacement Surgery and Skin Substitutes codes have been revised to assist users in understanding the intent of the add-on measurement codes that are found in this subsection. The guidelines have also been revised with the deletion and movement of the staged procedure instructions to the end of the guidelines, to indicate that use of modifier 58 for staged procedures was not intended to be limited to the listing of codes in the paragraph in which this was previously included.

Guideline revisions also address the need for clarification of the minimum requirements for reporting additional measurements over those described by the initial service codes. Guideline text has been added to clarify that, when the procedure performed is greater than that described in the initial service code, from 1 cm to the stated amount, the additional service should be reported. Revisions of the descriptors for codes 15003, 15005, 15201, 15221, 15241, 15261, and 15341 have also been made with the addition of "or part thereof" to clarify that the existing body surface measurements, whether by percentage or square centimeter, are intended to include repair of any additional portion of the measurement. These revisions were made to address confusion regarding reporting for repairs over the initial measured body surface and to convey consistency with other add-on integumentary codes that include measurement as a reporting mechanism.

The descriptor for code 15341 has also been editorially revised with the addition of the phrase, "(List separately in addition to code for primary procedure)," to convey consistency in CPT nomenclature for conventional add-on procedure descriptions.

FLAPS (SKIN AND/OR DEEP TISSUES)

The regions listed refer to the recipient area (not the donor site) when a flap is being attached in a transfer or to a final site.

The regions listed refer to a donor site when a tube is formed for later ▶transfer◀ or when a "delay" of flap ▶occurs◀ prior to the transfer.

Procedures 15570-15738 do not include extensive immobilization (eg, large plaster casts and other immobilizing devices are considered additional separate procedures).

A repair of a donor site requiring a skin graft or local flaps is considered an additional separate procedure.

(For microvascular flaps, see 15756-15758)

(For flaps without inclusion of a vascular pedicle, see 15570-15576)

(For adjacent tissue transfer flaps, see 14000-14300)

15570   Formation of direct or tubed pedicle, with or without transfer; trunk

 Rationale

The guideline instructions for the Flaps (Skin and/or Deep Tissues) have been revised to clarify the intent of the description of the timing of the tube formation in the flap donor site. Previously these instructions suggested, but did not specify, that transferring of the flap was intended when tube formation was performed.

Breast

INTRODUCTION

▲ **19296**   Placement of radiotherapy afterloading expandable catheter (single or multichannel) into the breast for interstitial radioelement application following partial mastectomy, includes imaging guidance; on date separate from partial mastectomy

+▲ **19297**   concurrent with partial mastectomy (List separately in addition to code for primary procedure)

 Rationale

Codes 19296 and 19297 were revised to assist reporting the use of cavity-conforming catheters in placement procedures and reflect new technology for the catheters described in this service. The revisions indicate that afterloading radiotherapy

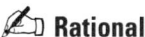=Revised Code   ●=New Code   ▶◀=New or Revised Text   ○=Reinstated Code

catheters are expandable, and include the use of either single or multichannel devices. The addition of "(single or multichannel)" assists in differentiation of this code from code 19298.

Code 19296 and add-on code 19297 describe interstitial radioelement application catheter placement for radiotherapy afterloading into the cavity created by an excisional biopsy or a lumpectomy procedure for the purpose of radioelement application. Code 19296 should be reported when the catheter is placed on a separate date from the partial mastectomy. Add-on code 19297 should be reported when the catheter is placed after the partial mastectomy during the same operative session (concurrent). A parenthetical instruction following code 19297 directs users to report code 19297 in conjunction with the concurrently performed partial mastectomy code (ie, 19301 or 19302).

Musculoskeletal System

General

INTRODUCTION OR REMOVAL

20550   Injection(s); single tendon sheath, or ligament, aponeurosis (eg, plantar "fascia")

▶(For injection of Morton's neuroma, see 64455, 64632)◀

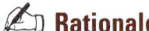 **Rationale**

In support of the addition of codes 64455 and 64632 to report injection and destruction by injection of the plantar common digital nerve for treatment of Morton's neuroma, a cross-reference has been added following code 20550 to direct users to the appropriate codes when these services are provided.

●**20696**   Application of multiplane (pins or wires in more than one plane), unilateral, external fixation with stereotactic computer-assisted adjustment (eg, spatial frame), including imaging; initial and subsequent alignment(s), assessment(s), and computation(s) of adjustment schedule(s)

▶(Do not report 20696 in conjunction with 20692, 20697)◀

⊘●**20697**   exchange (ie, removal and replacement) of strut, each

▶(Do not report 20697 in conjunction with 20692, 20696)◀

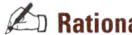 **Rationale**

Codes 20696 and 20697 were established to describe the application of external fixation using stereotactic computer-assisted adjustment. Computer-assisted external fixation provides the simultaneous correction of multiple axes of a fracture or deformity. This is possible because the fixation is dynamic, with multiple fixator struts. Code 20696 is reported for initial and subsequent alignment(s), assessment(s), and computation(s) of adjustment schedule(s). A parenthetical note was added following code 20696 instructing users not to report this code in conjunction with code 20692 or 20697. Code 20697 is reported for the exchange of each strut and includes both the removal of and replacement of each strut. A parenthetical note was added below code 26097 instructing users not to report this code in conjunction with code 20692 or 20696. Imaging is included in both codes.

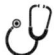
Clinical Example (20696)

A 33-year-old woman with a biplanar deformity and acquired limb length discrepancy with tibial nonunion undergoes reconstructive surgery using a computer-dependent multiplanar, tensioned wire external fixation system designed for gradual deformity correction and controlled mechanical distraction osteogenesis.

Note: Code 20696 includes application of the dynamic fixation device and all follow-up hospital and/or office patient work through the 90-day global period except the changing of a strut. A strut change, if necessary, is separately reported using new code 20697.

Description of Procedure (20696)
Under anesthesia, the external fixator is mounted orthogonal to each segment of bone. Each ring is mounted perpendicular to the bone on the anteroposterior (AP) and lateral (LAT) fluoroscopic projections as well as orthogonal in the axial plane with the centering bolts on the AP and LAT projections overlapping when the leg is held in the same "patella forward" position. This is accomplished by mounting the ring on an intraosseous wire placed perpendicular to the bone on the AP projection and a half pin placed perpendicular to the bone on the LAT projection. Each segment of bone has a ring mounted in this way with a wire and half pin. Additional wires and half pins (minimum of three per segment) are added to each bone segment once both rings are mounted to each segment. The bone is examined under fluoroscopy to assess whether the correction can be performed without cutting the bone. Once the frame is mounted with intraosseous wires and half pins, the six struts are connected. The mounting parameters are then assessed by determining where the LAT and AP centering bolts are in reference to the center of the ring. Radiographs are taken in the operating room while the surgeon positions the limb(s) to ensure complete accuracy of the mounting radiographs. The intraoperative mounting parameters, deformity parameters, and initial strut settings are inserted into a computer program prior to the patient's discharge. The rate of correction is determined from the "greatest structure at risk" while the deformity is being corrected. This rate of correction is also placed into the computer program to generate a safe daily schedule for the patient to perform gradual deformity correction, which would begin on postoperative day 5-7.

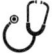
Clinical Example (20697)

A 33-year-old woman with a biplanar deformity and acquired limb length discrepancy with tibial nonunion while undergoing deformity correction requires exchange of strut.

Note: Initial placement of the dynamic external fixation system is separately reported using code 20696.

Description of Procedure (20697)

A spanning strut is placed onto the frame to stabilize the frame at the site of the strut change. The old strut is removed and a new strut with larger/smaller numbers is placed. Once the new strut is secured, the temporary strut can be removed.

GRAFTS (OR IMPLANTS)

(For spinal surgery bone graft[s] see codes 20930-20938)

+ **20930** Allograft for spine surgery only; morselized (List separately in addition to code for primary procedure)

(Use 20930 in conjunction with 22319, 22532, 22533, 22548-22558, 22590-22612, 22630, 22800-22812, ▶0195T, 0196T◀)

+ **20936** Autograft for spine surgery only (includes harvesting the graft); local (eg, ribs, spinous process, or laminar fragments) obtained from same incision (List separately in addition to code for primary procedure)

(Use 20936 in conjunction with 22319, 22532, 22533, 22548-22558, 22590-22612, 22630, 22800-22812, ▶0195T, 0196T◀)

+ **20937** morselized (through separate skin or fascial incision) (List separately in addition to code for primary procedure)

(Use 20937 in conjunction with 22319, 22532, 22533, 22548-22558, 22590-22612, 22630, 22800-22812, ▶0195T, 0196T◀)

(Use 20938 in conjunction with 22319, 22532, 22533, 22548-22558, 22590-22612, 22630, 22800-22812)

Rationale

To support the addition of two Category III codes, 0195T and 0196T, to report percutaneous lumbar discectomy and preparation of the interspace for fusion, the cross-references following the bone grafting codes 20930, 20936, and 20937 have been revised to instruct that grafting should be separately reported with Category III code 0195T or 0196T.

OTHER PROCEDURES

+ ▲ **20985** Computer-assisted surgical navigational procedure for musculoskeletal procedures, image-less (List separately in addition to code for primary procedure)

▶(Do not report 20985 in conjunction with 61795)◀

▶(20986, 20987 have been deleted)◀

▶(For computer-assisted navigational procedures with image guidance based on pre-operative and intraoperatively obtained images, see 0054T, 0055T)◀

✍ Rationale

Codes 20986 and 20987 and the parenthetical instructions associated with these codes have been deleted. Computer-assisted musculoskeletal surgical navigational preoperative and intraoperative imaging will now be reported with codes 0054T and 0055T, and differentiated solely by the type of imaging (fluoroscopic [0054T], computed tomography/magnetic resonance imaging [0055T]). Codes 0054T and 0055T will continue as Category III codes pending the availability of further information to demonstrate that the necessary criteria for Category I code status has been met.

For *CPT 2008*, three new Category I codes, 20985-20987, were added to report computer-assisted surgical navigational procedures. Of these codes, only code 20985 continues to meet the criteria for retention of this Category I code.

Spine (Vertebral Column)

SPINAL INSTRUMENTATION

+ 22840 Posterior non-segmental instrumentation (eg, Harrington rod technique, pedicle fixation across one interspace, atlantoaxial transarticular screw fixation, sublaminar wiring at C1, facet screw fixation) (List separately in addition to code for primary procedure)

(Use 22840 in conjunction with 22100-22102, 22110-22114, 22206, ▶22207,◀ 22210-22214, 22220-22224, 22305-22327, 22532, 22533, 22548-22558, 22590-22612, 22630, 22800-22812, 63001-63030, 63040-63042, 63045-63047, 63050-63056, 63064, 63075, 63077, 63081, 63085, 63087, 63090, 63101, 63102, 63170-63290, 63300-63307)

+ 22841 Internal spinal fixation by wiring of spinous processes (List separately in addition to code for primary procedure)

(Use 22841 in conjunction with 22100-22102, 22110-22114, 22206, ▶22207,◀ 22210-22214, 22220-22224, 22305-22327, 22532, 22533, 22548-22558, 22590-22612, 22630, 22800-22812, 63001-63030, 63040-63042, 63045-63047, 63050-63056, 63064, 63075, 63077, 63081, 63085, 63087, 63090, 63101, 63102, 63170-63290, 63300-63307)

+ 22842 Posterior segmental instrumentation (eg, pedicle fixation, dual rods with multiple hooks and sublaminar wires); 3 to 6 vertebral segments (List separately in addition to code for primary procedure)

(Use 22842 in conjunction with 22100-22102, 22110-22114, 22206, ▶22207,◀ 22210-22214, 22220-22224, 22305-22327, 22532, 22533, 22548-22558, 22590-22612, 22630, 22800-22812, 63001-63030, 63040-63042, 63045-63047, 63050-63056, 63064, 63075, 63077, 63081, 63085, 63087, 63090, 63101, 63102, 63170-63290, 63300-63307)

+ 22843 7 to 12 vertebral segments (List separately in addition to code for primary procedure)

(Use 22843 in conjunction with 22100-22102, 22110-22114, 22206, ▶22207,◀ 22210-22214, 22220-22224, 22305-22327, 22532, 22533, 22548-22558, 22590-22612, 22630, 22800-22812, 63001-63030, 63040-63042, 63045-63047, 63050-63056, 63064, 63075, 63077, 63081, 63085, 63087, 63090, 63101, 63102, 63170-63290, 63300-63307)

+ 22844 13 or more vertebral segments (List separately in addition to code for primary procedure)

(Use 22844 in conjunction with 22100-22102, 22110-22114, 22206, ▶22207,◀ 22210-22214, 22220-22224, 22305-22327, 22532, 22533, 22548-22558, 22590-22612, 22630, 22800-22812, 63001-63030, 63040-63042, 63045-63047, 63050-63056, 63064, 63075, 63077, 63081, 63085, 63087, 63090, 63101, 63102, 63170-63290, 63300-63307)

+ 22845 Anterior instrumentation; 2 to 3 vertebral segments (List separately in addition to code for primary procedure)

(Use 22845 in conjunction with 22100-22102, 22110-22114, 22206, ▶22207,◀ 22210-22214, 22220-22224, 22305-22327, 22532, 22533, 22548-22558, 22590-22612, 22630, 22800-22812, 63001-63030, 63040-63042, 63045-63047, 63050-63056, 63064, 63075, 63077, 63081, 63085, 63087, 63090, 63101, 63102, 63170-63290, 63300-63307)

+ 22846 4 to 7 vertebral segments (List separately in addition to code for primary procedure)

(Use 22846 in conjunction with 22100-22102, 22110-22114, 22206, ▶22207,◀ 22210-22214, 22220-22224, 22305-22327, 22532, 22533, 22548-22558, 22590-22612, 22630, 22800-22812, 63001-63030, 63040-63042, 63045-63047, 63050-63056, 63064, 63075, 63077, 63081, 63085, 63087, 63090, 63101, 63102, 63170-63290, 63300-63307)

+ 22847 8 or more vertebral segments (List separately in addition to code for primary procedure)

(Use 22847 in conjunction with 22100-22102, 22110-22114, 22206, ▶22207,◀ 22210-22214, 22220-22224, 22305-22327, 22532, 22533, 22548-22558, 22590-22612, 22630, 22800-22812, 63001-63030, 63040-63042, 63045-63047, 63050-63056, 63064, 63075, 63077, 63081, 63085, 63087, 63090, 63101, 63102, 63170-63290, 63300-63307)

+ 22848 Pelvic fixation (attachment of caudal end of instrumentation to pelvic bony structures) other than sacrum (List separately in addition to code for primary procedure)

(Use 22848 in conjunction with 22100-22102, 22110-22114, 22206, ▶22207,◀ 22210-22214, 22220-22224, 22305-22327, 22532, 22533, 22548-22558, 22590-22612, 22630, 22800-22812, 63001-63030, 63040-63042, 63045-63047, 63050-63056, 63064, 63075, 63077, 63081, 63085, 63087, 63090, 63101, 63102, 63170-63290, 63300-63307)

22849 Reinsertion of spinal fixation device

22850 Removal of posterior nonsegmental instrumentation (eg, Harrington rod)

+ 22851 Application of intervertebral biomechanical device(s) (eg, synthetic cage(s), threaded bone dowel(s), methylmethacrylate) to vertebral defect or interspace (List separately in addition to code for primary procedure)

(Use 22851 in conjunction with 22100-22102, 22110-22114, 22206, ▶22207,◀ 22210-22214, 22220-22224, 22305-22327, 22532, 22533, 22548-22558, 22590-22612, 22630, 22800-22812, 63001-63030, 63040-63042, 63045-63047, 63050-63056, 63064, 63075, 63077, 63081, 63085, 63087, 63090, 63101, 63102, 63170-63290, 63300-63307)

Rationale

The parenthetical instructions following the add-on spinal instrumentation codes 22840-22848 and 22851 have been revised to delete the reference to code 22208. As an add-on code, this code was inappropriately included in the parenthetical instructions following the instrumentation codes, and should not be reported in addition to these codes.

● **22856** Total disc arthroplasty (artificial disc), anterior approach, including discectomy with end plate preparation (includes osteophytectomy for nerve root or spinal cord decompression and microdissection), single interspace, cervical

▶(Do not report 22856 in conjunction with 22554, 22845, 22851, 63075 when performed at the same level)◀

▶(Do not report 22856 in conjunction with 69990)◀

▶(For additional interspace cervical total disc arthroplasty, use 0092T)◀

▲ **22857** Total disc arthroplasty (artificial disc), anterior approach, including discectomy to prepare interspace (other than for decompression), single interspace, lumbar

(Do not report 22857 in conjunction with 22558, 22845, 22851, 49010 when performed at the same level)

(For additional interspace, use Category III code 0163T)

● **22861** Revision including replacement of total disc arthroplasty (artificial disc), anterior approach, single interspace; cervical

▶(Do not report 22861 in conjunction with 22845, 22851, 22864, 63075 when performed at the same level)◀

▶(Do not report 22861 in conjunction with 69990)◀

▶(For additional interspace revision of cervical total disc arthroplasty, use 0098T)◀

▲ **22862** lumbar

(Do not report 22862 in conjunction with 22558, 22845, 22851, 22865, 49010 when performed at the same level)

(For additional interspace, use Category III code 0165T)

● **22864** Removal of total disc arthroplasty (artificial disc), anterior approach, single interspace; cervical

▶(Do not report 22864 in conjunction with 22861, 69990)◀

▶(For additional interspace removal of cervical total disc arthroplasty, use 0095T)◀

▲ **22865** lumbar

(Do not report 22865 in conjunction with 49010)

(For additional interspace, see Category III code 0164T)

(22856-22865 include fluoroscopy when performed)

✎ Rationale

Codes 22856, 22861, and 22864 were established to report artificial cervical total disc arthroplasty procedures. These services were previously reported with Category III codes 0090T, 0096T, and 0093T, respectively. These Category III codes have been deleted for *CPT 2009*. To accommodate the addition of the

Category I codes, the lumbar arthroplasty codes that were added for CPT 2007, 22857, 22862, and 22865, have been revised to indented codes.

These procedures are typically performed for treatment of cervical disc disease and are added to the list of options for treatment of cervical radiculopathy (hand, shoulder, or wrist pain resulting from nerve compression in the cervical spine), cervical spondylosis (cervical spine degeneration as a result of disc degeneration), or cervical myelopathy (loss of sensation due to spinal injury). The new artificial cervical total disc arthroplasty codes typically consist of an anterior cervical approach to include discectomy with decompression and removal of any osteophytes or other pathologic disc material. A total disc arthroplasty consists of a procedure in which all or most of the disc tissue is removed and a replacement device is implanted into the space between the vertebra to imitate the functions of a normal disc.

The use of the operating microscope and fluoroscopic guidance is inherent in these procedures and would not be separately reported. Interspace preparation (22554), anterior instrumentation (22845), intervertebral biomechanical device application (22851), and cervical anterior discectomy with decompression and osteophytectomy (63075) all describe procedures that are inherent in the arthroplasty procedure, which would not be separately reported with code 22856. Total cervical arthroplasty of an additional space should be separately reported with code 0092T, Total disc arthroplasty (artificial disc), anterior approach, including discectomy with end plate preparation (includes osteophytectomy for nerve root or spinal cord decompression and microdissection), each additional interspace, cervical (List separately in addition to code for primary procedure).

Anterior instrumentation (22845), intervertebral biomechanical device application (22851), and cervical anterior discectomy with decompression and osteophytectomy (63075) describe procedures that are inherent in the arthroplasty revision procedure, and would not be separately reported with code 22861. Revision and removal of an additional space for a total cervical arthroplasty should be separately reported with, respectively, code 0098T, Revision including replacement of total disc arthroplasty (artificial disc), anterior approach, each additional interspace, cervical (List separately in addition to code for primary procedure), and code 0095T, Removal of total disc arthroplasty (artificial disc), anterior approach, each additional interspace, cervical (List separately in addition to code for primary procedure).

Clinical Example (22856)

A 48-year-old man presents with right-sided cervical brachial pain refractory to multimodality conservative therapy. Examination shows findings of nerve root compression with cervical motion, C6 radiculopathy on neurologic examination, along with a magnetic resonance image showing a single degenerative C5-6 disc with focal right paracentral disc herniation and associated osteophyte formation with foraminal and canal compromise.

Description of Procedure (22856)
A skin incision is made and sharp and blunt dissection is used to dissect between the carotid sheath laterally and the esophagus and trachea medially, exposing the

prevertebral space. Vertebral level is identified using fluoroscopy and the edges of the longus coli muscles are dissected and elevated from the vertebral bodies. Self-retaining retractors are inserted beneath the edge of the longus coli. The disc space is incised and the disc material is removed with curettes and rongeurs to the posterior longitudinal ligament. Disc space distractor pins are introduced into the C5 and C6 vertebral bodies; the distractor is applied, and the space is opened up with end plates parallel to each other. The operating microscope is sterilely draped and brought into the field. The remainder of the procedure is performed utilizing standard microdissection techniques. The posterior ligament is opened and resected. The disc herniation is identified and removed from the epidural space decompressing the nerve root. A punch and/or high-speed drill is used to perform a foraminotomy on both sides to remove uncovertebral osteophytes. Hemostasis is achieved and the cartilaginous end plate is removed, sparing the bone. The implant trial is introduced into the disc space between the uncinate processes. The trial is then confirmed to be appropriately sized and located utilizing antero-posterior (AP) and lateral plane fluoroscopy. A drill guide is then introduced over the implant trial and tracts are created in the inferior and superior end plates and cleaned of bone debris. The trial is removed and the final implant is inserted into the tracts previously cut and tapped into position. Fluoroscopy is used to confirm position in AP and lateral projections; adjustments are made as necessary. Hemostasis is achieved, the retractors are removed, the incision is closed in layers, and a sterile dressing is placed.

Clinical Example (22861)

A 48-year-old man presents after having had anterior cervical disc arthroplasty several days previously. Follow-up X rays show migration of the implant, requiring revision.

Description of Procedure (22861)

A skin incision is made through the old incision. A sharp and blunt dissection is used to dissect through the scar tissue of the prior operation between the carotid sheath laterally and the esophagus and trachea medially, exposing the prevertebral space. The implant level is identified using fluoroscopy and the edges of the longus coli muscles are dissected and elevated from the vertebral bodies. Self-retaining retractors are inserted beneath the edge of the longus coli. The device is dissected free of the superior and inferior bone, and the device is removed from the endplates. Disc space distractor pins are introduced into the C5 and C6 vertebral bodies, the distractor is applied, and the space is opened up with end plates parallel to each other. The implant trial is introduced into the disc space between the uncinate processes. The trial is then confirmed to be appropriately sized and located on AP and lateral plane fluoroscopy. A drill guide is then introduced over the implant trial and, if needed, new tracts are created in the inferior and superior end plates and cleaned of bone debris. The trial is removed and the final implant is inserted into the tracts previously cut and tapped into position. Fluoroscopy is used to confirm position in AP and lateral projections, and adjustments are made as necessary. Hemostasis is achieved, the retractors are removed, the incision is closed in layers, and a sterile dressing is placed.

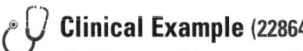 **Clinical Example (22864)**

A 48-year-old man with a previously implanted C5-6 total disc arthroplasty developed an infection and abscess and has demonstrated loosening of the implant, requiring removal.

Description of Procedure (22864)

A skin incision is made and sharp and blunt dissection is used to dissect through the scar tissue of the prior approach between the carotid sheath laterally and the esophagus and trachea medially, exposing the prevertebral space. Vertebral level is identified using fluoroscopy and the edges of the longus coli muscles are dissected and elevated from the vertebral bodies. Self-retaining retractors are inserted beneath the edge of the longus coli. The device is dissected free of the superior and inferior bone and the device is removed from the endplates. Additional procedures may be performed and reported separately as appropriate. Hemostasis is achieved; the retractors are removed, the incision is closed in layers, and a sterile dressing is placed.

Shoulder

FRACTURE AND/OR DISLOCATION

▲ **23585**   Open treatment of scapular fracture (body, glenoid or acromion) includes internal fixation, when performed

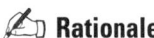 **Rationale**

The open treatment of scapular fracture code 23585 was revised with the removal of the terms "with or without" and the addition of the terms "includes" and "when performed" for consistency with current CPT nomenclature.

Pelvis and Hip Joint

INCISION

●**27027**   Decompression fasciotomy(ies), pelvic (buttock) compartment(s) (eg, gluteus medius-minimus, gluteus maximus, iliopsoas, and/or tensor fascia lata muscle), unilateral

▶(To report bilateral procedure, report 27027 with modifier 50)◀

EXCISION

27054   Arthrotomy with synovectomy, hip joint

●**27057**   Decompression fasciotomy(ies), pelvic (buttock) compartment(s) (eg, gluteus medius-minimus, gluteus maximus, iliopsoas, and/or tensor fascia lata muscle) with debridement of nonviable muscle, unilateral

▶(To report bilateral procedure, report 27057 with modifier 50)◀

Rationale

Codes 27027 and 27057 have been added to report decompressive buttock fasciotomies. As is noted in the parenthetical notes added following these codes, bilateral performance of these services should be identified by appending modifier 50. Debridement procedures identified by codes 11040-11043 are included as part of this service (27057) and are not separately reported.

Pelvic compartment fasciotomies described in code 27057 are performed for patients developing or having compartment syndrome involving one or more of the pelvic compartments (gluteus medius-minimus, gluteus maximus, iliopsoas, and/or tensor fascia lata muscle compartments). The most commonly recognized compartment for this syndrome is the gluteal "buttock" compartment, as its large muscle mass is confined by the tight inelastic fascia. The most common causes of pelvic compartment syndrome are musculoskeletal pelvic trauma, prolonged immobility with prolonged buttock pressure due to altered level of consciousness (eg, acute alcohol intoxication, drug overdose, drug-induced coma), Ehlers-Danlos syndrome, and sickle cell–associated muscle infarction.

If the compartment syndrome is unrecognized or untreated, it can lead to renal failure, sepsis, and death.

Clinical Example (27027)

A 23-year-old man involved in a motorcycle crash sustains fractures of the tibia and fibula, a pulmonary contusion, and contusions and significant skin abrasions to the buttocks and legs. There is a large left buttock contusion with no evidence of a pelvic fracture. Over the next 6 hours, the contusion and associated interstitial hemorrhage and edema expand, causing increasing pain down the left leg. The patient is taken to the operating room emergently for pelvic compartment fasciotomy(ies).

Description of Procedure (27027)

An incision is made on the superolateral thigh beginning at the greater trochanter and extending proximally and posteriorly into the buttock, ending 4 cm below the posterior superior iliac spine. Hemostasis is achieved in the dermal and subcutaneous tissues with electrocautery. The iliotibial band is identified and incised in line with the incision. Proximally, the gluteus maximus is bluntly split in the direction of its fibers. The inferior gluteal artery is identified and protected. The gluteus medius and the tensor fascia lata muscles are identified. The dissection is deepened to allow identification of the sciatic nerve and the piriformis, obturator internus, obturator externus, superior and inferior gemelli, and quadratus femoris muscles. Deep hematoma is identified and evacuated. The superior gluteal artery and nerve and the inferior gluteal artery and nerve are identified and, if injured, bleeding is controlled. The fascia overlying the gluteus medius, gluteus minimum, gluteus maximus (including gluteal aponeurosis), and tensor fascia lata muscles are released as required to provide decompression. All muscles are inspected and evaluated for viability, contractility, and/or injury. Epimysial and intramuscular hemorrhage is controlled. Complete hemostasis is achieved. The wound is packed and left open.

Clinical Example (27057)

A 75-year-old woman has fallen at home and been poorly mobilized for 72 hours. She presents with tenderness and discoloration over the left buttock. She is febrile with leukocytosis. The patient is taken to the operating room emergently for pelvic compartment fasciotomy(ies) and excisional debridement of necrotic muscle in the gluteal group.

Description of Procedure (27057)

An incision is made on the superolateral thigh beginning at the greater trochanter and extending proximally and posteriorly into the buttock, ending 4 cm below the posterior superior iliac spine. Hemostasis is achieved in the dermal and subcutaneous tissues with electrocautery. The iliotibial band is identified and incised in line with the incision. Proximally, the gluteus maximus is bluntly split in the direction of its fibers. The inferior gluteal artery is identified and protected. The gluteus medius and the tensor fascia lata muscles are identified. The dissection is deepened to allow identification of the sciatic nerve and the piriformis, obturator internus, obturator externus, superior and inferior gemelli, and quadratus femoris muscles. Deep hematoma is identified and evacuated. The superior gluteal artery and nerve and the inferior gluteal artery and nerve are identified and, if injured, bleeding is controlled. The fascia overlying the gluteus medius, gluteus minimum, gluteus maximus (including gluteal aponeurosis), and tensor fascia lata muscles are released as required to provide decompression. All muscles are inspected and evaluated for viability, contractility, and/or injury. All nonviable, necrotic gluteal muscles are excised. Epimysial and intramuscular hemorrhage is controlled. Complete hemostasis is achieved. The wound is packed and left open.

FRACTURE AND/OR DISLOCATION

▲ **27215** Open treatment of iliac spine(s), tuberosity avulsion, or iliac wing fracture(s), unilateral, for pelvic bone fracture patterns that do not disrupt the pelvic ring, includes internal fixation, when performed

▶(To report bilateral procedure, report 27215 with modifier 50)◀

▲ **27216** Percutaneous skeletal fixation of posterior pelvic bone fracture and/or dislocation, for fracture patterns that disrupt the pelvic ring, unilateral (includes ipsilateral ilium, sacroiliac joint and/or sacrum)

▶(To report bilateral procedure, report 27216 with modifier 50)◀

▲ **27217** Open treatment of anterior pelvic bone fracture and/or dislocation for fracture patterns that disrupt the pelvic ring, unilateral, includes internal fixation, when performed (includes pubic symphysis and/or ipsilateral superior/inferior rami)

▶(To report bilateral procedure, report 27217 with modifier 50)◀

▲ **27218** Open treatment of posterior pelvic bone fracture and/or dislocation, for fracture patterns that disrupt the pelvic ring, unilateral, includes internal fixation, when performed (includes ipsilateral ilium, sacroiliac joint and/or sacrum)

▶(To report bilateral procedure, report 27218 with modifier 50)◀

Rationale

Codes 27215-27218 were editorially revised to clarify the unilateral nature of these codes. This revision clarifies that these treatments pertain to unilateral services and, when performed concurrently on the pelvic ring on the left and right sides of the body, should be reported with modifier 50. A parenthetical note was also added following each code to support the descriptor revisions instructing users to report modifier 50 when the procedure is performed bilaterally.

Clinical Example (27215)

A 27-year-old female pedestrian is struck on her right side by a motorized vehicle and knocked to the ground. She has immediate pain over the iliac wing with ecchymosis and an obvious deformity. She complains of pain over the ilium with radiation to the anterolateral thigh, on ambulation and with respiration. Radiographs in the emergency department reveal a displaced iliac wing fracture with an intact pelvic ring. Due to the displaced fracture, dysfunction associated with activities of daily living and deformity, the patient undergoes open treatment of the fracture with internal fixation.

Description of Procedure (27215)

An extensile incision is made over the iliac crest. The muscles and fascia are incised; subperiosteal reflection from the bone is utilized to expose the injured segment(s). Care is taken to avoid injury to the lateral femoral cutaneous nerve, sciatic nerve and the superior gluteal vessels. The fracture site(s) is cleansed of hematoma and reduction achieved using a combination of direct and indirect techniques. Provisional fixation is maintained with bone clamps and K-wires. The reduction is confirmed with image intensification. Definitive fixation is then completed using a combination of plates, screws, wires, and sutures. The reduction and position of the implants is again assessed by fluoroscopy. The wound is irrigated and closed in layers over a drain.

Clinical Example (27216)

A 42-year-old man is involved in a motor vehicle crash and is transported to the emergency department. He complains of posterior left hip and buttock pain. He is unable to sit upright or stand due to pain. Radiographs reveal a dislocation of the left sacroiliac joint. The patient is taken to the operating room for repair using percutaneous skeletal fixation.

Description of Procedure (27216)

A small incision is made in the gluteal region based upon image guidance and preoperative planning. The muscles and fascia are incised. A guide pin is inserted through the ilium, across the sacroiliac joint, and into the sacrum. This is monitored by means of multiplanar images (anteroposterior, lateral inlet, and outlet views) to avoid injury to the lumbosacral nerve roots. Once appropriate position is confirmed, a cannulated screw is inserted. Depending upon the stability of the fracture, the quality of the bone, the morphology of the pelvis, and the size of the patient, additional screws are inserted by means of separate incisions and similar techniques. The reduction and position of the implants are confirmed with fluoroscopy. The wounds are irrigated and closed in layers.

Clinical Example (27217)
A 34-year-old man is involved in a motorcycle crash and complains of pain in his right hip and groin. He has pain with weight bearing and hip motion. Radiographs in the emergency department demonstrate disruption of the pelvic ring anteriorly with an oblique parasymphysial fracture exiting through the inferior pubic symphysis. The patient is taken to the operating room where he undergoes open treatment of the fracture-symphysial injury with internal fixation.

Description of Procedure (27217)
A curved transverse low anterior incision is made to the rectus fascia, which is then divided vertically and minimally elevated from the pubic rami. The bladder and urethra are identified and assessed for injury. The pelvic hematoma is evacuated and hemostasis obtained. The extent of the bony and ligamentous injury is identified. The fracture and symphysis are repositioned by a combination of direct manipulation and bone clamps; this is checked with fluoroscopy. Provisional fixation with wires is achieved and the alignment checked again with fluoroscopy. Definitive fixation is completed with plates and screws under image intensification. The wound is irrigated and closed over a drain.

Clinical Example (27218)
A 28-year-old man is involved in a motor vehicle crash. He is brought to the emergency department complaining of buttock, hip, and flank pain. He has pain on movement and with respiration and is unable to sit or stand. Radiographs reveal a break in the posterior pelvic ring with a displaced fracture of the left posterior ilium exiting anteriorly through the sacroiliac joint. The patient is taken to the operating room and undergoes open treatment of the left fracture-dislocation with internal fixation.

Description of Procedure (27218)
A vertically oriented posterior incision is made just lateral to the sacroiliac (SI) joint and carried to the gluteal fascia, which is then incised and carefully reflected. Care is taken to avoid injury to the sciatic nerve. The pelvic hematoma is evacuated and hemostasis obtained. The extent of the bony and ligamentous injury is identified. The fractured ilium and SI joint are repositioned by a combination of direct manipulation and bone clamps; this is checked with fluoroscopy. Provisional fixation with wires is achieved and the alignment checked again with fluoroscopy. Definitive fixation is completed with standard plates and screws for the iliac fracture. Cannulated screws are inserted over a guidewire from the ilium across the SI joint and into the sacrum under image intensification to stabilize the SI joint dislocation. The position of these screws is carefully monitored to avoid injury to the lumbosacral nerve roots. Once satisfactory fixation is completed, the wound is irrigated and closed over a drain.

Femur (Thigh Region) and Knee Joint

REPAIR, REVISION, AND/OR RECONSTRUCTION

▲ 27396   Transplant or transfer (with muscle redirection or rerouting), thigh (eg, extensor to flexor); single tendon

▲ 27397   multiple tendons

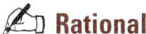 Rationale

Codes 27396 and 27397 have been editorially revised to report muscle transplant or transfer of muscles in the thigh. These code changes were made to allow performance of procedures beyond transplant from a hamstring tendon to the patella. Because the efforts of transfers to other areas of the thigh require an equal amount of work, these codes have been revised to reflect any transplant or transfer of muscles, including redirection or rerouting of muscles to any part of the thigh. This includes transplant or transfer for any tendon, whether an extensor or a flexor tendon.

Muscular imbalance in the thigh can lead to knee dysfunction and gait abnormality. Various tendon transfers in the thigh may be utilized to minimize the dysfunction by redirecting muscle forces.

Foot and Toes

FRACTURE AND/OR DISLOCATION

28446   Open osteochondral autograft, talus (includes obtaining graft[s])

(Do not report 28446 in conjunction with 27705, 27707)

(For arthroscopic osteochondral talus graft, use 29892)

(For open osteochondral allograft or repairs with industrial grafts, use ▶28899◀)

Rationale

The cross-reference following code 28446 has been revised to direct users to the appropriate unlisted procedure code.

Respiratory System

Trachea and Bronchi

ENDOSCOPY

31641 Bronchoscopy (rigid or flexible); with destruction of tumor or relief of stenosis by any method other than excision (eg, laser therapy, cryotherapy)

(For bronchoscopic photodynamic therapy, report 31641 in addition to 96570, 96571 as appropriate)

31643 with placement of catheter(s) for intracavitary radioelement application

(For intracavitary radioelement application, see 77761-77763, ▶77785-77787◀)

🖎 Rationale

In support of the deletion of radiation oncology codes 77781-77784 and the establishment of codes 77785-77787, the cross-reference following code 31643 has been revised to direct users to the appropriate codes for reporting intracavitary radioelement application.

Lungs and Pleura

INTRODUCTION

⊙**32550** Insertion of indwelling tunneled pleural catheter with cuff

▶(Do not report 32550 in conjunction with 32421, 32422)◀

🖎 Rationale

The exclusionary parenthetical following code 32550 has been revised with the removal of several codes from this instruction. This revision indicates that although these services were related to other catheter-based services, the services that were described by former code 32019 and current code 32550 are separate and not inclusive of the services reported with codes 32551, 32560, 36000, 36410, 62318, 62319, 64450, 64470, and 64475.

Cardiovascular System

Heart and Pericardium

PACEMAKER OR PACING CARDIOVERTER-DEFIBRILLATOR

(For electronic, telephonic analysis of internal pacemaker system, see ▶93279, 93280, 93288, 93293, 93294◀)

(For radiological supervision and interpretation with insertion of pacemaker, use 71090)

(33200, 33201 have been deleted)

33202 Insertion of epicardial electrode(s); open incision (eg, thoracotomy, median sternotomy, subxiphoid approach)

Rationale

In tandem with the changes to the Cardiovascular Device Monitoring section in Medicine, the parenthetical note following the Pacemaker or Pacing Cardioverter-Defibrillator guidelines was revised to reflect the correct codes to report for electronic, telephonic analysis of internal pacemaker systems.

ELECTROPHYSIOLOGIC OPERATIVE PROCEDURES

Incision

33250 Operative ablation of supraventricular arrhythmogenic focus or pathway (eg, Wolff-Parkinson-White, atrioventricular node re-entry), tract(s) and/or focus (foci); without cardiopulmonary bypass

▶(For intraoperative pacing and mapping by a separate provider, use 93631)◀

33254 Operative tissue ablation and reconstruction of atria, limited (eg, modified maze procedure)

33255 Operative tissue ablation and reconstruction of atria, extensive (eg, maze procedure); without cardiopulmonary bypass

33256 with cardiopulmonary bypass

(Do not report 33254-33256 in conjunction with 32100, 32551, 33120, 33130, 33210, 33211, 33400-33507, 33510-33523, 33533-33548, 33600-33853, 33860-▶33864◀, 33910-33920)

Rationale

A cross-reference has been added following code 33250 to instruct and assist users to locate the appropriate codes for intraoperative pacing and mapping vs operative ablation of an arrhythmogenic focus or pathway. These revisions are intended to assist in differentiating and reporting the services provided by a cardiac electrophysiologist vs those of a surgeon. It is not appropriate for both codes to be reported by a single provider for pacing/mapping and ablation for the same arrhythmogenic focus, since ablation of the focus by the same provider is included and not separately reported.

The exclusionary cross-reference included after code 33256 was revised to reflect exclusion of new code 33864 used to identify ascending aortic grafting. This code was added to the CPT codebook in 2008 and represents a more intensive ascending aortic grafting procedure that includes valve suspension, coronary reconstruction, and valve-sparing aortic annulus remodeling. Inclusion of this code within the exclusionary parenthetical note listing reflects the intent that this procedure code is mutually exclusive with the operative ablation with cardiopulmonary bypass procedure represented by codes 33254-33256.

PATIENT-ACTIVATED EVENT RECORDER

33282 Implantation of patient-activated cardiac event recorder

(Initial implantation includes programming. For subsequent electronic analysis and/or reprogramming, use ▶93285, 93291, 93298◀)

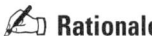
Rationale
In tandem with the changes to the Cardiovascular Device Monitoring section in Medicine, the parenthetical note following code 33282 has been revised to accurately reflect the codes to report for subsequent electronic analysis and/or reprogramming of a patient-activated cardiac event recorder.

THORACIC AORTIC ANEURYSM

33864 Ascending aorta graft, with cardiopulmonary bypass with valve suspension, with coronary reconstruction and valve-sparing aortic annulus remodeling (eg, David Procedure, Yacoub Procedure)

(Do not report 33864 in conjunction with 32551, 33210, 33211, 33400, ▶33860-33863◀)

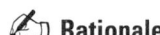
Rationale
The exclusionary parenthetical note following code 33864 has been revised to reflect the exclusion of use of all codes included in the series of codes used to report ascending aortic grafting (33860-33863).

CARDIAC ASSIST

▶(For percutaneous implantation of extracorporeal ventricular assist device or for removal of percutaneously implanted extracorporeal ventricular assist device, see Category III codes 0048T, 0049T, 0050T)◀

33960 Prolonged extracorporeal circulation for cardiopulmonary insufficiency; initial 24 hours

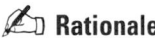
Rationale
In support of the deletion of Category III code 0049T, the cross-reference preceding code 33960 has been revised to instruct users regarding the appropriate codes for reporting placement or removal of a percutaneously implanted extracorporeal ventricular assist device.

Arteries and Veins

ENDOVASCULAR REPAIR OF ABDOMINAL AORTIC ANEURYSM

+▲ 34806 Transcatheter placement of wireless physiologic sensor in aneurysmal sac during endovascular repair, including radiological supervision and interpretation, instrument calibration, and collection of pressure data (List separately in addition to code for primary procedure)

(Use 34806 in conjunction with 33880, 33881, 33886, 34800-34805, 34825, 34900)

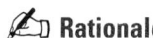 **Rationale**

Code 34806 was established for CPT 2008. It has been revised for CPT 2009 to include conventional descriptor add-on language to direct the use of this code with the codes listed in the parenthetical instruction.

BYPASS GRAFT

Vein

35501 Bypass graft, with vein; common carotid-ipsilateral internal carotid

●35535   hepatorenal

▶(Do not report 35535 in conjunction with 35221, 35251, 35281, 35500, 35536, 35560, 35631, 35636)◀

●35570   tibial-tibial, peroneal-tibial, or tibial/peroneal trunk-tibial

▶(Do not report 35570 in conjunction with 35256, 35286)◀

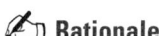 **Rationale**

Two new codes, 35535 and 35570, have been established in the vein bypass graft subsection (35500-35572) to report creation of bypass grafts for revascularization of the right kidney and the lower extremity.

While codes have been available for reporting the creation of an extra-anatomic bypass with vein from the splenic artery to the left renal artery (35536) and by direct splenic artery transposition onto the left renal artery (35636) to route blood around stenotic or occluded renal arteries for revascularization of the left kidney, revascularization procedures of the right kidney required these procedures to be previously reported with an unlisted code.

Code 35535 describes the creation of a bypass with vein (usually harvested from a lower extremity), similar to that described by code 35536. The bypass described by code 35535 originates on the hepatic artery and ends on the right renal artery. A typical indication for performing an extra-anatomic bypass to the right renal artery is for patients with chronic arterial occlusive disease with significant cardiac disease and in whom manipulation of the aorta might prove inappropriate or have excessive risk of morbidity.

Occasionally, code 35251 (Repair blood vessel with vein graft; intra-abdominal) may be used to report repair of a renal artery by creation of an arterial bypass between the hepatic and renal arteries. However, this code is more typically used to report repair of traumatic injuries, while the new code will be used to report treatment of chronic arterial occlusive disease. Surgical exposure for code 35251 extends proximal and distal to the injury site but is typically performed in a limited area in the abdomen. The difference between code 35535 and code 35251 is that the new code will typically require placement of a longer bypass conduit than code 35251 because chronic arterial occlusive disease is more extensive and diffuse than trauma. In addition, the traumatized artery (35251) is usually normal beyond the region of injury, while the chronically diseased artery (35535) is likely to have plaque at the anastomosis sites. This procedure actually focuses, then, on the evaluation of the vessel for the extent and distance of the occlusion to determine the necessary length of the graft.

Code 35535 and existing code 35560 (Bypass graft, with vein; aortorenal) are each appropriately reported for treatment of renal artery ischemia and require harvest of the vein conduit. However, the aortorenal bypass (35560) is performed using the aorta as inflow instead of the hepatic artery used for code 35535. Aortic cross-clamping, required for reporting code 35560, is inherently more stressful for the patient than temporary hepatic artery occlusion. Code 35535 requires mobilization of the hepatic artery with dissection in the right upper quadrant of the abdomen, protecting the portal vein and common bile duct, while exposing an adequate length of hepatic artery for creation of the proximal anastomosis.

An exclusionary parenthetical has been added following code 35535 to indicate that codes 35221 (Repair blood vessel, direct; intra-abdominal), 35251 (Repair blood vessel with vein graft; intra-abdominal), 35281 (Repair blood vessel with graft other than vein; intra-abdominal), 35500 (Harvest of upper extremity vein, one segment, for lower extremity or coronary artery bypass procedure), 35536 (Bypass graft, with vein; splenorenal), 35560 (Bypass graft, with vein; aortorenal), 35631 (Bypass graft, with other than vein; aortoceliac, aortomesenteric, aortorenal), and 35636 (Bypass graft, with other than vein; splenorenal) contain elements of the service that are integral to this code and should not be reported at the same session. The harvest of the vein graft is also included and not separately reported in addition to code 35535.

The lower extremity bypass graft CPT codes are typically organized and described on the basis of inflow artery, outflow artery, and the conduit used and, until the addition of code 35570, included the majority of inflow/outflow combinations except the three tibial arteries in the calf. These are the tibial-tibial, peroneal-tibial, and tibial/peroneal trunk–tibial combinations. The tibial bypass procedures are most typically performed for the patient in whom all three of the tibial calf arteries are occluded. Code 35570 was established to describe the creation of a lower extremity bypass with autogenous conduit for limb salvage for the tibial-tibial, peroneal-tibial, or tibial/peroneal trunk–tibial inflow/outflow combinations.

Codes that are similar to code 35570 include 35571 and 35256 (Repair blood vessel with vein graft; lower extremity).

Code 35571 is used to report a vein bypass when the inflow artery is the popliteal artery and the outflow artery is a tibial artery. For code 35570, however, the inflow artery would be another tibial or peroneal artery that is more proximal in the leg than the outflow distal tibial artery. The harvest of the vein conduit, usually from the lower extremity, is included and not separately reported.

While code 35570 will be used to report treatment of chronic arterial occlusive disease, code 35256 (Repair blood vessel with vein graft; lower extremity) can also be used to report tibial bypass procedures. However, these procedures will be repairs of traumatic injuries that extend proximal and distal to the injury site. Code 35570 will typically require placement of a longer bypass conduit than that required for completion of the graft typically reported with code 35256 because chronic arterial occlusive disease is more extensive and diffuse than trauma. In addition, the traumatized artery graft repair reported with code 35256 is usually normal beyond the region of injury while the chronically diseased artery repair reported with code 35570 is likely to involve plaque at the anastomosis sites and to affect the anastomotic process.

An exclusionary parenthetical has also been added following code 35570 to indicate that codes 35256 (Repair blood vessel with vein graft; lower extremity) and 35286 (Repair blood vessel with graft other than vein; lower extremity) contain elements of the service that are integral to this code and should not be reported at the same session.

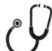

Clinical Example (35535)

A 70-year-old female smoker with hypercholesterolemia and significant coronary artery disease has chronic renal insufficiency and severe hypertension refractory to maximum doses of three medications. She underwent stent placement in the right renal artery origin 2 years ago. Duplex ultrasound confirms a recurrent stenosis, and arteriography reveals near occlusion of the right renal artery felt unsuitable for repeat percutaneous intervention. Her infrarenal aorta contains diffuse atherosclerotic plaque, and she is deemed high risk for aortic cross clamping. A hepatorenal bypass is performed using vein conduit.

Description of Procedure (35535)
A laparotomy is performed with a complete routine abdominal exploration. The soft tissue is dissected inferior to the liver to find the common hepatic artery. Soft tissue is then cleared from the common hepatic artery and gastroduodenal and proper hepatic artery origins, followed by exposure of adequate lengths of these three arteries to achieve proximal and distal control. An incision is made into the soft tissue over the right kidney and the right renal artery is located. Soft tissue from the renal artery is cleared to provide sufficient length for proximal and distal control.

An incision is made into the skin of the thigh and calf for saphenous vein harvest. Soft tissue is dissected to find the saphenous vein and then cleared from the surface of the saphenous vein for exposure of adequate length. All branch ends of the saphenous vein are ligated, divided, and removed from the thigh. The saphenous vein conduit is tested for leaks and repaired with vascular suture.

Systemic anticoagulant is administered with a wait for evidence of circulation. Proximal and distal clamps are placed on common hepatic, proper hepatic, and gastroduodenal arteries. Longitudinal arteriotomy is performed at the proximal anastomosis site. The vein conduit is anastomosed to the hepatic artery with vascular suture. The clamp is removed, a test is performed for leak detection, and any necessary additional sutures are applied to control hemorrhage.

Proximal and distal clamps are applied to the right renal artery and arteriotomy is performed at the anastomosis site. The vein is then cut to the appropriate length and the end of the vein conduit is anastomosed to the right renal artery.

The system is flushed to remove air and debris. Clamps are removed and additional sutures are applied as needed to achieve hemostasis. The distal pulses are palpated to check for restitution of blood flow. Audible Doppler evaluation is performed to ensure normal flow pattern throughout the reconstruction. The agent for anticoagulant neutralization is applied. The abdomen is irrigated and final hemostasis is evaluated. The site is irrigated with sterile saline and the fascia, subcutaneous tissue, and skin of the abdominal incision are closed. The saphenous harvest site is irrigated and closed.

Clinical Example (35570)

A 68-year-old cigarette-smoking woman with hypertension, diabetes, and coronary artery disease develops ischemic ulceration of the great toe. Diagnostic evaluation reveals minimal occlusive disease from the aorta to the proximal tibial arteries, but she has occlusion of all three tibial vessels soon after their origins. The distal anterior tibial artery reconstitutes. A proximal to distal anterior tibial artery bypass graft is performed using reversed vein conduit.

Description of Procedure (35570)

In proximal arterial dissection, the skin is incised overlying the proximal tibial artery. The soft tissue in the calf is dissected to expose and incise the fascia. Muscle bundles are separated to expose the proximal tibial artery, avoiding injury to multiple nearby nerves and veins. Soft tissue is cleared from 5-6 cm of the proximal tibial artery. A soft rubber loop is gently passed around this vessel. Quality of inflow is assessed by testing pulsatility and/or examining with handheld Doppler.

In distal dissection, the skin overlying the target distal tibial artery is incised. Dissection through soft tissue is performed, avoiding injury to surrounding structures. The appropriate muscle compartment fascia is incised. The dissection plane toward the tibial artery target is developed. Mechanical retractors are applied as needed to allow dissection to continue into deep compartments. The appropriate neurovascular bundle is identified. Tibial veins and nerves are carefully teased away from the target tibial artery, and 5-6 cm of the artery is exposed, avoiding injury to small branches. Hemostasis is achieved after unavoidable incidental division of small artery branches and larger veins. Visual and palpation examination of target artery is performed to determine whether it is soft enough to allow suture placement. If the target is acceptable, the next step is performed. If not, dissection is extended or moved to another artery. Soft rubber loops are passed around the exposed target artery for control. Depending on the distal target site, a tunnel/pathway is created for bypass conduit. The tunnel is confirmed to have no sharp turns or fascial planes that would compress or kink the bypass.

In vein harvest, the skin is incised over the segment of donor vein to be harvested (typically the ipsilateral greater saphenous vein). Dissection through soft tissue is performed to expose the entire length of vein required for bypass. All side branches of the donor vein are dissected, ligated, and divided, avoiding injury to saphenous nerve. Soft tissue from around entire length of the donor vein is completely dissected. The proximal and distal ends of the vein are ligated and divided once it is confirmed that sufficient length has been harvested. The vein is moved from limb to back table for preparation. Blood from the saphenous conduit is gently flushed with heparinized saline. The end of the vein is occluded and distended with pressurized saline, with the surgeon looking for untied branches and other sources of leaks. Leaks are repaired with vascular suture, with great caution not to reduce the caliber of the flow channel. The surgeon decides whether the vein will be reversed, thereby not requiring valve lysis, vs antegrade use. If antegrade use is required, valves are lysed with a range of valvulotome devices. Leaks are retested and repaired as needed with vascular suture, with great caution not to reduce caliber.

In proximal anastomosis, the patient is anticoagulated with intravenous anticoagulant. Mechanical retractors are inserted in the proximal calf to allow sufficient space to perform anastomosis. Vascular clamps are applied to inflow artery. Longitudinal arteriotomy is carefully performed. The vein conduit is brought onto the table to determine which end will be the inflow site. The proximal end of the vein is beveled to match the arteriotomy. Ninety percent of the anastomosis (vein conduit to tibial artery) is performed with fine vascular suture. The clamps are opened briefly to flush the system and therefore remove air and debris. Anastomosis is completed and arterial clamps are removed. Additional sutures are applied as needed to control hemorrhage. The vein is passed through the conduit through an appropriate plane to the distal tibial target artery, with care to avoid twists/kinks.

In distal anastomosis, the vein conduit is stretched to full length. The vascular clamp is opened momentarily to test quality of blood flow through the vein conduit. A mechanical retraction device is inserted to allow sufficient space to sew the distal anastomosis. Proximal and distal vascular clamps are applied to the target vessel with care to avoid nerves, veins, etc. Distal tibial arteriotomy is carefully performed. The vein conduit is cut and beveled to exactly match the length and size of the arteriotomy. Ninety percent of the vein to tibial anastomosis is performed with very fine vascular suture. Pen clamps are opened briefly to flush out air and debris. Anastomosis is completed and vascular clamps are removed. Additional sutures are applied as required to achieve hemostasis. Doppler is listened to and the distal pulses are palpated to ensure bypass patency. Other completion maneuvers are performed as required to ensure technical adequacy. This may include inserting an angiocatheter into the bypass for a completion study. The bypass is revised as required to achieve a technically adequate endpoint and good blood flow. All incisions and tunnels are irrigated copiously and heparin is reversed. Wound hemostasis is achieved as needed with cautery, sutures, or ties. All incisions are closed in multiple layers. Pulses are rechecked to ensure patency before the application of sterile dressings.

Other Than Vein

35601   Bypass graft, with other than vein; common carotid-ipsilateral internal carotid

●**35632**   ilio-celiac

▶(Do not report 35632 in conjunction with 35221, 35251, 35281, 35531, 35631)◀

●**35633**   ilio-mesenteric

▶(Do not report 35633 in conjunction with 35221, 35251, 35281, 35531, 35631)◀

●**35634**   iliorenal

▶(Do not report 35634 in conjunction with 35221, 35251, 35281, 35560, 35536, 35631)◀

Rationale

Three new codes, 35632, 35633, and 35634, have been established in the prosthetic bypass graft subsection (35600-35671) to report creation of bypass grafts for revascularization of the celiac, renal, and mesenteric arteries and treatment of chronic arterial occlusive disease.

Each of these grafts uses the iliac vein as the inflow vessel for the initial attachment of the prosthetic graft, with a distal anastomosis of the prosthetic conduit to the celiac, renal, or mesenteric arteries.

While ilioceliac, iliomesenteric, and iliorenal graft procedures may be reported with code 35281, this code is used for repair of traumatic injuries. This code is not appropriately reported for placement of a prosthetic graft for treatment of vessel occlusion on the ilioceliac, iliomesenteric, and iliorenal arteries, because this procedure must address the vascular plaque at the anastomotic site. Synthetic graft procedures are also performed for treatment of chronic arterial occlusive disease in the celiac, mesenteric, and renal arteries and reported with code 35631 (Bypass graft, with other than vein; aorto-celiac, -mesenteric, or -renal). However, as indicated by the descriptor, this code is reported for prosthetic graft procedures that are directly attached to the aorta and use it as the inflow vessel. Codes 35632-35634 use the iliac artery as the inflow vessel for the graft attachment. Aortoceliac, aortorenal, and aortomesenteric grafting is also a shorter and more direct bypass than the iliac graft bypasses (35632-35634) that require mobilization of the iliac artery and dissection in the lower abdomen with a medial visceral rotation of the abdominal contents, allowing for appropriate tunneling of a long bypass graft in the retroperitoneum with a curving technique to avoid graft kinking or occlusion.

Codes 35531 (Bypass graft, with other than vein; aorto-celiac, -mesenteric, or -renal) and code 35536 (Bypass graft, with vein; splenorenal) are also reported for treatment of arterial ischemia in the celiac, mesenteric, and renal arteries using the aorta as inflow, but they would not be reported in this case, because in addition to the wrong inflow source (aorta), these procedures are reported when a vein is utilized for the graft.

Exclusionary parentheticals have been added following each of the iliac artery graft codes to indicate that codes 35221 (Repair blood vessel, direct; intra-abdominal), 35251 (Repair blood vessel with vein graft; intra-abdominal), 35281 (Repair blood vessel with graft other than vein; intra-abdominal), and code 35631 (Bypass graft, with other than vein; aortoceliac, aortomesenteric, aortorenal) contain elements of the service that are integral to this code and should not be reported at the same session. Other codes included in the exclusionary parentheticals include code 35531 (Bypass graft, with vein; aortoceliac or aortomesenteric), which should not be separately reported with the iliocelic (35632) and iliomesentery (35633) artery graft procedures, and codes 35536 (Bypass graft, with vein; splenorenal) and 35560 (Bypass graft, with vein; aortorenal), which should not be reported with code 35634.

Clinical Example (35632)

A 70-year-old female smoker with hypercholesterolemia and significant coronary artery disease has severe postprandial abdominal pain and a 40-pound weight loss over the last few months due to food fear. Upper endoscopy reveals ischemic gastric ulcers. Arteriography reveals occlusion of the celiac artery origin. Her superior mesenteric artery is patent, but there are no collaterals feeding the celiac system. Her aorta is aneurysmal and cannot be clamped safely for a proximal anastomosis. Her common iliac arteries contain plaque but are adequate to serve as inflow. An iliocelic bypass is performed with synthetic conduit.

Description of Procedure (35632)

A long midline laparotomy is performed, with a routine abdominal exploration. The small bowel is mobilized to expose the distal intrarenal aorta and one common iliac artery. The retroperitoneum is incised and the soft tissue is cleared from these arteries. Adequate length of the common iliac artery is exposed to achieve proximal and distal control with enough space to sew the anastomosis. The liver is retracted upward and an incision is made in the soft tissue overlying the celiac axis. The celiac, common hepatic, splenic, and left gastric arteries are gently dissected out and passed soft loops for control. The exact pathway of proposed graft from common iliac to celiac is determined. Appropriate tunnels for the graft, possibly including retropancreatic or transmesenteric, are created. A Teflon tie is passed through tunnels to preserve exact location. The appropriate diameter synthetic conduit is chosen. A systemic anticoagulant is administered and time for circulation is observed. Proximal and distal clamps are placed on the inflow common iliac artery. An incision is made at the inflow iliac longitudinally at the proximal anastomosis site. The end of the synthetic conduit is appropriately beveled and anastomosed to the inflow iliac with vascular suture. Clamps are removed and the anastomosis is tested for leaks. Additional sutures are applied as needed to control any hemorrhaging. The common iliac is isonated with Doppler to ensure that flow beyond the anastomosis has been restored. The conduit is passed through premade tunnels, taking care to avoid kinks. Geometry of the graft-to-celiac proposed anastomosis is examined to determine optimal lie of graft. Proximal and distal clamps are applied to the celiac artery beyond the occlusion, as well as splenic, hepatic, and gastric arteries. An incision is made at the celiac artery longitudinally at the distal anastomosis site. The synthetic conduit is cut to appropriate length and the end is beveled to optimize geometry. The end of the synthetic conduit to celiac artery is anastomosed. The system is flushed to remove air and debris. Clamps are removed and additional sutures are applied as needed to achieve hemostasis. Pulses in celiac, common hepatic, and splenic vessels are palpated to assess restitution of blood flow. These vessels and liver are listened to with a Doppler to ensure that normal flow has been restored. The anticoagulant is reversed with protamine. The abdomen is irrigated and a final check for hemostasis is conducted. The abdominal incision is closed and then the subcutaneous tissue is irrigated and the skin is closed.

Clinical Example (35633)

A 70-year-old female smoker with hypercholesterolemia and significant coronary artery disease has severe postprandial abdominal pain and a 40-pound weight loss due to food fear. She has had previous gastric surgery. Arteriography reveals near occlusion of the celiac artery and a long-segment superior mesenteric artery (SMA) occlusion. Her infrarenal aorta harbors a small aortic aneurysm and cannot be used for inflow. Her common iliac arteries are diseased but acceptable inflow sources. An ilio-SMA bypass is performed with the use of synthetic conduit.

Description of Procedure (35633)

A long midline laparotomy is performed, with a routine abdominal exploration. The small bowel is mobilized to expose the distal intrarenal aorta and one common iliac artery. The retroperitoneum is incised and the soft tissue is cleared from these arteries. Adequate length of the common iliac artery is exposed to achieve proximal and distal control with enough space to sew the anastomosis. The transverse mesocolon is retracted upward and an incision is made in the soft tissue overlying the SMA. The SMA and proximal branches are gently dissected out and soft loops are passed for control. The exact pathway of the proposed graft from common iliac to SMA is determined. Appropriate tunnels for graft are created, with options considered including transmesenteric and retroperitoneal approaches. A Teflon tie is passed through the tunnels to preserve exact location. The appropriate diameter synthetic conduit is chosen. A systemic anticoagulant is administered and time for circulation is observed. Proximal and distal clamps on inflow common iliac artery are placed. Arteriotomy is performed at the inflow iliac longitudinally at the proximal anastomosis site. The end of the conduit is beveled appropriately and the synthetic conduit is anastomosed to the inflow iliac with vascular suture. Clamps are removed and the anastomosis is tested for leaks. Additional sutures are applied as needed to achieve hemostasis. The common iliac is isonated with Doppler to ensure that flow beyond the anastomosis has been restored. The conduit is passed through premade tunnels, taking care to avoid kinks. Geometry of the graft-to-SMA proposed anastomosis is examined to determine the optimal lie of the graft. Proximal and distal clamps are applied to the SMA beyond occlusion, as well as to adjacent branch arteries. Longitudinal arteriotomy of the SMA at the distal anastomosis site is performed. The synthetic conduit is cut to the appropriate length and the end is beveled to optimize geometry. The end of the synthetic conduit to the SMA is anastomosed. The system is flushed to remove air and debris. Clamps are removed and additional sutures are applied as needed to achieve hemostasis. Pulses in the SMA are palpated to assess restitution of blood flow. The SMA and branches are listened to with a Doppler to confirm that normal flow has been restored. The graft is revised as needed to optimize blood flow, then the anticoagulant is reversed with protamine. The abdomen is irrigated and a final check for hemostasis is conducted. The abdominal incision is closed and then the subcutaneous tissue is irrigated and the skin is closed.

Clinical Example (35634)

A 70-year-old female smoker with hypercholesterolemia and coronary artery disease has chronic renal insufficiency and severe hypertension refractory to maximum doses of three medications. She underwent renal stent placement 3 years ago, but her hypertension has now recurred. Duplex ultrasound confirms recurrent renal artery stenosis. Arteriogram reveals near occlusion of the artery felt unlikely to respond to repeat percutaneous intervention. She has a small infrarenal aortic aneurysm that precludes aortorenal bypass. An iliorenal bypass graft is performed using prosthetic conduit.

Description of Procedure (35634)

A long midline laparotomy is performed, with a routine abdominal exploration. The small bowel is mobilized to expose the distal intrarenal aorta and one common iliac artery. The retroperitoneum is incised and the soft tissue is cleared from these arteries. Adequate length of the common iliac artery is exposed to achieve proximal and distal control with enough space to sew the anastomosis. Overlying the kidney is Gerota's fascia, which is to be revascularized. This is incised. The renal artery is gently dissected out, avoiding injury to vena cava and associated structures and soft loops are passed around the artery for control. The exact pathway of the proposed graft from common iliac to renal artery is determined. Appropriate tunnels for the graft, with options including a transabdominal or retroperitoneal approach, are created. A Teflon tie is passed through the tunnels to preserve the exact location. The appropriate diameter synthetic conduit is chosen. Administration of renal protective agents is requested by anesthesia. A systemic anticoagulant is administered and the time for circulation is observed. Proximal and distal clamps are placed on the inflow common iliac artery. Arteriotomy is performed at the inflow iliac longitudinally at the proximal anastomosis site. The end of the conduit is beveled appropriately and synthetic conduit is anastomosed to the inflow iliac with vascular suture. Clamps are removed and the anastomosis is tested for leaks. Additional sutures are applied as needed to achieve hemostasis. The common iliac is isonated with a handheld Doppler to ensure that flow beyond anastomosis has been restored. The conduit is passed through premade tunnels, taking care to avoid kinks. The geometry of the graft-to-renal artery anastomosis is examined to determine the optimal lie of the graft. Proximal and distal clamps are applied to the renal artery, as well as to adjacent branch arteries. A longitudinal arteriotomy of the renal artery at the distal anastomosis site is performed. The synthetic conduit is cut to the appropriate length and the end is beveled to optimize geometry. The end of the synthetic conduit to the renal artery is anastomosed. The system is flushed to remove air and debris. Clamps are removed and additional sutures are applied as needed to achieve hemostasis. Pulses in the renal artery are palpated to assess restitution of blood flow. The renal and branches are listened to with a Doppler to ensure that normal flow has been restored. The graft is revised as needed to optimize blood flow, and then the anticoagulant is reversed with protamine. The abdomen is irrigated and a final check for hemostasis is conducted. The abdominal incision is closed, the subcutaneous tissue is irrigated, and the skin is closed.

VASCULAR INJECTION PROCEDURES

Venous

36475 Endovenous ablation therapy of incompetent vein, extremity, inclusive of all imaging guidance and monitoring, percutaneous, radiofrequency; first vein treated

+ 36476 second and subsequent veins treated in a single extremity, each through separate access sites (List separately in addition to code for primary procedure)

(Use 36476 in conjunction with 36475)

(Do not report 36475, 36476 in conjunction with 36000-36005, 36410, 36425, 36478, 36479, 37204, 75894, 76000, 76001, 76937, 76942, ▶76998◄, 77022, 93970, 93971)

36478 Endovenous ablation therapy of incompetent vein, extremity, inclusive of all imaging guidance and monitoring, percutaneous, laser; first vein treated

+ 36479 second and subsequent veins treated in a single extremity, each through separate access sites (List separately in addition to code for primary procedure)

(Use 36479 in conjunction with 36478)

(Do not report 36478, 36479 in conjunction with 36000-36005, 36410, 36425, 36475, 36476, 37204, 75894, 76000, 76001, 76937, 76942, ▶76998◄, 77022, 93970, 93971)

Rationale

The parenthetical notes following the endovenous ablation therapy (EVAT) family of codes 36475-36479 and diagnostic ultrasound code 76998 have been revised to clarify that intraoperative ultrasound is not separately reportable in conjunction with the EVAT codes.

Codes 36475, 37476, 37468, and 36479 include all imaging required in performance of the service. The code descriptors specifically describe inclusion of "all imaging guidance and monitoring," but to address confusion with respect to the use of code 76998, the parenthetical notes following 36475-36479 and 76988 have been revised to clarify that "all imaging guidance and monitoring" includes intraoperative ultrasound.

TRANSCATHETER PROCEDURES

Arterial Mechanical Thrombectomy

⊙**37184** Primary percutaneous transluminal mechanical thrombectomy, noncoronary, arterial or arterial bypass graft, including fluoroscopic guidance and intraprocedural pharmacological thrombolytic injection(s); initial vessel

(Do not report 37184 in conjunction with 76000, 76001, ▶96374◄, 99143-99150)

+⊙37185 second and all subsequent vessel(s) within the same vascular family (List separately in addition to code for primary mechanical thrombectomy procedure)

(Do not report 37185 in conjunction with 76000, 76001, ▶96375◀)

+⊙37186 Secondary percutaneous transluminal thrombectomy (eg, nonprimary mechanical, snare basket, suction technique), noncoronary, arterial or arterial bypass graft, including fluoroscopic guidance and intraprocedural pharmacological thrombolytic injections, provided in conjunction with another percutaneous intervention other than primary mechanical thrombectomy (List separately in addition to code for primary procedure)

(Do not report 37186 in conjunction with 76000, 76001, ▶96375◀)

Venous Mechanical Thrombectomy

⊙37187 Percutaneous transluminal mechanical thrombectomy, vein(s), including intraprocedural pharmacological thrombolytic injections and fluoroscopic guidance

(Do not report 37187 in conjunction with 76000, 76001, ▶96375◀)

⊙37188 Percutaneous transluminal mechanical thrombectomy, vein(s), including intraprocedural pharmacological thrombolytic injections and fluoroscopic guidance, repeat treatment on subsequent day during course of thrombolytic therapy

(Do not report 37188 in conjunction with 76000, 76001, ▶96375◀)

Rationale

In support of the deletion, relocation, and renumbering of codes 90760-90779, the instructional notes following codes 37184, 37185, 37186, 37187, and 37188 have been revised to reflect the new code numbers.

LIGATION

▶(For ligation, division, and stripping of the greater saphenous vein, use 37722. For ligation, division, and stripping of the short saphenous vein, use 37718)◀

37735 Ligation and division and complete stripping of long or short saphenous veins with radical excision of ulcer and skin graft and/or interruption of communicating veins of lower leg, with excision of deep fascia

Rationale

The parenthetical note preceding code 37735 was editorially revised to remove the reference to previously deleted code 37730.

Digestive System

Tongue and Floor of Mouth

INCISION

41019 Placement of needles, catheters, or other device(s) into the head and/or neck region (percutaneous, transoral, or transnasal) for subsequent interstitial radioelement application

(For imaging guidance, see 76942, 77002, 77012, 77021)

(For stereotactic insertion of intracranial brachytherapy radiation sources, use 61770)

(For interstitial radioelement application, see 77776-▶77787◀)

Rationale

In support of the deletion of codes 77781-77784 and the establishment of codes 77785-77787, the parenthetical note following code 41019 has been revised to include the appropriate codes to report.

OTHER PROCEDURES

●**41512** Tongue base suspension, permanent suture technique

▶(For fixation of tongue, mechanical, other than suture, use 41500)◀

▶(For suture of tongue to lip for micrognathia, use 41510)◀

●**41530** Submucosal ablation of the tongue base, radiofrequency, one or more sites, per session

Rationale

Code 41512 has been established to report tongue base suspension that utilizes a permanent suture technique for treatment of snoring and obstructive sleep apnea. Code 41512 differs from code 41500, as 41500 describes nonsuture (eg, K-wire) tongue base suspension.

A cross-reference parenthetical note was added following code 41512 to direct users to code 41510 for suture of tongue to lip for micrognathia.

Code 41530 has been established to report submucosal radiofrequency tissue volume reduction of the tongue base. Concurrently, Category III code 0088T, which previously described this procedure, has been deleted. A parenthetical note has been placed in the Category III section directing users to the new Category I code.

Radiofrequency tongue base tissue volume reduction is a procedure in which a larger oropharyngeal airway is created to prevent obstruction during sleep. The procedure is typically performed in the outpatient setting with the patient under local and topical anesthesia. Several treatment sessions may be necessary to adequately remove the obstructive tissue. Code 41530 is reported one time per session, regardless of the number of sites of the tongue base that are treated.

Clinical Example (41512)

A 57-year-old, hypertensive man with a body mass index of 35 kg/m² is diagnosed with severe obstructive sleep apnea by polysomnography. He exhibits an apnea-hypopnea index of 52/hr and concomitant severe oxygen desaturation. Both continuous positive airway pressure and bilevel positive airway pressure have failed due to noncompliance. Prior nasal surgery and uvulopalatopharyngoplasty also failed to produce subjective or objective improvement of his sleep apnea. Examination shows macroglossia, and fiberoptic laryngoscopy demonstrates retrolingual airway narrowing and collapse.

Description of Procedure (41512)

After general anesthesia with nasotracheal intubation, appropriate landmarks are marked to maintain orientation and to determine the position of the neurovascular bundles. The planned incision site is injected with a local anesthetic with epinephrine.

An incision is made in either the floor of mouth or the submental area to access the posterior cortex of the anterior mandible. Other than the minor differences associated with the intraoral vs external submental approach to the mandible, the procedure is virtually identical regardless of access incision.

If the procedure is performed through the floor of mouth, an incision is made a few millimeters posterior to Wharton's ducts, along the lingual frenulum. Blunt dissection is performed in the midline to gain access to the posterior cortex of the mandible. Periosteum is elevated from the mandible just superior to the genioglossus tubercle and inferior to the dental roots. A drill system is used to attach a screw or metal plate to the cortex of the mandible. A suture(s) is attached to the screw or plate. One end of the permanent suture is then passed with a suture passer from the floor of mouth incision, through tongue muscle, into the posterior aspect of the base of tongue. The suspension suture may attach to the base of tongue tissue by means of suture triangulation or other means. The suture(s) is tightened and the base of tongue is suspended anteriorly. Anterior tongue movement is verified. Bleeding is controlled and the mucosal incision is closed.

When the procedure is performed from the submental area, the incision is made through skin, subcutaneous tissue, and platysma muscle. Periosteum is elevated off the mandibular cortex and the screw or plate is attached to the mandibular cortex just inferior to the genioglossus tubercle. The suspension sutures are placed in an identical fashion. At the end of the procedure, the incision is copiously irrigated, hemostasis is obtained, and the incision is closed with sutures and dressed with a sterile dressing.

Clinical Example (41530)

A 57-year-old, hypertensive man with a body mass index of 35 kg/m² is diagnosed with severe obstructive sleep apnea by polysomnography. He exhibits an apnea-hypopnea index of 52/hr and concomitant severe oxygen desaturation. Both continuous positive airway pressure and bilevel positive airway pressure have failed due to noncompliance. Prior nasal surgery and uvulopalatopharyngoplasty also failed to produce subjective or objective improvement of his sleep apnea.

Examination shows macroglossia, and fiberoptic laryngoscopy demonstrates retrolingual airway narrowing and collapse.

Description of Procedure (41530)

After topical oral and pharyngeal anesthesia is administered, the surgeon has the patient rinse his mouth with an antibacterial rinse. The mouth is secured open with bite blocks and the tongue is protruded, held in position, and immobilized. The tongue midline and circumvallate papillae are marked with a skin marker to maintain orientation. Planned probe insertion sites are similarly marked. Planned treatment sites are injected with an anesthetic agent. For each treatment site, the physician injects saline, inserts the probe, and verifies proper position away from the neurovascular bundle, and radiofrequency energy is delivered to the submucosal tissues. The surgeon actively monitors the treatment sites as energy is delivered to ensure complete submucosal application and no mucosal overlap of applied energy. This procedure is performed on each subsequent target site until all planned sites have been treated for this session.

Esophagus

ENDOSCOPY

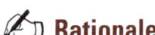**43273**   Endoscopic cannulation of papilla with direct visualization of common bile duct(s) and/or pancreatic duct(s) (List separately in addition to code(s) for primary procedure)

▶(Use 43273 in conjunction with 43260, 43261, 43263-43265, 43267-43272)◀

🖉 Rationale

Add-on code 43273 was established to report endoscopic cannulation of the papilla of Vater with direct visualization of the common bile duct(s) and/or the pancreatic duct(s). Cholangioscopy/pancreatoscopy is the direct visualization of the biliary and/or pancreatic ducts. Direct visualization of the pancreaticobiliary tree allows for inspection and treatment of abnormalities that may not be detected radiographically. After endoscopic retrograde cholangiopancreatography (ERCP) is performed, a thin cholangioscope is introduced into the side-viewing duodenoscope and is passed through the scope until it reaches the papilla. The cholangioscope cannulates the papilla and is maneuvered up through the biliary and/or pancreatic ducts. Subsequently, the areas of interest are observed through direct visualization.

The addition of code 43273 for cannulation and direct visualization of the bile duct differentiates this new procedure from code 43260 for ERCP, which provides fluoroscopic images of the papilla and common bile ducts and is performed in the interventional endoscopy or radiology suite. The standard therapeutic duodenoscope is inserted into the patient's mouth and is passed through the esophagus and stomach and into the duodenum until it reaches the papilla of Vater. At this point, a catheter is inserted through the duodenoscope and used to inject contrast dye into the biliary and pancreatic ducts. To examine the areas of interest, a series of fluoroscopic X rays are taken as the dye moves through the ducts and fluoroscopy images are viewed.

Code 43273 would not be reported in addition to the therapeutic ERCP code 43262 (papillotomy) since access to the ducts is inherent in code 43273 and should not be reported twice.

Clinical Example (43273)

A 60-year-old male presents with severe epigastric pain with radiation to the back. An abdominal ultrasound shows a normal gallbladder without stones and normal gallbladder wall thickness. An abdominal computed tomographic scan reveals a markedly dilated pancreatic duct at 1 cm in diameter and a normal biliary tree. An ERCP reveals an enlarged ampulla of Vater with a markedly dilated opening and mucin in the orifice. Pancreatoscopy is performed to evaluate a presumed intraductal papillary mucinous neoplasm.

Description of Procedure (43273)

After informed consent is obtained, the patient is brought to the therapeutic endoscopy suite. Sedation is administered intravenously, and the duodenoscope is introduced through the mouth with inspection of the esophagus, stomach, and duodenum. Selective cannulation of the bile duct is obtained followed by multiple views of the cholangiogram under fluoroscopy. A guidewire is passed such that the tip is in the proximal biliary tree, and a standard biliary sphincterotomy is performed.

The cholangioscope is passed through the duodenoscope and into the biliary tree. Direct visualization is performed with careful inspection of the biliary and pancreatic epithelium. The mass lesion is identified and multiple biopsies are taken. The right and left intrahepatic biliary tree, common hepatic duct, and common bile duct are all viewed. The cholangioscope is then withdrawn and then passed into the pancreatic duct. At the conclusion of the procedure, the cholangioscope is withdrawn and the physician proceeds with the remainder of the ERCP procedure.

LAPAROSCOPY

Surgical laparoscopy always includes diagnostic laparoscopy. To report a diagnostic laparoscopy (peritoneoscopy) (separate procedure), use 49320.

●43279 Laparoscopy, surgical, esophagomyotomy (Heller type), with fundoplasty, when performed

▶(For open approach, see 43330, 43331)◀

▶(Do not report 43279 in conjunction with 43280)◀

43280 Laparoscopy, surgical, esophagogastric fundoplasty (eg, Nissen, Toupet procedures)

▶(Do not report 43280 in conjunction with 43279)◀

REPAIR

43330 Esophagomyotomy (Heller type); abdominal approach

▶(For laparoscopic esophagomyotomy procedure, use 43279)◀

Rationale

Code 43279 was established to report the Heller-type laparoscopic esophagomyotomy and includes fundoplasty when fundoplasty is concurrently performed. This procedure is typically performed for treatment of achalasia, a condition in which food remains stuck in the esophagus at the terminal end near the cardioesophageal junction due to improper esophageal motility. Achalasia is frequently caused by an autonomic nerve response in the esophagus. Code 43279 was added to specify the laparoscopic performance of this procedure, since existing codes were available only to report the thorascopic, laparoscopic fundoplication, and open abdominal procedures.

Cross-references and exclusionary parenthetical notes have been added to direct users to the open procedure codes (43330, 43331) and to restrict use of code 43279 when a laparoscopic fundoplication procedure is performed (code 43280). A cross-reference following code 43330 directs users to the correct code for the new procedure.

Clinical Example (43279)

A 45-year-old man presents with a history of progressive dysphagia to solid and liquid food. After extensive evaluation, a diagnosis of achalasia is confirmed. A laparoscopic esophagomyotomy with fundoplication is performed.

Description of Procedure (43279)

After induction of general anesthesia, prepping, and draping, pneumoperitoneum is induced by insertion of a needle, bladeless optical trocar, open insertion of the first port, or other appropriate technique. Additional trocars are placed on the basis of the patient's anatomy and need for exposure.

The left lateral segment of the liver is retracted to allow visualization of the esophageal hiatus. The proposed myotomy site is inspected for evidence of scarring resulting from prior nonsurgical treatment for the achalasia. If the stomach is dilated, it is emptied with a gastric tube; introduction of the tube into the stomach may be impossible and another method such as needle aspiration may be necessary.

The peritoneum overlying the phrenoesophageal ligament is incised and the distal esophagus is mobilized into the mediastinum. Caudal retraction is maintained on the stomach to allow further development of the esophagus into the chest. A site is selected on the anterior surface of the esophagus to initiate the myotomy. The longitudinal muscle fibers are split at the starting point, exposing the circular fibers, which are carefully divided to unroof the submucosal layer.

The myotomy is then extended cephalad into the mediastinum, exposing the submucosa up to and above the level of the muscular hypertrophy. Care is taken to protect the vagus nerve during the dissection. The myotomy is then extended distally below the gastroesophageal junction 2 cm onto the stomach. The oblique muscle fibers in the stomach wall are divided to expose the gastric submucosa. The length and adequacy of the myotomy are confirmed and the myotomy is extended cephalad or caudad as needed. Should a tear in the submucosa occur, it is meticulously repaired. Before proceeding, the absence of leaks from the exposed submucosal floor of the myotomy is confirmed.

If an esophagogastric fundoplication is deemed necessary, it is then performed per the surgeon's preference. Possible configurations are an anterior or posterior partial fundoplication, total fundoplication, or other maneuver designed to prevent reflux of gastric content into the esophagus. This may also include positioning of adjacent gastric fundus over or around the myotomy and fixation with multiple sutures to the stomach, esophagus, edge of the myotomy, and crura of the diaphragm.

The operative field is carefully inspected to ensure hemostasis. The liver retraction is released and the trocars are removed. The incisions are closed and sterile dressings applied.

MANIPULATION

▲ **43460** Esophagogastric tamponade, with balloon (Sengstaken type)

 Rationale

Code 43460 has been revised to correct the misspelling of Sengstaken.

Stomach

INTRODUCTION

43752 Naso- or oro-gastric tube placement, requiring physician's skill and fluoroscopic guidance (includes fluoroscopy, image documentation and report)

(For percutaneous placement of gastrostomy tube, use 49440)

(For enteric tube placement, see 44500, 74340)

(Do not report 43752 in conjunction with critical care codes 99291-99292, neonatal critical care codes ▶99468, 99469◀, pediatric critical care codes ▶99471, 99472◀ or low birth weight intensive care service codes ▶99478, 99479◀)

 Rationale

In support of the extensive editorial revisions in the Neonatal and Pediatric Critical Care section, the parenthetical note following code 43752 has been revised to include the new neonatal and critical care codes 99468 and 99469, the pediatric critical care codes 99471 and 99472, and the low-birth-weight intensive care codes 99478 and 99479.

OTHER PROCEDURES

43882 Revision or removal of gastric neurostimulator electrodes, antrum, open

(For laparoscopic approach, see 43647, 43648)

(For insertion of gastric neurostimulator pulse generator, use 64590)

(For revision or removal of gastric neurostimulator pulse generator, use 64595)

(For electronic analysis and programming of gastric neurostimulator pulse generator, ▶see 95980-95982)◀

Rationale

One of the parenthetical notes following code 43882 has been revised to reflect the addition of codes to identify electronic analysis and programming of gastric neurostimulator pulse generators. It directs users to use codes 95980-95982 for these services. For more information regarding these procedures, see the Rationale for codes 95980-95982.

Rectum

EXCISION

45170   Excision of rectal tumor, transanal approach

▶(For transanal endoscopic microsurgical [ie, TEMS] excision of rectal tumor, use 0184T)◀

Rationale

A parenthetical note has been added following code 45170 to direct users to the appropriate code for transanal endoscopic microsurgical excision of rectal tumor (eg, 0184T).

Anus

EXCISION

46260   Hemorrhoidectomy, internal and external, complex or extensive;

46261   with fissurectomy

46262   with fistulectomy, with or without fissurectomy

(For injection of hemorrhoids, use 46500; for destruction, ▶use 46930;◀ for ligation, see 46945, 46946; for hemorrhoidopexy, use 46947)

Rationale

A parenthetical note has been included following codes 46260-46262 to direct users to the appropriate codes to use to identify the injection of hemorrhoids with sclerosing solution (46500), destruction (46930), ligation of hemorrhoids (46945-46946), and hemorrhoidopexy (46947). Similar notes have been placed after these procedures to allow users to correctly code for those procedures and to identify the correct codes to be used to identify complex or extensive internal and external hemorrhoidectomy.

INTRODUCTION

46500 Injection of sclerosing solution, hemorrhoids

(For excision of hemorrhoids, see 46250-46262; for destruction, ▶use 46930;◀ for ligation, see 46945, 46946; for hemorrhoidopexy, use 46947)

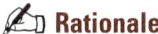 **Rationale**

A parenthetical note has been included following code 46500 to direct users to the appropriate codes to use to identify hemorrhoidal excision procedures (46250-46262), destruction procedures (46930), ligations (46945-46946), and hemorrhoidopexy procedures (46947). Similar notes have been placed after these procedures to allow users to correctly code for those procedures and to identify the correct codes to use to identify complex or extensive internal and external hemorrhoidectomy.

DESTRUCTION

●**46930** Destruction of internal hemorrhoid(s) by thermal energy (eg, infrared coagulation, cautery, radiofrequency)

▶(Codes 46934-46936 have been deleted. For incision of external thrombosed hemorrhoid(s), use 46083; for destruction of internal hemorrhoid(s) by thermal energy, use 46930; for destruction of hemorrhoid(s) by cryosurgery, use 46999; for excision of hemorrhoid(s), see 46250-46262, 46320; for injection, use 46500; for ligation, see 46221, 46945, 46946; for hemorrhoidopexy, use 46947)◀

SUTURE

46947 Hemorrhoidopexy (eg, for prolapsing internal hemorrhoids) by stapling

(For excision of hemorrhoids, see 46250-46262; for injection, use 46500; for destruction, ▶use 46930)◀

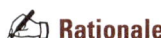 **Rationale**

Code 46930 has been added to report various thermal energy destruction procedures for hemorrhoids. Establishment of this code is accompanied by the deletion of codes 46934, 46935, and 46936, since these codes are redundant and do not identify multiple hemorrhoid destruction. Because other codes may be used to identify nonthermal hemorrhoid destruction (46221, Hemorrhoidectomy, by simple ligature [eg, rubber band]; 46945, Ligation of internal hemorrhoids; single procedure; 46946, Ligation of internal hemorrhoids; multiple procedures; and 46947, Hemorrhoidopexy [eg, for prolapsing internal hemorrhoids] by stapling), the addition of code 46930 allows for identification of all methods of hemorrhoid destruction. A parenthetical note has been included following code 46930 to direct users to the appropriate codes to use to report the different methods of removal and destruction for hemorrhoids.

Note: Codes 46934-46936 have been deleted. For incision of external thrombosed hemorrhoid(s), see code 46083; for destruction of internal hemorrhoid(s) by thermal energy, use code 46933; for destruction of hemorrhoid(s) by cryosurgery, use code 46999; for excision of hemorrhoid(s), see codes 46230-46262; for injection, use code 46500; for ligation, see codes 46945 and 46946; for hemorrhoidopexy, use code 46947.

Clinical Example (46930)

A 32-year-old man, with no past medical history, has had intermittent bright-red rectal bleeding into the commode for the past 6 months. Office examination including anoscopy and/or sigmoidoscopy reveals grade I internal hemorrhoids in the left lateral, right posterior, and right anterior quadrants that exhibit friability and contact bleeding. He undergoes thermal energy ablation of the hemorrhoid(s).

Description of Procedure (46930)

The patient is placed in a kneeling position on a Ritter table. The patient's buttocks are effaced. Visual inspection of the perineum is performed. A lubricated anoscope is then placed in the anal canal. Once in the anal canal, the anoscope is rotated 180 degrees and the obturator is removed. Thermal energy ablation (eg, infrared coagulation) is applied four to five times in an arc at the apex of the hemorrhoid complex(es). The anoscope is removed.

Abdomen, Peritoneum, and Omentum

REPAIR

Hernioplasty, Herniorrhaphy, Herniotomy

 49568   Implantation of mesh or other prosthesis for open incisional or ventral hernia repair or mesh for closure of debridement for necrotizing soft tissue infection (List separately in addition to code for the incisional or ventral hernia repair)

Rationale

Add-on code 49568 was revised, adding the word "open" to the descriptor. This was done to accommodate development of the codes used to identify laparoscopic provision of hernia repair (the addition of the word "open" to this code specifically identifies this code as an open procedure and restricts use of this code for laparoscopic procedures). The new codes used to identify laparoscopic provision of hernia repair specifically include language that identifies use of those codes for laparoscopic hernia procedures.

LAPAROSCOPY

●49652   Laparoscopy, surgical, repair, ventral, umbilical, spigelian or epigastric hernia (includes mesh insertion, when performed); reducible

▶(Do not report 49652 in conjunction with 44180, 49568)◀

●49653   incarcerated or strangulated

▶(Do not report 49653 in conjunction with 44180, 49568)◀

●**49654**   Laparoscopy, surgical, repair, incisional hernia (includes mesh insertion, when performed); reducible

▶(Do not report 49654 in conjunction with 44180, 49568)◀

●**49655**   incarcerated or strangulated

▶(Do not report 49655 in conjunction with 44180, 49568)◀

●**49656**   Laparoscopy, surgical, repair, recurrent incisional hernia (includes mesh insertion, when performed); reducible

▶(Do not report 49656 in conjunction with 44180, 49568)◀

●**49657**   incarcerated or strangulated

▶(Do not report 49657 in conjunction with 44180, 49568)◀

Rationale

Codes 49652-49657 were added to report laparoscopic repairs performed for hernias. Parenthetical notes have been added following codes 49656 and 49657 to restrict use of these codes with open procedures for mesh insertion and lysis of adhesions. Instead, the laparoscopic provision of the previously noted laparoscopic services includes mesh insertion and adhesiolysis when performed. As is true with many other surgical procedures, diagnostic laparoscopy, which includes collection of specimens and brushings or washings, is also inherently included as part of the surgical services included in these new codes. For other hernia repairs performed laparoscopically, the unlisted code 49659 should continue to be used. In addition, a parenthetical note has been added to restrict use of these codes with open mesh placement.

Clinical Example (49652)

A 35-year-old obese man presents with a new abdominal wall bulge first noted after exercise, which has been increasing in size over the last few months. It is occasionally painful, with tender edges. The hernia is reducible on examination. He is referred for a laparoscopic repair.

Description of Procedure (49652)

If hernia contents are present, they are manually reduced. Pneumoperitoneum is induced by insertion of a needle, bladeless optical trocar, open insertion of the first port (described below), or other appropriate technique.

Starting at a distance from the hernia location, for open insertion the first skin incision is made and carried through the subcutaneous tissues. Hemostasis is obtained. The fascia is exposed and incised, and the peritoneum is opened carefully under direct vision, avoiding underlying bowel, omentum, or adhesions. The first trocar is inserted and secured with stay sutures as needed. The abdomen is then insufflated while physiologic changes are monitored. The appropriate camera is inserted, and a preliminary visual exploration of the abdominal cavity is made before subsequent cannulae are placed. With the camera viewing placement of each port, typically two more are positioned to allow two-handed surgical technique while remaining at a distance from the hernia. A thorough visual examination of the abdominal cavity is then undertaken with the aid of instruments inserted through the other ports, viewing where possible the liver, small bowel, colon, stomach, spleen, and pelvic organs. At any stage in this initial process, adhesions may require sharp and/or blunt lysis to allow adequate exposure.

The hernia defect is identified and, if necessary, its contents are reduced. An appropriate margin around the defect to accommodate overlapping mesh is cleared by lysing adhesions or mobilizing structures such as the falciform ligament. Hemostasis is secured before continuing, and intestine that has been handled or freed by adhesiolysis is carefully checked to confirm that it is intact. Sites on the abdominal wall are selected for the transfascial fixation sutures if used. The size of the defect is measured and an appropriate-sized mesh patch is selected. The mesh is rolled and introduced though the largest available cannula or abdominal puncture and, once inside, is unfurled and positioned with the correct surface facing the abdominal wall. The entire periphery of the mesh is secured at appropriate intervals to the abdominal wall with a combination of any or all of the following: tacks, staples, transfascial or intracorporeal stitches, or other permanent fixation devices. A fourth or subsequent port may be necessary to permit access of instrumentation for fixation of an inaccessible corner of the mesh. The number and position of these fixation points is intended to achieve adequate overlap of flat-lying mesh beyond the edge of the defect, and prevent both movement of the mesh and protrusion of intestine, omentum, or other abdominal structures between the mesh and the abdominal wall. A second or subsequent concentric inner ring of fixation points between the outer ring and the edge of the defect may be inserted according to surgeon preference. The mesh is inspected for gaps, large ripples, and other defects, with and without insufflation, and corrected as needed.

The secondary cannulae are removed, carbon dioxide is allowed to escape from the abdomen, and the fascial defects of all port punctures are repaired as appropriate. Local anesthetic is injected once again to all trocar sites and transfascial fixation points. If needed, the subcutaneous tissues of the larger punctures are approximated with interrupted sutures to eliminate a dead space. The skin incisions are closed according to surgeon preference. Sponge, needle, and instrument counts are obtained and confirmed prior to closure.

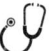

Clinical Example (49653)

A 50-year-old woman with no past surgical history presents with a large abdominal wall mass. She reports that it has been slowly increasing in size over the last 3-4 years. It would initially go away when she laid down but has been nonreducible for the last year. It is increasingly tender and often painful. She has occasional nausea but no vomiting associated with it. On examination she is afebrile with normal vital signs. She has a chronically incarcerated ventral hernia and is referred for a laparoscopic repair.

Description of Procedure (49653)

An attempt is made to reduce the hernia contents manually. Pneumoperitoneum is induced by insertion of a needle, bladeless optical trocar, open insertion of the first port (described below), or other appropriate technique.

Starting at a distance from the hernia location, for open insertion the first skin incision is made and carried through the subcutaneous tissues. Hemostasis is obtained. The fascia is exposed and incised and the peritoneum opened carefully under direct vision, avoiding underlying bowel, omentum, or adhesions. The first trocar is inserted and secured with the stay sutures as needed. The abdomen is then insufflated while physiologic changes are monitored. The appropriate camera is inserted, and a preliminary visual exploration of the abdominal cavity is made before subsequent cannulae are placed. With the camera viewing placement of each port, typically two more are positioned to allow two-handed surgical technique while remaining at a distance from the hernia. A thorough visual examination of the abdominal cavity is then undertaken with the aid of instruments inserted through the other ports, viewing where possible the liver, small bowel, colon, stomach, spleen, and pelvic organs. At any stage in this initial process, adhesions may require sharp and/or blunt lysis to allow adequate exposure.

The hernia defect is identified and, if necessary, its contents are reduced by a combination of external pressure, careful traction with the laparoscopic instruments, and judicious adhesiolysis as necessary. An appropriate margin around the defect to accommodate overlapping mesh is cleared by lysing adhesions or mobilizing structures such as the falciform ligament. Hemostasis is secured before continuing, and intestine that has been reduced, handled, or freed by adhesiolysis is carefully checked to confirm that it is intact. Devitalized tissue such as fat or omentum is excised and removed. Sites on the abdominal wall are selected for the transfascial fixation sutures if used. The size of the defect is measured and an appropriate-sized mesh patch is selected. The mesh is rolled and introduced though the largest available cannula or abdominal puncture and, once inside, is unfurled and positioned with the correct surface facing the abdominal wall. The entire periphery of the mesh is secured at appropriate intervals to the abdominal wall with a combination of any or all of the following: tacks, staples, transfascial or intracorporeal stitches, or other permanent fixation devices. A fourth or subsequent port may be necessary to permit access of instrumentation for fixation of an inaccessible corner of the mesh. The number and position of these fixation points are intended to achieve adequate overlap of flat-lying mesh beyond the edge of the defect, and prevent both movement of the mesh and protrusion of intestine, omentum, or other abdominal structures between the mesh and the abdominal wall. A second or subsequent concentric inner ring of fixation points between the outer ring and the edge of the defect may be inserted according to surgeon preference. The mesh is inspected for gaps, large ripples, and other defects, with and without insufflation, and corrected as needed.

The secondary cannulae are removed, carbon dioxide is allowed to escape from the abdomen, and the fascial defects of all port punctures are repaired as appropriate. Local anesthetic is injected once again to all trocar sites and transfascial fixation points. If needed, the subcutaneous tissues of the larger punctures are approximated with interrupted sutures to eliminate dead space. The skin incisions are closed according to surgeon preference. Sponge, needle, and instrument counts are obtained and confirmed prior to closure.

🩺 Clinical Example (49654)

A 60-year-old man with a prior laparotomy for a colectomy has developed a bulge in the midline incision. The defect has been increasing in size during follow-up. He has symptoms of pain and local tenderness. He has had no history of incarceration or bowel obstruction. On examination, he is found to have a reducible incisional hernia. He is referred for laparoscopic repair.

Description of Procedure (49654)

If hernia contents are present, they are gently reduced. Pneumoperitoneum is induced by open insertion of the first port (described below) or other appropriate technique.

Starting at a distance from the hernia location for open insertion, the first skin incision is made and carried through the subcutaneous tissues. Hemostasis is obtained. The fascia is exposed and incised, and the peritoneum is opened carefully under direct vision, avoiding underlying bowel, omentum, or adhesions. The first trocar is inserted and secured with the stay sutures as needed. The abdomen is then insufflated while physiologic changes are monitored. The appropriate camera is inserted, and a preliminary visual exploration of the abdominal cavity to identify the pattern of adhesions is made before subsequent cannulae are placed. The camera views placement of each port. Typically, two more cameras are positioned to allow two-handed surgical technique while remaining at a distance from the hernia. A thorough visual examination of the abdominal cavity is then undertaken with the aid of instruments inserted through the other ports, viewing where possible the liver, small bowel, colon, stomach, spleen, and pelvic organs. At any stage in this initial process, adhesions may require sharp and/or blunt lysis to allow adequate exposure. There are several defects adjacent to each other containing suture loops from the first wound closure. Adhesions to the abdominal wall between loops of bowel, and between bowel and other structures, are meticulously lysed to free the entire anterior abdominal fascia.

The hernia defects are identified and, if necessary, their contents reduced. An appropriate margin around the ensemble of defects to accommodate overlapping mesh is cleared by lysing adhesions or mobilizing structures such as the falciform ligament. Hemostasis is secured before continuing, and intestine that has been handled or freed by adhesiolysis is carefully checked to confirm that it is intact. Sites on the abdominal wall are selected for the transfascial fixation sutures, if used. The distribution of the defects is measured and an appropriate-sized mesh patch is selected. The mesh is rolled and introduced though the largest available cannula or abdominal puncture and, once inside, is unfurled and positioned with the correct surface facing the abdominal wall. The entire periphery of the mesh is secured at appropriate intervals to the abdominal wall with a combination of any or all of the following: tacks, staples, transfascial or intracorporeal stitches, or other permanent fixation devices. A fourth or subsequent port may be necessary to permit access of instrumentation for fixation of an inaccessible corner of the mesh. The number and position of these fixation points are intended to achieve adequate overlap of flat-lying mesh beyond the edge of the defect, and prevent both movement of the mesh and protrusion of intestine, omentum, or other abdominal structures between the mesh and the abdominal wall. A second or subsequent concentric inner ring of fixation points between the outer ring and the edge of the defect may be inserted according to the surgeon's preference. The mesh is inspected for gaps, large ripples, and other defects, with and without insufflation, and corrected as needed.

The secondary cannulae are removed; carbon dioxide is allowed to escape from the abdomen and the fascial defects of all port punctures are repaired as appropriate. Local anesthetic is injected once again to all trocar sites and transfascial fixation points. If needed, the subcutaneous tissues of the larger punctures are approximated with interrupted sutures to eliminate dead space. The skin incisions are closed according to surgeon preference. Sponge, needle, and instrument counts are obtained and confirmed prior to closure.

Clinical Example (49655)

A 54-year-old man has a surgical history of a partial gastrectomy for ulcer disease. He has developed an incisional hernia in the midline incision. During the past few months, it has become chronically protuberant. He reports increasing pain and discomfort associated with it. He has had episodes of worsening distention and occasionally vomiting with the episodes of pain. He is not able to reduce the hernia even when lying down. He is referred for laparoscopic repair.

Description of Procedure (49655)

If hernia contents are present, they are gently reduced, if possible. Pneumoperitoneum is induced by open insertion of the first port (described below) or other appropriate technique.

Starting at a distance from the hernia location for open insertion, the first skin incision is made and carried through the subcutaneous tissues. Hemostasis is obtained. The fascia is exposed and incised, and the peritoneum is opened carefully under direct vision, avoiding underlying bowel, omentum, or adhesions. The first trocar is inserted and secured with the stay sutures as needed. The abdomen is then insufflated while physiologic changes are monitored. The appropriate camera is inserted and a preliminary visual exploration of the abdominal cavity to identify the pattern of adhesions is made before subsequent cannulae are placed. There are many adhesions to the anterior abdominal wall involving the small and large intestine. The hernia contains both omentum and multiple loops of small bowel. The small bowel entering the hernia appears chronically dilated; the loops leaving it are flat and decompressed. The camera views placement of each port; typically two more cameras are positioned to allow two-handed surgical technique while remaining at a distance from the hernia. A thorough visual examination of the abdominal cavity is then undertaken with the aid of instruments inserted through the other ports, viewing where possible the liver, small bowel, colon, stomach, spleen, and pelvic organs. At any stage in this initial process, adhesions may require sharp and/or blunt lysis to allow adequate exposure.

The hernia defect or defects are identified and, if necessary, the contents are reduced. Adhesions to the hernia(s), to the abdominal wall, between loops of bowel, and between bowel and other structures are slowly and meticulously lysed to free the entire anterior abdominal fascia. An appropriate margin around the defect(s) to accommodate overlapping mesh is cleared by lysing adhesions or mobilizing structures such as the falciform ligament or adjacent colon. Hemostasis is secured before continuing, and intestine that has been handled or freed by adhesiolysis is carefully checked to confirm that it is intact. Sites on the abdominal wall are selected for the transfascial fixation sutures, if used. The size/distribution of the defects is measured and an appropriate-sized mesh patch is selected. The mesh is rolled and introduced though the largest available cannula or abdominal puncture and, once inside, is unfurled and positioned with the correct surface facing the abdominal wall. The entire periphery of the mesh is secured at appropriate intervals to the abdominal wall with a combination of any or all of the following: tacks, staples, transfascial or intracorporeal stitches, or other permanent fixation devices. A fourth or subsequent port may be necessary to permit access of instrumentation for fixation of an inaccessible corner of the mesh. The number and position of these fixation points are intended to achieve adequate overlap of flat-lying mesh beyond the edge of the defect and prevent both movement of the mesh and protrusion of intestine, omentum, or other abdominal structures between the mesh and the abdominal wall. A second or subsequent concentric inner ring of fixation points between the outer ring and the edge of the defect(s) may be inserted according to surgeon preference. The mesh is inspected for gaps, large ripples, and other defects, with and without insufflation, and corrected as needed.

The secondary cannulae are removed; carbon dioxide is allowed to escape from the abdomen and the fascial defects of all port punctures are repaired as appropriate. Local anesthetic is injected once again to all trocar sites and transfascial fixation points. If needed, the subcutaneous tissues of the larger punctures are approximated with interrupted sutures to eliminate dead space. The skin incisions are closed according to surgeon preference. Sponge, needle, and instrument counts are obtained and confirmed prior to closure.

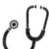

Clinical Example (49656)
A 65-year-old woman has a surgical history of an open cholecystectomy 20 years ago. She developed an incisional hernia. She underwent a surgical repair of that hernia 10 years ago because of increasing size and symptoms. That repair was performed as laparotomy with implantation of a synthetic mesh as an inlay for closure. The patient has developed a recurrence of the hernia with new defects of varying sizes at multiple points around the margins of the inlay mesh. She has symptoms of pain and tenderness at the sites. She is referred for laparoscopic repair of a recurrent incisional hernia.

Description of Procedure (49656)
If hernia contents are present, they are gently reduced. Pneumoperitoneum is induced by open insertion of the first port (described below) or other appropriate technique.

Starting at a distance from the hernia location for open insertion, the first skin incision is made and carried through the subcutaneous tissues. Hemostasis is obtained. The fascia is exposed and incised, and the peritoneum is opened carefully under direct vision, avoiding underlying bowel, omentum, or adhesions. The first trocar is inserted and secured with the stay sutures as needed. The abdomen is then insufflated while physiologic changes are monitored. The appropriate camera is inserted, and a preliminary visual exploration of the abdominal cavity to identify the pattern of adhesions is made before subsequent cannulae are placed. Extensive adhesions of varying thickness and vascularity are found to the anterior abdominal wall and especially to the mesh inlay. These involve the omentum, stomach, and small and large intestine. The camera views placement of each port; typically two more cameras are positioned to allow two-handed surgical technique while remaining at a distance from the hernia. A thorough visual examination of the abdominal cavity is then undertaken with the aid of instruments inserted through the other ports, viewing where possible the liver, small bowel, colon, stomach, spleen, and pelvic organs. At any stage in this initial process, adhesions may require sharp and/or blunt lysis to allow adequate exposure.

The hernia defects are identified and, if necessary, the contents are reduced. Adhesions to the hernias, to the abdominal wall, between loops of bowel, and between bowel and other structures are meticulously lysed to free the entire anterior abdominal fascia. An appropriate margin around the defects to accommodate overlapping mesh is cleared by lysing adhesions or mobilizing structures such as the falciform ligament or adjacent colon. Hemostasis is secured before continuing, and intestine that has been handled or freed by adhesiolysis is carefully checked to confirm that it is intact. Sites on the abdominal wall are selected for the transfascial fixation sutures, if used. The size of the defect is measured and an appropriate-sized mesh patch is selected. The mesh is rolled and introduced through the largest available cannula or abdominal puncture and, once inside, is unfurled and positioned with the correct surface facing the abdominal wall. The entire periphery of the mesh is secured at appropriate intervals to the abdominal wall with a combination of any or all of the following: tacks, staples, transfascial or intracorporeal stitches, or other permanent fixation devices. A fourth or subsequent port may be necessary to permit access of instrumentation for fixation of an inaccessible corner of the mesh. The number and position of these fixation points are intended to achieve adequate overlap of flat-lying mesh beyond the edge of the defect, and prevent both movement of the mesh and protrusion of intestine, omentum, or other abdominal structures between the mesh and the abdominal wall. A second or subsequent concentric inner ring of fixation points between the outer ring and the edge of the defect may be inserted according to surgeon preference. The mesh is inspected for gaps, large ripples, and other defects, with and without insufflation, and corrected as needed.

The secondary cannulae are removed; carbon dioxide is allowed to escape from the abdomen and the fascial defects of all port punctures are repaired as appropriate. Local anesthetic is injected once again to all trocar sites and transfascial fixation points. If needed, the subcutaneous tissues of the larger punctures are approximated with interrupted sutures to eliminate dead space. The skin incisions are closed according to surgeon preference. Sponge, needle, and instrument counts are obtained and confirmed prior to closure.

Clinical Example (49657)

A 60-year-old man presents with an irreducible mass in the midline of the abdomen. He has a history of a laparotomy for repair of a perforated gastric ulcer in the distant past. He had an incisional hernia from that operation that was repaired electively with a mesh 5 years ago. He developed a recurrence from that repair that was being observed. During the last few months, it has been slowly increasing in size. It is now irreducible and tender. He is referred for laparoscopic repair of an incarcerated, recurrent incisional hernia.

Description of Procedure (49657)

If hernia contents are present, they are gently reduced if possible. Pneumoperitoneum is induced by open insertion of the first port (described below) or other appropriate technique.

Starting at a distance from the hernia location for open insertion, the first skin incision is made and carried through the subcutaneous tissues. Hemostasis is obtained. The fascia is exposed and incised, and the peritoneum is opened carefully under direct vision, avoiding underlying bowel, omentum, or adhesions. The first trocar is inserted and secured with the stay sutures as needed. The abdomen is then insufflated while physiologic changes are monitored. The appropriate camera is inserted, and a preliminary visual exploration of the abdominal cavity to identify the pattern of adhesions is made before subsequent cannulae are placed. The camera views placement of each port; typically two more cameras are positioned to allow two-handed surgical technique while remaining at a distance from the hernia. A thorough visual examination of the abdominal cavity is then undertaken with the aid of instruments inserted through the other ports, viewing where possible the liver, small bowel, colon, stomach, spleen, and pelvic organs.

There are many adhesions to the anterior abdominal wall from the small and large intestine. The hernia contains multiple loops of small bowel with adhesions from the intestine to the prior mesh inlay. There are also adhesions from the omentum and colon to the exposed areas of mesh. Careful adhesiolysis proceeds very slowly to fully expose the hernia defect and the incarcerated contents. The viscera are gently reduced with a combination of intra-abdominal traction and extra-abdominal pressure. The area of recurrence is dissected free, and all the intra-abdominal adhesions are taken down to allow for deployment of a new mesh. After all the contents are reduced, the entire small and large bowel is carefully inspected to assess for any injury. Hemostasis is secured before continuing, and intestine that has been handled or freed by adhesiolysis is carefully checked to confirm that it is intact. Sites on the abdominal wall are selected for the transfascial fixation sutures, if used. The size of the defect is measured and an appropriate-sized mesh patch is selected. The mesh is rolled and introduced though the largest available cannula or abdominal puncture and, once inside, is unfurled and positioned with the correct surface facing the abdominal wall. The entire periphery of the mesh is secured at appropriate intervals to the abdominal wall with a combination of any or all of the following: tacks, staples, transfascial or intracorporeal stitches, or other permanent fixation devices. A fourth or subsequent port may be necessary to permit access of instrumentation for fixation of an inaccessible corner of the mesh. The number and position of these fixation points are intended to achieve adequate overlap of flat-lying mesh beyond the edge of the defect and prevent both movement of the mesh and protrusion of intestine, omentum, or other abdominal structures between the mesh and the abdominal wall. A second or subsequent concentric inner ring of fixation points between the outer ring and the edge of the defect may be inserted according to surgeon preference. The mesh is inspected for gaps, large ripples, and other defects, with and without insufflation, and corrected as needed.

The secondary cannulae are removed; carbon dioxide is allowed to escape from the abdomen and the fascial defects of all port punctures are repaired as appropriate. Local anesthetic is injected once again to all trocar sites and transfascial fixation points. If needed, the subcutaneous tissues of the larger punctures are approximated with interrupted sutures to eliminate dead space. The skin incisions are closed according to the surgeon's preference. Sponge, needle, and instrument counts are obtained and confirmed prior to closure.

Urinary System

Bladder

TRANSURETHRAL SURGERY

Urethra and Bladder

52214 Cystourethroscopy, with fulguration (including cryosurgery or laser surgery) of trigone, bladder neck, prostatic fossa, urethra, or periurethral glands

▶(For transurethral fulguration of prostate tissue performed within the postoperative period of 52601 or 52630 performed by the same physician, append modifier 78)◀

▶(For transurethral fulguration of prostate tissue performed within the postoperative period of a related procedure performed by the same physician, append modifier 78)◀

▶(For transurethral fulguration of prostate for postoperative bleeding performed by the same physician, append modifier 78)◀

Rationale

A series of parenthetical notes have been added following code 52214 to direct users regarding the appropriate method of reporting transurethral fulguration that requires a return to the operating room and services from the same physician during the postoperative period. For transurethral fulguration of the prostate performed by the same physician during the postoperative period of codes 52601 or 52630, users are directed to use code 52214, appending modifier 78 to identify provision of this service by the same physician. Users are also directed to append modifier 78 to code 52214 for transurethral fulguration of prostate procedures performed during the postoperative period of a related procedure. Finally, transurethral fulguration of the prostate for postoperative bleeding performed by the same physician is reported by appending modifier 78 to code 52214.

VESICAL NECK AND PROSTATE

52601 Transurethral electrosurgical resection of prostate, including control of postoperative bleeding, complete (vasectomy, meatotomy, cystourethroscopy, urethral calibration and/or dilation, and internal urethrotomy are included)

▶(52606 has been deleted. For transurethral fulguration of prostate, use 52214)◀

▶(52612, 52614, 52620 have been deleted. For first stage transurethral partial resection of prostate, use 52601. For second stage partial resection of prostate, use 52601 with modifier 58. For transurethral resection of residual or regrowth of obstructive prostate tissue, use 52630)◀

▲ **52630** Transurethral resection; residual or regrowth of obstructive prostate tissue including control of postoperative bleeding, complete (vasectomy, meatotomy, cystourethroscopy, urethral calibration and/or dilation, and internal urethrotomy are included)

▶(For resection of residual prostate tissue performed within the postoperative period of a related procedure performed by the same physician, append modifier 78)◀

52640 of postoperative bladder neck contracture

Urethra

MANIPULATION

53605 Dilation of urethral stricture or vesical neck by passage of sound or urethral dilator, male, general or conduction (spinal) anesthesia

▶(For dilation of urethral stricture, male, performed under local anesthesia, see 53600, 53601, 53620, 53621)◀

53665 Dilation of female urethra, general or conduction (spinal) anesthesia

(For urethral catheterization, see 51701-51703)

▶(For dilation of urethra performed under local anesthesia, female, see 53660, 53661)◀

OTHER PROCEDURES

▶(53853 has been deleted. To report, use 55899)◀

53899 Unlisted procedure, urinary system

Rationale

The transurethral prostate resection and thermotherapy destruction of prostate tissue codes have been reformatted to reflect current medical practice for prostate resection and destruction of prostate tissue. With advances in endoscopic resection of prostate tissue, performance of a two-stage prostate resection has become obsolete. As a result, codes 52612 and 52614 have been deleted with addition of an instruction that first- and second-stage transurethral resection of the prostate procedures be reported with code 52601. Modifier 58 should be reported in conjunction with code 52601 when the resection (partial) of the prostate is performed as a second-stage procedure. See Appendix A: Modifiers for the definition and instructions for use of this modifier.

In addition, code 52606 has been deleted and the service previously identified with this code should now reported with code 52214 with modifier 78 appended. Similarly, it was found that physician work and operative technique are equivalent in resecting residual vs regrowth of obstructing tissue. Therefore, code 52620 has also been deleted and code 52630 revised to report this service.

Related to this topic is the use of code 53853 to report the destruction of prostatic tissue. The technology of utilizing heated water to destroy prostate tissue has also become obsolete, with use of microwave and radiofrequency techniques increasing for heat destruction of prostate tissue. As a result, code 53853 has been deleted. An instructional note indicates that the service previously identified by this code should be reported with unlisted code 55899, Unlisted procedure, male genital system. Parenthetical notes that reflect these changes have been placed in appropriate locations to direct users to the correct codes and modifiers to use to identify the specific procedure that is being performed.

Parenthetical notes were also added following codes 53605 and 53665 to instruct correct reporting for dilation of a urethral stricture or dilation of the urethra performed with the patient under local anesthesia.

Male Genital System

Prostate

INCISION

55700 Biopsy, prostate; needle or punch, single or multiple, any approach

(If imaging guidance is performed, use 76942)

(For fine needle aspiration, see 10021, 10022)

(For evaluation of fine needle aspirate, see 88172, 88173)

▶(For transperineal stereotactic template guided saturation prostate biopsies, use 55706)◀

●**55706** Biopsies, prostate, needle, transperineal, stereotactic template guided saturation sampling, including imaging guidance

▶(Do not report 55706 in conjunction with 55700)◀

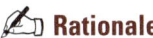 **Rationale**

Code 55706 was established to report transperineal biopsies of the prostate using stereotactic template guidance. This service was previously reported with code 0137T, which has been deleted. To notify users of this change, parenthetical notes have been added following code 55700 that direct users to use code 55706 to report transperineal stereotactic template-guided saturation prostate biopsies.

An exclusionary parenthetical note instructs the inappropriate use of code 55706 in conjunction with code 55700.

Prostate biopsy is performed to verify the presence of cancer, allowing determination of the level of tumor aggressiveness (Gleason score). This procedure is used in the management of prostate cancer, using biopsy data supplemented by clinical (age, general health) and biochemical (prostate-specific antigen [PSA]) data.

Transperineal saturation prostate biopsy procedures are not lesion-oriented but rather systematic collections of samples in those areas of the gland where tumors are most frequent. The whole gland is sampled to address the multicentric nature of prostate cancer and for accurate diagnosis of cancer of the prostate.

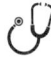

Clinical Example (55706)
A 58-year-old man presented 4 months ago with a PSA of 5.8 ng/mL and a normal digital rectal examination. At that time, he underwent a standard 12-core transrectal biopsy, which revealed high-grade prostatic intraepithelial neoplasia (PIN) involving the right mid-base and mid-apex of his prostate. He was followed carefully, and a repeat PSA has now increased to 8.6 ng/mL. His digital rectal examination remains normal. Given his increasing PSA and prior history of high-grade PIN, the patient elects to undergo a transperineal stereotactic template-guided saturation sampling of his prostate under general anesthesia.

Description of Procedure (55706)
The patient is placed under general or spinal anesthesia and is then placed in the lithotomy position. The digital rectal examination is repeated, the anus is dilated and any feces are manually removed, and the rectum is irrigated. The patient is prepped and draped and a Foley catheter is placed in the bladder. The scrotum is placed out of the operative field by suturing it to the lower abdominal wall.
A preliminary transrectal ultrasound is carried out and the biopsy template (grid) is positioned so that precise and exact coordinates for the prostate biopsies can be taken. The urologist transperineally inserts the needle of the biopsies 35-60 times and cores are taken at intervals through the template (grid). Each specimen is removed from the biopsy needle and placed on nonadherent dressing, the gun is reloaded, and the needle is then carefully reinserted through the biopsy template. Each core is then placed in a container with formalin and the bottle is labeled. Each time the biopsy needle is reintroduced through the biopsy template, sagittal and transverse ultrasound images are taken to ensure precise localization of the biopsy needle. Upon completion of the biopsies, the transrectal ultrasound probe is removed. The biopsy template and sled are disassembled. Perineal and rectal pressure is applied to the prostate and sutures are removed between the scrotum and abdominal wall. The patient is taken out of the lithotomy position.

OTHER PROCEDURES

55875 Transperineal placement of needles or catheters into prostate for interstitial radioelement application, with or without cystoscopy

(For placement of needles or catheters into pelvic organs and/or genitalia [except prostate] for interstitial radioelement application, use 55920)

(For interstitial radioelement application, see 77776-77787)

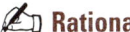 **Rationale**

In support of the deletion of codes 77781-77784 and the establishment of codes 77785-77787, the parenthetical note following code 55875 has been revised to include the appropriate codes to report.

Female Genital System

Vagina

INTRODUCTION

57155 Insertion of uterine tandems and/or vaginal ovoids for clinical brachytherapy

(For placement of needles or catheters into pelvic organs and/or genitalia [except prostate] for interstitial radioelement application, use 55920)

(For insertion of radioelement sources or ribbons, see 77761-77763, ▶77785-77787◀)

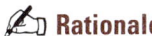 **Rationale**

In support of the deletion of codes 77781-77784 and the establishment of codes 77785-77787, the parenthetical note following code 57155 has been revised to include the appropriate codes to report.

REPAIR

+57267 Insertion of mesh or other prosthesis for repair of pelvic floor defect, each site (anterior, posterior compartment), vaginal approach (List separately in addition to code for primary procedure)

(Use 57267 in conjunction with 45560, 57240-57265, ▶57285◀)

Rationale

The parenthetical note following code 57267 has been revised with the addition of code 57285. Code 57267 is an add-on code that describes the insertion of mesh or other prosthesis through a vaginal approach and is always used in conjunction with certain primary procedures. Code 57285 was added for 2008 and was subsequently identified to be appropriately reported in addition to code 57267 when paravaginal defect repair requires insertion of mesh.

MANIPULATION

▲ **57400** Dilation of vagina under anesthesia (other than local)

▲ **57410** Pelvic examination under anesthesia (other than local)

▲ **57415** Removal of impacted vaginal foreign body (separate procedure) under anesthesia (other than local)

Rationale
Codes 57400, 57410, and 57415 have been revised with the addition of "other than local" to clarify the intent of the references to anesthesia services and the circumstances under which these services would be reported.

Corpus Uteri

INTRODUCTION

58346 Insertion of Heyman capsules for clinical brachytherapy

(For placement of needles or catheters into pelvic organs and/or genitalia [except prostate] for interstitial radioelement application, use 55920)

(For insertion of radioelement sources or ribbons, see 77761-77763, ▶77785-77787◀)

Rationale
In support of the deletion of codes 77781-77784 and the establishment of codes 77785-77787, the parenthetical note following code 58346 has been revised to include the appropriate codes to report.

Nervous System

Skull, Meninges, and Brain

CRANIECTOMY OR CRANIOTOMY

+ **61517** Implantation of brain intracavitary chemotherapy agent (List separately in addition to code for primary procedure)

(Use 61517 only in conjunction with 61510 or 61518)

(Do not report 61517 for brachytherapy insertion. For intracavitary insertion of radioelement sources or ribbons, see ▶77785-77787◀)

Rationale
In support of the deletion of codes 77781 through 77784 and the establishment of codes 77785 through 77787, the parenthetical note following code 61517 has been revised to include the appropriate codes to report.

STEREOTAXIS

61790   Creation of lesion by stereotactic method, percutaneous, by neurolytic agent (eg, alcohol, thermal, electrical, radiofrequency); gasserian ganglion

61791   trigeminal medullary tract

▶(61793 has been deleted. To report, see 61796-61800, 63620-63621)◀

▶STEREOTACTIC RADIOSURGERY (CRANIAL)◀

▶Cranial stereotactic radiosurgery is a distinct procedure that utilizes externally generated ionizing radiation to inactivate or eradicate defined target(s) in the head without the need to make an incision. The target is defined by and the treatment is delivered using high-resolution stereotactic imaging. Stereotactic radiosurgery codes and headframe application procedures are reported by the neurosurgeon. The radiation oncologist reports the appropriate code(s) for clinical treatment planning, physics and dosimetry, treatment delivery, and management from the **Radiation Oncology** section (77261-77790). Any necessary planning, dosimetry, targeting, positioning, or blocking by the neurosurgeon is included in the stereotactic radiation surgery services. The same physician should not report stereotactic radiosurgery services with radiation treatment management codes (77427-77435).

Cranial stereotactic radiosurgery is typically performed in a single planning and treatment session, using a rigidly attached stereotactic guiding device, other immobilization technology and/or a stereotactic image-guidance system, but can be performed with more than one planning session and in a limited number of treatment sessions, up to a maximum of five sessions. Do not report stereotactic radiosurgery more than once per lesion per course of treatment when the treatment requires more than one session.

Codes 61796 and 61797 involve stereotactic radiosurgery for simple cranial lesions. Simple cranial lesions are lesions less than 3.5 cm in maximum dimension that do not meet the definition of a complex lesion provided below. Report code 61796 when all lesions are simple.

Codes 61798 and 61799 involve stereotactic radiosurgery for complex cranial lesions and procedures that create therapeutic lesions (eg, thalamotomy or pallidotomy). All lesions 3.5 cm in maximum dimension or greater are complex. When performing therapeutic lesion creation procedures, report code 61798 only once regardless of the number of lesions created. Schwannomas, arterio-venous malformations, pituitary tumors, glomus tumors, pineal region tumors and cavernous sinus/parasellar/petroclival tumors are complex. Any lesion that is adjacent (5mm or less) to the optic nerve/optic chasm/optic tract or within the brainstem is complex. If treating multiple lesions, and any single lesion treated is complex, use 61798.

Do not report codes 61796-61800 in conjunction with code 20660.

Codes 61796-61799 include computer-assisted planning. Do not report codes 61796-61799 in conjunction with 61795.◀

▶(For intensity modulated beam delivery plan and treatment, see 77301, 77418. For stereotactic body radiation therapy of lesions that are neither cranial nor spinal, use 77435)◀

+61795   Stereotactic computer-assisted volumetric (navigational) procedure, intracranial, extracranial, or spinal (List separately in addition to code for primary procedure)

● **61796** Stereotactic radiosurgery (particle beam, gamma ray, or linear accelerator); 1 simple cranial lesion

▶(Do not report 61796 more than once per course of treatment)◀

▶(Do not report 61796 in conjunction with 61798)◀

+ ● **61797** each additional cranial lesion, simple (List separately in addition to code for primary procedure)

▶(Use 61797 in conjunction with 61796, 61798)◀

▶(For each course of treatment, 61797 and 61799 may be reported no more than once per lesion. Do not report any combination of 61797 and 61799 more than 4 times for entire course of treatment regardless of number of lesions treated)◀

● **61798** 1 complex cranial lesion

▶(Do not report 61798 more than once per course of treatment)◀

▶(Do not report 61798 in conjunction with 61796)◀

+ ● **61799** each additional cranial lesion, complex (List separately in addition to code for primary procedure)

▶(Use 61799 in conjunction with 61798)◀

▶(For each course of treatment, 61797 and 61799 may be reported no more than once per lesion. Do not report any combination of 61797 and 61799 more than 4 times for entire course of treatment regardless of number of lesions treated)◀

+ ● **61800** Application of stereotactic headframe for stereotactic radiosurgery (List separately in addition to code for primary procedure)

▶(Use 61800 in conjunction with 61796, 61798)◀

Rationale

For 2009, significant changes have been made to the CPT coding system for reporting stereotactic radiosurgery (SRS). When code 61793 was added to the CPT codebook, the technology and technique of SRS was first emerging. Since that time, broader indications have been developed for SRS. Due to these changes in the technology, code 61793 no longer adequately describes the physician work involved in the procedures. To accurately reflect the current practice of SRS, code 61793 has been deleted and seven new codes have been established. These new codes are listed under new subheadings, with guidelines to provide education for reporting these codes.

The new codes are divided between cranial procedures and spinal procedures. Codes 61796-61800 are listed under the new subheading, Stereotactic Radiosurgery (Cranial). Codes 63620 and 63621 are listed in the Spinal section under the new subheading, Stereotactic Radiosurgery (Spinal). Rationale for the spinal codes 63620 and 63621 follows the Stereotactic Radiosurgery (Spinal) heading.

It is important to note that these new codes are not intended to report stereotactic body radiation therapy for lesions that are neither cranial nor spinal. Instead, code 77435 should be reported. Parenthetical notes have been added to the two new subsections to clarify this.

Code 61796 describes SRS performed on one simple cranial lesion. Simple lesions, as defined in the guidelines, are lesions less than 3.5 cm in maximum dimension that do not meet the definition of a complex lesion (also defined in the guidelines). Code 61797 is an add-on code that describes SRS performed on each additional simple cranial lesion. Code 61797 is reported in addition to either code 61796 or 61798, as appropriate.

Code 61798 describes SRS performed on a complex cranial lesion, as well as procedures that create therapeutic lesions. A complex lesion is 3.5 cm in maximum dimension or greater. When SRS is performed to create therapeutic lesions, code 61798 is reported one time, regardless of the number of therapeutic lesions created. Code 61799 is an add-on code that describes SRS performed on each additional complex cranial lesion and is reported in addition to code 61798. Parenthetical notes following codes 61797 and 61799 instruct users to report codes 61797 and 61799 only one time per lesion, and no more than four times for the entire course of treatment, regardless of the number of lesions that are treated.

It is important to note that, in the event when both a simple cranial lesion and a complex cranial lesion are treated, code 61798 should be reported for the complex lesion with code 61797 for the simple lesion. As stated in the guidelines, codes 61796-61799 include computer-assisted planning and should not be reported in conjunction with code 61795. Code 61800 describes the application of a stereotactic head frame for SRS. As stated in the guidelines, codes 61796-61800 should not be reported in conjunction with code 20660.

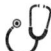

Clinical Example (61796)

A 75-year-old man with a history of renal cell carcinoma, metastatic to the right cerebellum, has headaches, dizziness, and compression of the fourth ventricle as seen on magnetic resonance imaging (MRI). No other lesions are evident, and the chest examination is normal. The lesion enhances and is 2 cm in diameter. He undergoes SRS of the lesion.

Description of Procedure (61796)

The intraservice work begins with the patient being transported to Radiology, where stereotactic computerized imaging studies are obtained. These may be either MRI or angiography. (Radiology services are reported separately.) The neurosurgeon must position and secure the patient on the imaging table and attach an appropriate stereotactic localizer. He or she then works with a radiologist or technician to identify the precise areas to be imaged by adjustment of the scanning geometry and by timing of the contrast injection(s). Finally, the neurosurgeon verifies that the target is optimally imaged. Dosimetry planning follows in conjunction with radiation oncology and a radiation physicist as well a computer programmer. The computer programmer processes all of the stereotactic images into the dose planning computer program during this phase. This dose planning involves use of a computer-based planning module to achieve an optimal dosimetry plan for the patient. A test is then done using the radiosurgical device to ensure correct targeting and dosimetry. The patient is placed in the device while still in the frame. Positioning is more complex due to the use of a stereotactic head frame that requires coordinate indexing to the patient table. The treatment is then delivered.

For each isocenter treated, the neurosurgeon must set the stereotactic coordinates, which are verified by other team members. The frame is removed at the end of the service period.

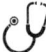
Clinical Example (61797)
A 37-year-old woman presents with a history of breast cancer and two tumors metastatic to her brain. Both tumors are in the right frontal lobe and are 1.5 cm in diameter. They are 3 cm from each other. She has undergone SRS for the first tumor and now during the same session undergoes SRS for the second tumor.

Description of Procedure (61797)
During the course of stereotactic radiosurgery treatment planning for multiple lesions, the patient has already undergone application of the stereotactic head frame under local anesthesia. The patient has previously been transported to Radiology, where stereotactic computerized imaging studies were obtained. The neurosurgeon works with a radiologist or technician to identify the additional area to be imaged by adjustment of the scanning geometry and by timing of the contrast injection(s). The neurosurgeon verifies that the additional target is optimally imaged. Additional dosimetry planning for the additional lesion follows in conjunction with radiation oncology and a radiation physicist. The computer processes all of the stereotactic images in a dose planning program during this phase. This dose planning involves use of a computer-based planning module to achieve an optimal dosimetry plan for the patient. Because of the existing treatment plan for the first lesion, several plans are developed for the additional lesion using different prescribed doses and delivery geometry. The plan that achieves the greatest radiation dose to the additional lesion (taking into account the treatment plan for the first lesion) with the least radiation to the brainstem, retinas, optic nerve, and optic tract is finally chosen. A test is then done using the radiosurgical device to ensure correct targeting and dosimetry. The patient is then placed in the device while still in the frame for stereotactic radiosurgery of both lesions. Positioning is more complex due to the multiple lesions and more complex treatment geometry required. The treatment is then delivered. For the additional lesion, the neurosurgeon must set the stereotactic coordinates, verified by other team members.

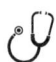
Clinical Example (61798)
A 47-year-old woman has a residual suprasellar meningioma after partial resection of the tumor. The tumor is 3 mm from the optic chiasm. She undergoes SRS of the tumor.

Description of Procedure (61798)
The patient is transported to Radiology, where stereotactic computerized imaging studies are obtained. This may be either MRI or angiography. (Radiology services are reported separately.) The neurosurgeon must position and secure the patient on the imaging table and attach an appropriate stereotactic localizer. He or she then works with a radiologist or technician to identify the precise areas to be imaged by adjustment of the scanning geometry and by timing of the contrast injection(s). Finally, the neurosurgeon verifies that the target is optimally imaged. Complex dosimetry planning follows in conjunction with radiation oncology and a radiation

physicist. The computer processes all of the stereotactic images in a dose planning program during this phase. This dose planning involves use of a computer-based planning module to achieve an optimal dosimetry plan for the patient. Because of the complex nature of the lesion and its proximity to critical radiosensitive structures, several plans are developed using different prescribed doses and delivery geometry. The plan that achieves the greatest radiation dose to the target with the least radiation to the brainstem, retinas, optic nerve, and optic tract is finally chosen. A test is then done using the radiosurgical device to ensure correct targeting and dosimetry. The patient is then placed in the device while still in the frame. Positioning is more complex due to the use of a stereotactic frame that requires coordinate indexing to the patient table. The treatment is then delivered. For each isocenter treated, the neurosurgeon must set the stereotactic coordinates, which are verified by other team members. The frame is removed at the end of the service period.

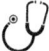

Clinical Example (61799)

A 33-year-old man presents with neurofibromatosis type 2 and bilateral vestibular schwannomas (acoustic neuromas). He has undergone SRS for the first tumor and now during the same session undergoes SRS for the second tumor.

Description of Procedure (61799)

During the course of SRS treatment planning for multiple lesions, the patient has already undergone application of the stereotactic head frame under local anesthesia. The patient has previously been transported to Radiology, where stereotactic computerized imaging studies were obtained. The neurosurgeon works with a radiologist or technician to identify the additional area to be imaged by adjustment of the scanning geometry and by timing of the contrast injection(s). The neurosurgeon verifies that the additional target is optimally imaged. Additional complex dosimetry planning for the additional complex lesion follows in conjunction with radiation oncology and a radiation physicist. The computer processes all of the stereotactic images in a dose planning program during this phase. This dose planning involves use of a computer-based planning module to achieve an optimal dosimetry plan for the patient. Because of the complex nature of the additional lesion and its proximity to critical radiosensitive structures, and because of the existing treatment plan for the first complex lesion, several plans are developed for the additional complex lesion using different prescribed doses and delivery geometry. The plan that achieves the greatest radiation dose to the additional lesion (taking into account the treatment plan for the first lesion) with the least radiation to the brainstem, retinas, optic nerve, and optic tract is finally chosen. A test is then done using the radiosurgical device to ensure correct targeting and dosimetry. The patient is then placed in the device while still in the frame for SRS of both lesions. Positioning is more complex due to the multiple lesions and more complex treatment geometry required. The treatment is then delivered. For the additional lesion, the neurosurgeon must set the stereotactic coordinates, which are verified by other team members.

Clinical Example (61800)

A 50-year-old man with a left occipital arteriovenous malformation is to undergo SRS for obliteration of the lesion. The frame is applied prior to the radiosurgery procedure.

Description of Procedure (61800)

In the radiosurgery clinic, the surgeon's assistant stabilizes the head ring. The skin is prepared, local anesthesia is injected into the scalp, and the ring is rigidly attached to the patient's skull.

Spine and Spinal Cord

INJECTION, DRAINAGE, OR ASPIRATION

▶Injection of contrast during fluoroscopic guidance and localization is an inclusive component of 62263, 62264, 62267, 62270-62273, 62280-62282, 62310-62319.◀ Fluoroscopic guidance and localization is reported with 77003, unless a formal contrast study (myelography, epidurography, or arthrography) is performed, in which case the use of fluoroscopy is included in the supervision and interpretation codes.

For radiologic supervision and interpretation of epidurography, use 72275. Code 72275 is only to be used when an epidurogram is performed, images documented, and a formal radiologic report is issued.

▶Code 62263 describes a catheter-based treatment involving targeted injection of various substances (eg, hypertonic saline, steroid, anesthetic) via an indwelling epidural catheter. Code 62263 includes percutaneous insertion and removal of an epidural catheter (remaining in place over a several-day period), for the administration of multiple injections of a neurolytic agent(s) performed during serial treatment sessions (ie, spanning two or more treatment days). If required, adhesions or scarring may also be lysed by mechanical means. Code 62263 is **not** reported for each adhesiolysis treatment, but should be reported **once** to describe the entire series of injections/infusions spanning two or more treatment days.◀

Code 62264 describes multiple adhesiolysis treatment sessions performed on the same day. Adhesions or scarring may be lysed by injections of neurolytic agent(s). If required, adhesions or scarring may also be lysed mechanically using a percutaneously-deployed catheter.

Codes 62263 and 62264 include the procedure of injections of contrast for epidurography (72275) and fluoroscopic guidance and localization (77003) during initial or subsequent sessions.

(Report 01996 for daily hospital management of continuous epidural or subarachnoid drug administration performed in conjunction with 62318-62319)

●**62267** Percutaneous aspiration within the nucleus pulposus, intervertebral disc, or paravertebral tissue for diagnostic purposes

▶(For imaging, see 77003, 77012)◀

▶(Do not report 62267 in conjunction with 10022, 20225, 62287, 62290, 62291)◀

▲ **62287** Decompression procedure, percutaneous, of nucleus pulposus of intervertebral disc, any method, single or multiple levels, lumbar (eg, manual or automated percutaneous discectomy, percutaneous laser discectomy)

(For fluoroscopic guidance, use ▶77003◀)

▶(Do not report 62287 in conjunction with 62267)◀

Rationale

Code 62267 was established to report percutaneous aspiration within the nucleus pulposus, intervertebral disc, or paravertebral tissue for diagnostic purposes. This code is intended to report the aspiration of fluid and/or cells of a percutaneous disc, nucleus pulposus, or paravertebral diagnostic purposes. This service is provided to evaluate cervical, thoracic, or lumbar infectious discitis; to evaluate spinal and/or paravertebral fluid accumulations; or to harvest cells for diagnostic or therapeutic purposes. A parenthetical note was added to instruct that codes 77003 and 77012 should be separately reported when (computed tomographic and fluoroscopic) imaging guidance is required and performed. An exclusionary parenthetical note was also added to exclude reporting code 62267 in conjunction with other aspiration codes 10022, 20225, 62287, 62290 and 62291. Code 62267 has significant preprocedure and postprocedure physician service and therefore is considered a stand-alone code.

The Injection, Drainage, or Aspiration guidelines were revised to include the new code 62267 to instruct that contrast injection during fluoroscopic guidance and localization is an inclusive component of code 62267 and not separately reported.

Code 62287 was editorially revised to exclude "aspiration" to distinguish this therapeutic procedure from the diagnostic aspiration reported with code 62267. An exclusionary parenthetical note excludes reporting code 62287 in conjunction with code 62267.

Clinical Example (62267)

A 70-year-old diabetic woman developed increasing, severe low back pain during the past 3 weeks. Lumbar magnetic resonance imaging with contrast is consistent with possible discitis of the L5-S1 disc, with some fluid seen around the disc and adjacent soft tissue. The patient wishes to proceed with a percutaneous needle aspiration of the disc fluid to determine whether a bacterial infection exists and to help guide future treatment options.

Description of Procedure (62267)

The local anesthesia is administered at the proposed puncture site. A needle is inserted under image guidance (separately coded). The needle is advanced and adjusted until positioned in the disc or surrounding paraspinal tissue. The fluid and/or tissue are then aspirated. The needle is again adjusted and additional samples are taken. The cultures collected are inoculated. The needle is withdrawn and dressing is applied.

POSTERIOR EXTRADURAL LAMINOTOMY OR LAMINECTOMY FOR EXPLORATION/DECOMPRESSION OF NEURAL ELEMENTS OR EXCISION OF HERNIATED INTERVERTEBRAL DISCS

▲ **63020** Laminotomy (hemilaminectomy), with decompression of nerve root(s), including partial facetectomy, foraminotomy and/or excision of herniated intervertebral disc, including open and endoscopically-assisted approaches; 1 interspace, cervical

(For bilateral procedure, report 63020 with modifier 50)

▲ **63030** 1 interspace, lumbar

(For bilateral procedure, report 63030 with modifier 50)

+▲ **63035** each additional interspace, cervical or lumbar (List separately in addition to code for primary procedure)

Rationale

Codes 63020, 63030, and 63035 have been revised to include open and endoscopically assisted approach for cervical and lumbar nerve root decompression procedures. This change clarifies appropriate application of this code in both open and endoscopic posterior cervical and lumbar discectomy and decompression.

►STEREOTACTIC RADIOSURGERY (SPINAL)◄

►Spinal stereotactic radiosurgery is a distinct procedure that utilizes externally generated ionizing radiation to inactivate or eradicate defined target(s) in the spine without the need to make an incision. The target is defined by and the treatment is delivered using high-resolution stereotactic imaging. These codes are reported by the surgeon. The radiation oncologist reports the appropriate code(s) for clinical treatment planning, physics and dosimetry, treatment delivery and management from the **Radiation Oncology** section (77261-77790). Any necessary planning, dosimetry, targeting, positioning, or blocking by the neurosurgeon is included in the stereotactic radiation surgery services. The same physician should not report stereotactic radiosurgery services with radiation treatment management codes (77427-77432).

Spinal stereotactic radiosurgery is typically performed in a single planning and treatment session using a stereotactic image-guidance system, but can be performed with a planning session and in a limited number of treatment sessions, up to a maximum of five sessions. Do not report stereotactic radiosurgery more than once per lesion per course of treatment when the treatment requires greater than one session.

Stereotactic spinal surgery is only used when the tumor being treated affects spinal neural tissue or abuts the dura mater. Arteriovenous malformations must be subdural. For other radiation services of the spine, see **Radiation Oncology** services.

Codes 63620, 63621 include computer-assisted planning. Do not report 63620, 63621 in conjunction with 61795.◄

►(For intensity modulated beam delivery plan and treatment, see 77301, 77418. For stereotactic body radiation therapy for lesions that are neither cranial nor spinal, use 77435)◄

● **63620** Stereotactic radiosurgery (particle beam, gamma ray, or linear accelerator); 1 spinal lesion

▶(Do not report 63620 more than once per course of treatment)◀

+ ●63621   each additional spinal lesion (List separately in addition to code for primary procedure)

▶(Report 63621 in conjunction with 63620)◀

▶(For each course of treatment, 63621 may be reported no more than once per lesion. Do not report 63621 more than 2 times for entire course of treatment regardless of number of lesions treated)◀

Rationale

For 2009, significant changes have been made to the CPT coding system for reporting stereotactic radiosurgery (SRS). When code 61793 was added to the CPT codebook, the technology and technique of SRS was first emerging. Since that time, broader indications have been developed for SRS. Due to these changes in the technology, code 61793 no longer adequately describes the physician work involved in the procedures. To accurately reflect the current practice of SRS, code 61793 has been deleted and seven new codes have been established. These new codes are listed under two new subheadings, with guidelines to provide education about the reporting of these codes.

It is important to note that these new codes are not intended to report stereotactic body radiation therapy for lesions that are neither cranial nor spinal. Instead, code 77435 should be reported. Parenthetical notes have been added to the two new subsections to clarify this.

The new codes are divided between cranial procedures and spinal procedures. Codes 61796-61800 are listed under the new subheading, Stereotactic Radiosurgery (Cranial). Codes 63620 and 63621 are listed in the Spinal section under the new subheading, Stereotactic Radiosurgery (Spinal). Rationale for the cranial codes 61796-61880 is listed under Stereotactic Radiosurgery (Cranial).

Code 63620 describes SRS performed on one spinal lesion. A parenthetical note was added following code 63620 instructing users not to report code 63620 more than once per course of treatment. Code 63621 is an add-on code that describes SRS performed on each additional spinal lesion and is reported in addition to code 63620 as appropriate. A parenthetical note was added following code 63621 instructing users that this code may not be reported more than once per lesion and no more than two times per each course of treatment, regardless of the number of lesions treated.

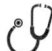

Clinical Example (63620)

A 65-year-old man presents with prostate cancer metastatic to the C4 vertebral body and epidural space, resulting in mild narrowing of the central canal. He undergoes stereotactic spinal radiosurgery for the single metastatic tumor.

Description of Procedure (63620)

The patient has already been transported to Radiology, where stereotactic computerized imaging studies are obtained. These may be either magnetic resonance images or angiography. (Radiology services are reported separately.) The neurosurgeon then works with a radiologist to verify that the target is optimally imaged. Complex dosimetry planning follows in conjunction with radiation oncology and a radiation physicist. The computer processes all of the stereotactic images in a dose planning program during this phase. The neurosurgeon carefully outlines the target lesion where it appears on each consecutive image. The neurosurgeon also outlines the spinal cord on the same images. This dose planning involves use of a computer-based planning module to achieve an optimal dosimetry plan for the patient. Because of the nature of the lesion and its proximity to the spinal cord, several plans are developed using different prescribed doses and delivery geometry. The plan that achieves the greatest radiation dose to the target with the least radiation to the spinal cord is finally chosen. The patient is then brought to the treatment device and positioned on the treatment table. The neurosurgeon is available to make changes in the treatment plan if optimal positioning cannot be achieved. The device automatically obtains positioning radiographs and compensates for the patient's actual position in the treatment device so that the expected treatment geometry matches the actual treatment geometry based on the bony landmarks of the spine. The neurosurgeon is available to make more changes in the treatment plan if this image fusion resulting in registration of the spine fails. The treatment is then delivered.

Clinical Example (63621)

A 45-year-old woman presents with breast cancer metastatic to the vertebral body and epidural space of T2 and T5. She has undergone stereotactic spinal radiosurgery for the first tumor and now, during the same session, undergoes stereotactic spinal radiosurgery for the second tumor.

Description of Procedure (63621)

The patient has already been transported to Radiology, where stereotactic computerized imaging studies are obtained. These may be either magnetic resonance images or angiography. (Radiology services are reported separately.) The neurosurgeon then works with a radiologist to verify that the additional target is optimally imaged. Complex dosimetry planning follows in conjunction with radiation oncology and a radiation physicist. The computer processes all of the stereotactic images in a dose planning program during this phase. The neurosurgeon carefully outlines the additional target lesion where it appears on each consecutive image. The neurosurgeon also outlines the spinal cord on the same images. This dose planning involves use of a computer-based planning module to achieve an optimal dosimetry plan for the patient. Because of the multiple lesions and their proximity to each other and to the spinal cord, several plans are developed using different prescribed doses and delivery geometry. The plan that achieves the greatest radiation dose to the additional lesion (taking into account the treatment plan for the first lesion) without interfering with the first lesion treatment plan and achieves the least radiation to the spinal cord is finally chosen. The patient is then brought to the treatment device and positioned on the treatment table. The neurosurgeon is available to make changes in the treatment plan for the additional lesion if optimal positioning cannot be achieved. The device automatically obtains positioning radiographs and compensates for the patient's actual position in the treatment device for the additional lesion so that the expected treatment geometry matches the actual treatment geometry based on the bony landmarks of the spine. The neurosurgeon is available to make more changes in the treatment plan for the additional lesion if this image fusion resulting in registration of the spine fails. The treatment is then delivered.

Extracranial Nerves, Peripheral Nerves, and Autonomic Nervous System

INTRODUCTION/INJECTION OF ANESTHETIC AGENT (NERVE BLOCK), DIAGNOSTIC OR THERAPEUTIC

Somatic Nerves

64400	Injection, anesthetic agent; trigeminal nerve, any division or branch
▲ **64416**	brachial plexus, continuous infusion by catheter (including catheter placement)
▲ **64446**	sciatic nerve, continuous infusion by catheter (including catheter placement)
▲ **64448**	femoral nerve, continuous infusion by catheter (including catheter placement)
▲ **64449**	lumbar plexus, posterior approach, continuous infusion by catheter (including catheter placement)
64450	other peripheral nerve or branch

(For phenol destruction, see 64622-64627)

(For subarachnoid or subdural injection, see 62280, 62310-62319)

(For epidural or caudal injection, see 62273, 62281-62282, 62310-62319)

▶(For injection of Morton's neuroma, see 64455, 64632)◀

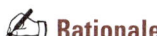
Rationale

Codes 64416, 64446, 64448, and 64449 were all revised to eliminate subsequent days of daily management for these codes. Previously, the descriptors for these codes included language that identified reference to the inclusion of " . . . daily management for anesthetic agent administration." The change was made largely due to the shift in the site of service for these procedures as these procedures are no longer performed predominantly in the inpatient setting. The change regarding the site of service for this procedure inherently affects the follow-up efforts for this service and, as a result, the language identifying inclusion of follow-up days for these procedures has been removed.

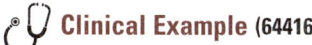
Clinical Example (64416)

A 36-year-old man suffered traumatic amputation of his thumb and forefinger on the right hand in an automobile accident. He has had these digits replanted under a general anesthetic and 5 hours of surgery. The digits are ischemic in appearance and cold with poor capillary filling despite a good surgical repair and anastomoses of the digital arteries. The surgeon requests a block with continuous infusion to manage postoperative pain and provide vasodilation to the arterial supply to the hand and digits in an effort to improve survival of the reimplanted digits. A continuous brachial plexus block using a catheter placed in the brachial plexus at the axilla and the infusion of local anesthetic is planned to provide pain relief and to provide vasodilation of the arterial supply to the hand and digits.

Description of Procedure (64416)
An intravenous infusion is initiated and supplemental oxygen is provided. The patient's right arm is abducted at the shoulder and flexed at the elbow with his hand positioned above his right shoulder. The infraclavicular and supraclavicular regions are prepared with an antiseptic solution, and the skin is anesthetized with a small amount of local anesthetic via a small-gauge needle (27G). A stimulating needle is inserted into either the infraclavicular or supraclavicular area and advanced until the proper location of the needle is ascertained with the use of a nerve stimulator, the elicitation of paresthesias, and/or the use of an ultrasound image (ultrasound guidance, when used, is separately reported). At that point, a nerve block catheter is inserted into the brachial plexus sheath. The needle is removed and the plastic cannula left in position. Next, an epidural-type plastic catheter is inserted through the cannula into the brachial plexus sheath and secured in place. A bacterial filter is attached. A brachial plexus block using the injection of about 30-40 mL of local anesthetic (usually 1-1.5% lidocaine, 0.25-0.375% bupivacaine, or 1-1.5% mepivacaine) is now performed after using a small test dose of the local anesthetic and frequent aspiration during the injection. The density and function of the block is then assessed over the next 30 minutes, as are signs and symptoms of local anesthetic toxicity. A continuous infusion of local anesthetic is now started (0.25% bupivacaine at 5-10 mL/hr.). Movement of the head and neck after placement make scrupulous attention to patient comfort in the choice of tunneling length, direction, and technique important in affixing the brachial plexus catheter.

Clinical Example (64446)
A 30-year-old man suffers a crushed left foot in an automobile accident. He undergoes major reconstruction of his left foot and ankle under general anesthesia. The surgeon requests a block with continuous infusion to manage postoperative pain and facilitate rehabilitation. To provide postoperative pain control, a continuous sciatic nerve block is performed at the end of surgery.

Description of Procedure (64446)
An intravenous infusion is initiated and supplemental oxygen is provided. The thigh is flexed on the hip to 45 degrees. The greater femoral trochanter and ischial tuberosity are marked and a line is drawn from the popliteal fossa to midway between the two landmarks. After antiseptic skin preparation and placement of a small amount of local anesthetic via a small-gauge needle (eg, 27G), a 20-gauge insulated needle is introduced vertically to the skin, just medial to the upper end of the marked line, to determine the depth of the sciatic nerve. A brisk motor response in the ankle, foot, or toes is noted with less than 0.4 mA of stimulation. It is possible to use ultrasound imaging to guide needle placement. When performed, this is separately reported. Next, an insulated epidural needle is advanced from approximately 5 cm cephalad and angled to intersect the tip of the first needle. Nerve stimulation is again noted, and a catheter is then advanced through the epidural needle and 50-100 mm beyond its tip. The

electrical connection is then transferred to the catheter and nerve stimulation is again evaluated. The epidural needle is removed, the catheter is secured in place, a bacterial filter is attached, and 15-20 mL of 0.5% bupivacaine is injected through the catheter. Block of the sciatic nerve is then assessed over the next 15-30 minutes and an infusion of 0.375% bupivacaine at 0.1 mL/kg/hr (~7 mL/hr) is started. Required infusion rates typically range from 2-12 mL/hr. Occasionally bolus injections (10-15 mL) are required. Subcutaneous tunneling, fixation, and dressing of the catheter must be done carefully, as this area is prone to bacterial contamination both during and after the procedure.

Clinical Example (64448)

A 65-year-old man undergoes a right total knee replacement (code 27447) under general anesthesia. The surgeon requests a block with continuous infusion to manage postoperative pain and facilitate rehabilitation. To provide postoperative pain control and increased mobility in the knee, a continuous femoral nerve block is performed.

Description of Procedure (64448)

An intravenous infusion is initiated and supplemental oxygen is provided. The patient's right groin is prepared with an antiseptic solution, and a 22-gauge short-bevel 10-cm insulated needle is inserted into an 18-gauge long plastic cannula. To access the femoral nerve sheath, a small amount of local anesthetic is injected with a small-gauge needle at a point located approximately 1 cm lateral to the femoral artery and 1 cm caudad from the inguinal ligament. The needle is placed through the wheal of local anesthetic, and proper location of the needle is ascertained with the use of a nerve stimulator, the elicitation of paresthesias, or both. An ultrasound imaging system may also improve the ability to discover the femoral sheath's location. When performed, ultrasound guidance is separately reported. The plastic cannula is then advanced over the needle into the sheath of the femoral nerve. Next, between 20 and 30 mL of 0.25% to 0.5% bupivacaine or other long-acting anesthetic with epinephrine 1:200,000 is injected carefully through the cannula and with frequent aspiration and monitoring of the electrocardiogram and pulse oximeter to avoid the possibility of intravascular injection. A 20-gauge epidural catheter is threaded through the cannula and the cannula is removed. The catheter is secured in place and sterilely dressed, and a bacterial filter is attached. Bupivacaine 0.25-0.125% at 0.14 mL/kg/hr (~10 mL/hr) is then infused. Subcutaneous tunneling, fixation, and dressing of the catheter must be done carefully, as this area is prone to bacterial contamination both during and after the procedure.

Clinical Example (64449)

A 62-year-old woman undergoes a left total knee replacement (code 27447) under general anesthesia. The surgeon requests a block with a continuous infusion to manage postoperative pain and facilitate rehabilitation. To provide postoperative pain control and increased mobility in her knee, a continuous lumbar plexus block is performed.

Description of Procedure (64449)

An intravenous infusion is initiated and supplemental oxygen is provided. A line is drawn between the iliac crests (eg, Tuffier's line). A second line is made 3-5 cm parasagittally to the left. A mark for the needle insertion is made where the two lines intersect. The low back is prepared with a topical antiseptic. After the skin and deeper tissues are infiltrated with local anesthetic with a small-gauge needle (eg, 27G), a 19-gauge, 10-cm needle, designed to allow the introduction of a catheter through the needle and connected to a peripheral nerve stimulator, is advanced to obtain stimulation of the lumbar plexus. When a transverse process is encountered, the needle is partially withdrawn and advanced slightly cephalad until it slides past the transverse process of the lumbar vertebra.

When the needle tip is in the psoas compartment and in the proper location, stimulation of the lumbar plexus is recognized by observing the rise of the patella and contraction of the quadriceps and sartorius muscles. Generally, current of 0.6-0.8 mA indicates stimulation of the femoral nerve when the needle is correctly positioned. Ultrasound imaging may be useful in this needle placement. When performed, ultrasound guidance is separately reported.

At this point, careful aspiration for blood and cerebrospinal fluid is performed. A test dose of local anesthetic (3 mL of 2% lidocaine with epinephrine 1:200,000) is administered to rule out intravenous or intrathecal injection. Between 15-30 mL of dilute local anesthetic (eg, 0.25% bupivacaine, 0.2% ropivacaine) is slowly injected through the needle, followed by insertion of an infusion catheter through the needle (about 5 cm past the tip of the needle). The patient is observed for signs of undesired epidural spread and associated hemodynamic changes, and for analgesia of the left leg and hip. The catheter is checked for intravascular and intrathecal placement and secured in place. Once correct function of the catheter is confirmed, a bacterial filter is attached and a continuous infusion of dilute concentration of local anesthetic (eg, 0.2% ropivacaine, 0.25% bupivacaine) is started at 8-10 mL/hr. Alternatively, a patient-controlled infusion may be started at 5 mL/hr with a bolus of 10 mL per 30-60 minutes. Assistance at the time of ambulation is essential.

●**64455** Injection(s), anesthetic agent and/or steroid, common digital nerve(s) (eg, Morton's neuroma)

▶(Do not report 64455 in conjunction with 64632)◀

(Codes 64470-64484 are unilateral procedures. For bilateral procedures, use modifier 50)

(For fluoroscopic guidance and localization for needle placement and injection in conjunction with 64470-64484, use 77003)

64470 Injection, anesthetic agent and/or steroid, paravertebral facet joint or facet joint nerve; cervical or thoracic, single level

DESTRUCTION BY NEUROLYTIC AGENT (EG, CHEMICAL, THERMAL, ELECTRICAL OR RADIOFREQUENCY)

Codes 64600-64681 include the injection of other therapeutic agents (eg, corticosteroids). ▶(For therapies that are not destructive of the target nerve [eg, pulsed radiofrequency]), use 64999)◀

Somatic Nerves

64630 Destruction by neurolytic agent; pudendal nerve

●**64632** plantar common digital nerve

▶(Do not report 64632 in conjunction with 64455)◀

64640 other peripheral nerve or branch

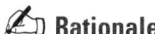 **Rationale**

Codes 64455 and 64632 were established to report injection of the plantar digital nerve (64455) and the destruction of a plantar common digital nerve by neurolytic agent injection (64632). These services are commonly provided for Morton's neuroma and are reported only for injections and nerve destruction to the lower extremity. Code 64455 is reported one time only, regardless of the number of injections provided during a session, as indicated by the optional plural forms for "injection" and "nerve." Exclusionary parenthetical notes have been added following each of these codes (64455, 64632) to preclude reporting these therapies at the same session.

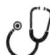 **Clinical Example (64455)**

A 46-year-old woman presents with a painful neuroma in the third intermetatarsal space of her right foot. The decision is made to proceed with a therapeutic intermetatarsal neuroma injection.

Description of Procedure (64455)

The intermetatarsal space is palpated and the point of maximal tenderness is identified. A dorsal approach is utilized and the needle is inserted top to bottom without penetrating the plantar skin. A portion of the injectable material is deposited. The needle is redirected distally and medially without exiting the dorsal site and a portion of the injectable material is deposited. The needle is again redirected distally and laterally without exiting the dorsal site and the final portion of the injectable material is deposited.

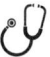 **Clinical Example (64632)**

A 35-year-old man presents with a painful neuroma in the second intermetatarsal space of his left foot, for which typical conservative measures have failed. The decision is made to proceed with neurolytic injection of the intermetatarsal neuroma.

Description of Procedure (64632)

The intermetatarsal space is palpated and the point of maximal tenderness is identified. A dorsal approach is utilized and the needle is inserted top to bottom without penetrating the plantar skin. A portion of the injectable material is deposited. The needle is redirected distally and medially without exiting the dorsal site and a portion of the injectable material is deposited. The needle is again redirected distally and laterally without exiting the dorsal site and the final portion of the injectable material is deposited.

Eye and Ocular Adnexa

Anterior Segment

CORNEA

Keratoplasty

Corneal transplant includes use of fresh or preserved grafts. ▶The preparation of donor material is included for penetrating or anterior lamellar keratoplasty, but reported separately for endothelial keratoplasty. Do not report 65710-65757 in conjunction with 92025.◀

(Keratoplasty excludes refractive keratoplasty procedures, 65760, 65765, and 65767)

▲ 65710   Keratoplasty (corneal transplant); anterior lamellar

▲ 65730   penetrating (except in aphakia or pseudophakia)

65750   penetrating (in aphakia)

65755   penetrating (in pseudophakia)

●65756   endothelial

+●65757   Backbench preparation of corneal endothelial allograft prior to transplantation (List separately in addition to code for primary procedure)

▶(Use 65757 in conjunction with 65756)◀

Rationale

Code 65756 has been established to report endothelial keratoplasty, which is offered to some patients as a substitute for full-thickness corneal transplants (65730, 65750, 65755). Unlike the classic transplant, which requires replacing the full-thickness of the cornea with donor tissue, endothelial keratoplasty involves replacement of only the innermost layer of the cornea containing the corneal endothelium. The surgical procedure is very different from the full-thickness (penetrating keratoplasty) procedures (65730, 65750, 65755) and requires different surgical skills. Existing code 65730 was revised to distinguish it from code 65755 by adding the term "pseudophakia" to the parenthetical exclusionary note. Code 65710 was revised for clarification to include the term "anterior," as the procedure it represents is performed for scarring of the anterior cornea and includes replacement of the anterior layers of the cornea only, with limited intraocular incisions or manipulations required, whereas endothelial keratoplasty involves replacement of the endothelium that has become dysfunctional through aging or disease. The eye is entered during surgery, and most of the manipulations are intraocular.

Add-on code 65757 for the transplant preparation was established to be used in conjunction with the endothelial keratoplasty code when the surgeon performs the preparation of the graft at the time of implant vs obtaining the graft material from an eye bank. The introductory language for the keratoplasty codes was revised to reflect current practice in which the work of the graft preparation is typically performed by the operating surgeon, whereas for endothelial keratoplasty the work is done, on estimate, only about 50% of the time by the surgeon. A parenthetical note was added to direct the user to report the primary procedure (endothelial keratoplasty) in conjunction with code 65757.

Clinical Example (65756)

A 65-year-old man develops pseudophakic corneal edema in his left eye 7 years after cataract surgery. Visual acuity is reduced to 20/80 and there is significant glare disability due to the edema, limiting his ability to drive, read, and watch television. A well-positioned posterior chamber intraocular lens is present, and the posterior segment examination is unremarkable.

Description of Procedure (65756)

Antibiotic and anesthetic agents are applied topically to the eye. White-to-white distance is measured with a caliper and a trephine size is selected. Superior and inferior silk sutures are placed and clamped. The epithelium of the recipient cornea is marked with the trephine.

The donor graft is punched with the same trephine used to mark the recipient. The lamellar disc is inspected and trimmed if it is full thickness in areas. The donor graft is covered with preservation media.

The temporal cornea is marked with calipers painted with stain. A conjunctival peritomy is performed temporally. Bleeding is controlled with cautery. A scleral tunnel is made temporally and carried forward to clear cornea with a crescent blade. A paracentesis is made to the right of the scleral tunnel, inside the trephine mark. Anesthetic is placed in the anterior chamber. A needle attached to irrigation is passed through clear cornea inside the trephine mark to the left of the scleral tunnel and used to maintain the anterior chamber and stabilize eye position throughout the procedure. Anterior chamber air is removed with a cannula through the paracentesis. Descemet's membrane is lightly scored with a reverse hook inside the epithelial trephine mark. Irrigation is turned off. Dye is placed in the anterior chamber to stain the endothelium. A small incision is made through the scleral tunnel into the anterior chamber with a 15-degree blade. Irrigation is turned on and excess dye is irrigated from the eye. A Descemet's membrane scraper is placed through the tunnel incision and used to scrape/detach Descemet's membrane, avoiding the central cornea. Descemet's membrane is removed with forceps and unfolded on the surface of the cornea to check for complete removal. Additional dye is placed and additional scraping is performed in cases of incomplete removal. The periphery of the recipient stroma is gently roughened with the scraper. The incision is opened to the full width of the tunnel with a 15-degree blade. The infusion needle is removed.

The donor graft is removed from the punch block with a spatula and transferred to the surface of the recipient cornea, endothelial side up. A small amount of cohesive viscoelastic is placed on the left side of the donor endothelium.

The epithelial lamella of the donor tissue is fixed with forceps, while the endothelial lamella is folded to the left with additional forceps so that the top half overlaps the bottom in a "taco" fashion. The folded posterior lamella is grasped with special insertion forceps and is inserted into the anterior chamber. The forceps are opened and removed without pulling out the donor graft. The anterior chamber is filled with balanced saline solution through the right-sided paracentesis without dislodging the donor graft. The scleral tunnel is sutured with three radial nylon sutures, which are tied and trimmed. A needle is placed through a limbal stab incision peripheral to the donor on the left, and air is slowly injected between the posterior and anterior halves of the folded donor graft. If the donor graft moves out of position prior to unfolding, a backhanded nylon suture is placed through the limbus on the left, through the anterior edge of the folded donor graft, and out through the recipient cornea and tied. Air is added slowly to unfold the donor graft. If the tissue does not unfold, a bent needle-tip is placed through a limbal paracentesis on the right and used to engage the stromal side of the inferior portion of the donor. The nylon donor suture is removed once the donor graft is unfolded and in position. Air is added until the eye is firm and left in place for 10 minutes. During this time, the surface is compressed with a roller to remove interface fluid and secure proper donor position. A midperipheral incision is placed in each of the four quadrants of the recipient cornea and used to release interface fluid. The conjunctiva is closed with cautery. A subconjunctival injection of steroid is administered inferonasally. A final paracentesis is made at the limbus, peripheral to the donor graft, with a 15-degree blade. Balanced saline solution is injected and air is removed, leaving a deep chamber and a 4-5–mm air bubble. The final paracentesis incision is hydrated with balanced saline solution. Cycloplegic and antibiotic agents are applied topically. The lid speculum and drapes are removed.

Clinical Example (65757)

An endothelial graft is required for an endothelial keratoplasty. The surgeon prepares this in the operating room prior to performing the intraocular surgery.

Description of Procedure (65757)

The endothelial graft is prepared in the operating room. The temperature of the artificial anterior chamber (AAC) on which the donor cornea will be mounted is checked, an infusion system is attached, and all air bubbles are removed. The donor cornea is secured to the AAC with a screw-top mechanism while reintroduction of air into the system is prevented. Alignment of the donor material is then checked under the operating microscope and the tissue is repositioned if necessary. The pressure in the system is measured. The corneal epithelium is removed under the microscope and a reference mark is applied to the donor cornea to allow alignment of the segments after the cornea has been cut. The central corneal thickness (pachymetry) is measured after the material has been hydrated, and the microkeratome, which splits the donor button into two pieces, is set for the appropriate depth to cut based on the pachymetry measurement. After the pressure settings of the AAC are rechecked and the cornea is rewetted, the microscope is used to inspect the microkeratome and then the corneal cap is cut from the donor material. Under the microscope, the cap is retrieved from the microkeratome and realigned on the donor bed by using the previously placed marker, and the cap is measured to be sure that the endothelial graft is of sufficient diameter to be used. The screw top of the AAC is then removed, the infusion is restarted, and the donor material is carefully removed from the AAC, making certain that there is no collapse of the chamber (which would damage the graft) during the process.

Other Procedures
▶Do not report 65760-65771 in conjunction with 92025.◀

65760 Keratomileusis

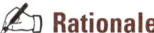 **Rationale**

A guideline has been added preceding the keratoplasty codes 65760-65771 to indicate that, when computerized corneal topography is performed with keratoplasty procedures, code 92025 is included in these codes and is not separately reported.

Posterior Segment

VITREOUS

67036 Vitrectomy, mechanical, pars plana approach;

▶(For application of intraocular epiretinal radiation with 67036, use 0190T)◀

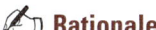 **Rationale**

In support of the establishment of Category III code 0190T, a cross reference was added following code 67036 directing users to 0190T for reporting application of intraocular epiretinal radiation.

Operating Microscope

The surgical microscope is employed when the surgical services are performed using the techniques of microsurgery. Code 69990 should be reported (without modifier 51 appended) in addition to the code for the primary procedure performed. Do not use 69990 for visualization with magnifying loupes or corrected vision. Do not report 69990 in addition to procedures where use of the operating microscope is an inclusive component (15756-15758, 15842, 19364, 19368, 20955-20962, 20969-20973, ▶22856-22861◀, 26551-26554, 26556, 31526, 31531, 31536, 31541, 31545, 31546, 31561, 31571, 43116, 43496, 49906, 61548, 63075-63078, 64727, 64820-64823, 65091-68850, ▶0184T◀).

+69990 Microsurgical techniques, requiring use of operating microscope (List separately in addition to code for primary procedure)

Rationale

In support of the establishment of codes 22856-22861 and code 0184T, the guidelines for use of the operating microscope code 69990 were revised to indicate that code 69990 should not be reported in conjunction with these new codes.

Radiology

Revisions of the Radiology section are minimal and include the deletion and addition of new codes for high dose rate brachytherapy and the addition of a code for injection for of a diagnostic radiopharmaceutical for localization with non-imaging gamma probes.

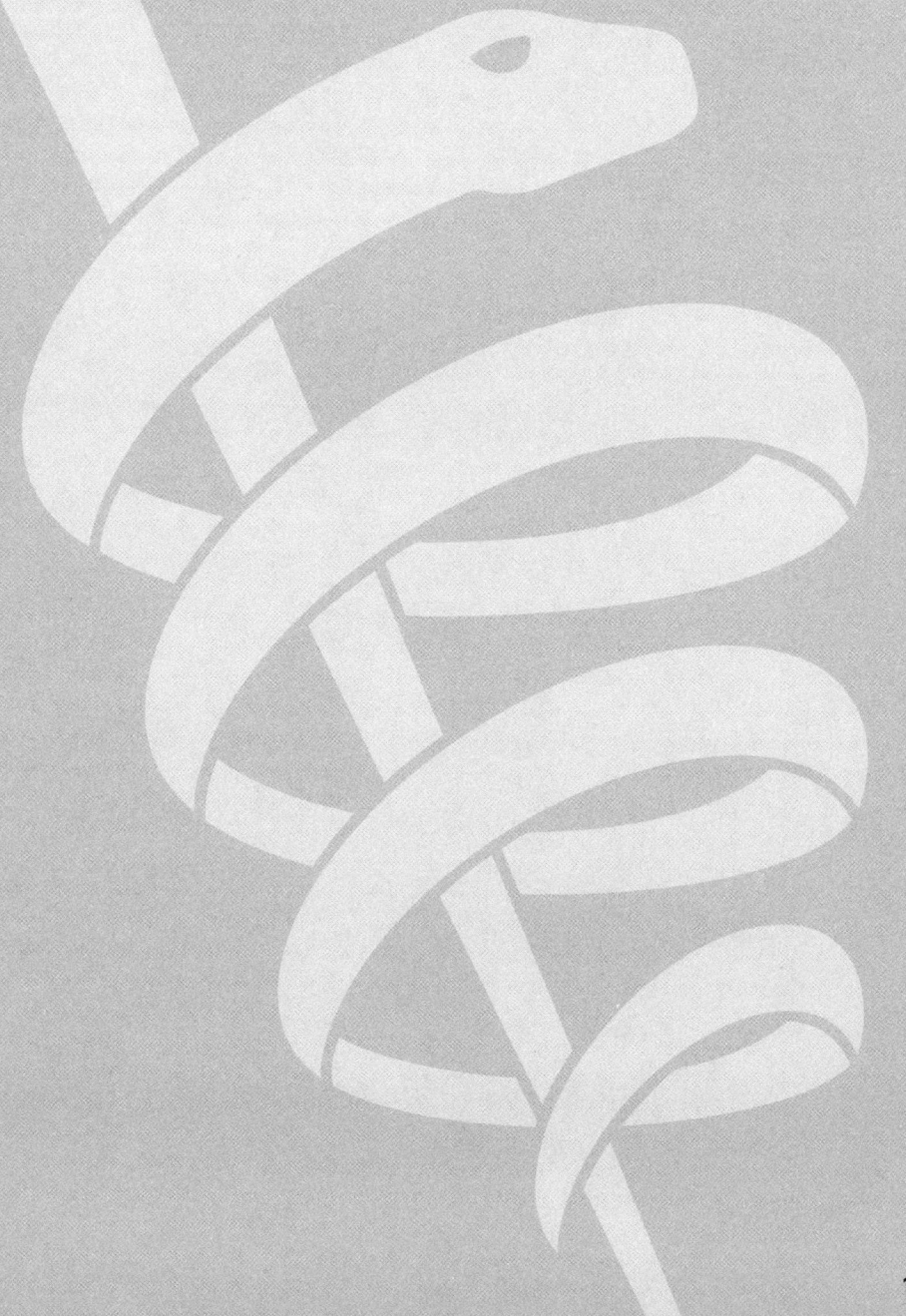

Radiology

Diagnostic Radiology (Diagnostic Imaging)

Spine and Pelvis

72275 Epidurography, radiological supervision and interpretation

(72275 includes 77003)

▶(For injection procedure, see 62280-62282, 62310-62319, 64479-64484)◀

Rationale

In support of the deletion of Category III code 0027T, the parenthetical note following code 72275 has been revised to include the appropriate codes to report for injection procedures.

Gastrointestinal Tract

▲ **74270** Radiologic examination, colon; contrast (eg, barium) enema, with or without KUB

Rationale

Code 74270 has been editorially revised to include the term "contrast" and to give barium as an example to clarify that this code may be used to report an enema study of the colon done with any type of contrast.

The previous code descriptor limited the use of code 74270 to barium enema contrast studies only. The addition of "eg," to the descriptor supports the intent of the descriptor to be applicable to any type of contrast enema, such as barium or water-soluble contrast and not be limited to a barium study. The intent of code 74270 is to describe a diagnostic enema study of the colon after the administration of a contrast, regardless of the type of contrast agent used.

Diagnostic Ultrasound

Evaluation of vascular structures using both color and spectral Doppler is separately reportable. To report, see **Noninvasive Vascular Diagnostic Studies** (93875-93990). However, color Doppler alone, when performed for anatomic structure identification in conjunction with a real-time ultrasound examination, is not reported separately.

Head and Neck

76506 Echoencephalography, real time with image documentation (gray scale) (for determination of ventricular size, delineation of cerebral contents, and detection of fluid masses or other intracranial abnormalities), including A-mode encephalography as secondary component where indicated

76510 Ophthalmic ultrasound, diagnostic; B-scan and quantitative A-scan performed during the same patient encounter

76511 quantitative A-scan only

76512 B-scan (with or without superimposed non-quantitative A-scan)

76513 anterior segment ultrasound, immersion (water bath) B-scan or high resolution biomicroscopy

▶(For scanning computerized ophthalmic diagnostic imaging of the anterior and posterior segments using technology other than ultrasound, see 92135, 0187T)◀

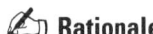 **Rationale**
A cross-reference has been added following code 76513 to direct users to codes 92135 and 0187T to report scanning computerized ophthalmic diagnostic imaging services.

Other Procedures

76998 Ultrasonic guidance, intraoperative

(Do not report 76998 in conjunction with 47370-47382▶, 36475-36479◀)

(For ultrasound guidance for open and laparoscopic radiofrequency tissue ablation, use 76940)

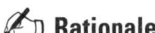 **Rationale**
The parenthetical note following code 76998 was revised to clarify that endovenous ablation therapy codes 36475-36479 are inclusive of ultrasound procedure code 76988 and should not be reported separately.

Radiologic Guidance

Fluoroscopic Guidance

77003 Fluoroscopic guidance and localization of needle or catheter tip for spine or paraspinous diagnostic or therapeutic injection procedures (epidural, transforaminal epidural, subarachnoid, paravertebral facet joint, paravertebral facet joint nerve, or sacroiliac joint), including neurolytic agent destruction

(Injection of contrast during fluoroscopic guidance and localization [77003] is included in 22526, 22527, 62263, 62264, ▶62267◀, 62270-62282, 62310-62319)

(Fluoroscopic guidance for subarachnoid puncture for . . .

(For epidural or subarachnoid needle or . . .

(For sacroiliac joint arthrography, see 27096, . . .

(For paravertebral facet joint injection, see . . .

(For destruction by neurolytic agent, see . . .

(For percutaneous or endoscopic lysis of epidural adhesions, 62263, 62264 include fluoroscopic guidance and localization)

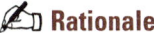

Rationale

The cross-reference following code 77003 was revised to include new code 62267 to instruct that contrast injection during fluoroscopic guidance and localization is an inclusive component of code 62267 and not separately reported.

Breast, Mammography

77057   Screening mammography, bilateral (2-view film study of each breast)

(Use 77057 in conjunction with 77052 for computer-aided detection applied to a screening mammogram)

▶(For electrical impedance breast scan, use 76499)◀

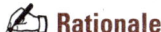

Rationale

In support of the deletion of code 0060T, a cross-reference has been added following code 77057 to direct users to the appropriate code to report an electrical impedance breast scan.

Bone/Joint Studies

77080   Dual-energy X-ray absorptiometry (DXA), bone density study, 1 or more sites; axial skeleton (eg, hips, pelvis, spine)

77081   appendicular skeleton (peripheral) (eg, radius, wrist, heel)

77082   vertebral fracture assessment

(For dual-energy X-ray absorptiometry [DEXA] body composition study, use 76499)

Rationale

A parenthetical note has been added following code 77082 to direct users to the appropriate code to report a dual-energy X-ray absorptiometry (DEXA) body composition study.

Radiation Oncology

Radiation Treatment Management

77432 Stereotactic radiation treatment management of cranial lesion(s) (complete course of treatment consisting of 1 session)

▶(The same physician should not report both stereotactic radiosurgery services [61796-61800] and radiation treatment management [77432 or 77435] for cranial lesions)◀

(For stereotactic body radiation therapy treatment, use 77435)

77435 Stereotactic body radiation therapy, treatment management, per treatment course, to 1 or more lesions, including image guidance, entire course not to exceed 5 fractions

(Do not report 77435 in conjunction with 77427-77432)

▶(The same physician should not report both stereotactic radiosurgery services [63620, 63621] and radiation treatment management [77435] for extracranial lesions)◀

Rationale

In support of the deletion of code 61793 and the establishment of codes 61796-61800, 63620, and 63621, the parenthetical notes following codes 77432 and 77435 have been revised. The first parenthetical note following code 77432 now indicates that the same physician should not report both stereotactic radiosurgery (SRS) services and radiation treatment management for cranial lesions. The second note following code 77435 now indicates that the physician should not report both SRS services and radiation treatment management for extracranial lesions.

Clinical Brachytherapy

▶(77781 has been deleted. To report, see 77785, 77786)◀

▶(77782-77784 have been deleted. To report, see 77785-77787)◀

●**77785** Remote afterloading high dose rate radionuclide brachytherapy; 1 channel

●**77786** 2-12 channels

●**77787** over 12 channels

Rationale

Radiation oncology codes 77781-77784 have been deleted because the nomenclature of these codes no longer accurately describes provision of high dose radiation brachytherapy. Instead, codes 77785-77787 have been established to report high dose rate (HDR) brachytherapy. These codes more accurately describe the current nomenclature and the differences between the parameters of each service.

Existing low dose rate (LDR) brachytherapy codes 77761-77763 and 77776-77778 involve a process in which the work or service is defined by the number of radioactive sources utilized. These procedures, however, are distinctly different from the

HDR codes 77785-77787, where the physician's work is measured by the number of catheters or channels used.

The new series of codes describe high dose radiation brachytherapy including 1 channel (77785), 2-12 channels (77786), and over 12 channels (77787). Four instructional parenthetical notes have been added to direct the user to the appropriate high dose radiation brachytherapy codes.

Brachytherapy has a long history starting in 1910 when low dose rate sources were used. Improved surgical and medical physics techniques dramatically increased its use in the late 1970s and early 1980s. All patients receiving LDR required hospitalization for isolation for radiation protection reasons, and medical personnel caring for the patients received radiation exposure. The introduction of robotic (machine-controlled) radioactive source loading devices made it possible to use HDR radiation sources to deliver radiation doses to patients with reduced treatment times and improved radiation safety. The introduction of HDR brachytherapy afterloading devices in the 1980s offered the advantage of improved radiation protection as well as an increase in the number of patients who could be treated on an outpatient basis.

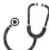

Clinical Example (77785)

A 65-year-old female status post hysterectomy, pelvic lymph node dissection, and periaortic lymph node sampling is found to have stage I C endometrial carcinoma, grade 2, 0/15 pelvic nodes and 0/4 periaortic lymph node positive. Vaginal cuff radiation is prescribed. A vaginal cylinder is inserted and simulation, computer planning, and medical physics preparation are performed (reported separately). HDR brachytherapy is then delivered.

Description of Procedure (77785)

An applicator is inspected for size, position, and stability following transport and adjusted as needed. The channel length is measured by the physicist and noted. A transfer tube is selected and connected to the channel applicator. The HDR afterloader device is positioned and locked. The transfer tube is connected to the indexer ring and locked in place. The afterloader device position is adjusted to minimize kinking. The emergency source retraction handle is exposed on the afterloader. The patient is examined for comfort; transfer tube and applicator stability are examined. The treatment vault is exited after ensuring that the patient, applicator, and afterloader emergency panel are visible on the remote camera monitor. Computer control console parameters are reviewed to correlate with approved computer plan. Fraction size, dose, source strength (additional decay calculation for afternoon treatments), retractions, channel number, and dwell time/total time are approved. Check cable is run through all source positions (connection in room to transfer tubes, etc, is adjusted as needed). Radioactive source is deployed. Dwell position and times are monitored. Patient monitoring is maintained by visual and verbal contact for the duration of treatment; variances, computer prompts, and error messages are acted upon promptly. The patient's condition, vitals, and any interruptions are monitored until end of treatment. Source retraction into safe position is confirmed (room radiation detector, first in room with Geiger counter, and survey patient). A disconnect is made from the afterloader and applicator position is reconfirmed. Applicator and Foley catheter are removed from patient, and the treatment site is examined.

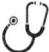
Clinical Example (77786)
A 68-year-old man with a history of heavy tobacco use presents with a 2.5-cm squamous cell cancer in the floor of mouth, T2 N0. The tumor and regional lymph nodes are treated with external beam irradiation. An interstitial implant boost of the oral tongue and floor of mouth is performed (reported separately). Following simulation, computer planning and medical physics preparation (reported separately) are performed, and high dose radiation (HDR) boost is administered.

Description of Procedure (77786)
The catheters/applicator are inspected for number, position, and integrity. Verification that no change in anatomy since insertion (eg, edema), position, and stability following transport is made; number and diagram are adjusted as needed. The channel stabilizers are removed from each catheter. The catheter lengths are measured (with source ruler), confirmed by the physicist, and noted. Individually numbered transfer tubes are selected and connected to similarly numbered catheter in patient. The HDR afterloader device is positioned and locked. The transfer tubes are connected to similarly numbered indexer ring and locked in place. Consistent numbering is verified. The position of the afterloader device is adjusted to minimize kinking, traction, or pressure on patient, etc. The emergency source retraction handle is exposed on afterloader. Patient comfort, airway, transfer tube, and applicator stability are evaluated and confirmed. The treatment vault is exited. Visibility of the patient, monitoring equipment, applicator, and afterloader emergency panel on the remote camera monitor is confirmed. The computer control console parameters are reviewed and correlated with approved computer plan as is the name, fraction, dose, source strength, retractions, channel numbers, and dwell times/total time. Cable through all channels and source positions is checked. Connection in room to transfer tubes, etc, is adjusted as identified by faults. Radioactive source is deployed. Active channel, dwell positions, and times are monitored. Patient is monitored by maintaining visual and verbal contact for duration of treatment; variances, computer prompts, and error messages are acted upon promptly. Patient's condition, vitals, and any interruptions are monitored until end of treatment. Source retraction into safe position is confirmed (room radiation detector, first in room with Geiger counter, and survey patient). Steps 4-15 are repeated for a second hook-up if needed. The afterloader is disconnected and the treatment site examined. Applicator is removed from the patient. Pain is managed, bimanual direct pressure is applied to control bleeding, and the incision is cleaned and dressed.

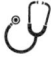
Clinical Example (77787)
A 70-year-old man presents with T2c Gleason 7, PSA 11 prostate cancer. He receives external beam radiation to the prostate and periprostatic lymph nodes. An interstitial implant boost of prostate is performed (reported separately). Following simulation, computer planning, and medical physics preparation (reported separately), a high dose radiation (HDR) boost is administered.

Description of Procedure (77787)

Catheters/applicator are inspected for number, position, and integrity. Confirmation is made that no change has occurred in anatomy since insertion (eg, edema). Position and stability following transport are ensured and adjustments made as needed. The site is numbered and diagramed. The channel stabilizers are removed from each catheter. The catheter lengths are measured (with source ruler), confirmed by the physicist, and noted. Individually numbered transfer tubes are selected and connected to similarly numbered catheter in patient. The HDR afterloader device is positioned and locked. Transfer tubes are connected to similarly numbered indexer ring and locked in place. Consistent numbering is verified. The afterloader device position is adjusted to minimize kinking, traction, or pressure on the patient, etc. The emergency source retraction handle is exposed on afterloader. Patient comfort and transfer tube and applicator stability are ensured. The treatment vault is exited. Visibility of the patient, monitoring equipment, applicator, and afterloader emergency panel on the remote camera monitor is confirmed. Computer control console parameters are reviewed and correlated with approved computer plan, as is name, fraction, dose, source strength, retractions, channel numbers, and dwell times/total time. Cable through all channels and source positions is checked. Connection in room to transfer tubes, etc, as identified by faults, is adjusted. Radioactive source is deployed. Active channel, dwell positions, and times are monitored. Patient is monitored by maintaining visual and verbal contact for duration of treatment; variances, computer prompts, and error messages are acted upon promptly. Patient's condition, vitals, and any interruptions are monitored until end of treatment. Source retraction into safe position is confirmed (room radiation detector, first in room with Geiger counter, and survey patient). Steps 4-15 are repeated for a second hook-up. The disconnect from afterloader is made. The treatment site is examined and the applicator is removed from the patient. Pain is managed, bimanual direct pressure is applied to control bleeding, the Foley catheter is irrigated, and the incision is cleaned and dressed.

Nuclear Medicine

Diagnostic

OTHER PROCEDURES

●**78808** Injection procedure for radiopharmaceutical localization by non-imaging probe study, intravenous (eg, parathyroid adenoma)

▶(For sentinel lymph node identification, use 38792)◀

🖉 Rationale

Nuclear medicine code 78808 was established to report an injection for radiopharmaceutical localization by non-imaging probe study. This code reflects the resources required to provide those radioactive drugs by intravenous routes prior to gamma probe localization (eg, parathyroid tumors).

Non-imaging gamma probe procedures in which a radiopharmaceutical is prepared, injected, and handled in accordance with acceptable regulatory and safety requirements are done during surgery as part of and during neck exploration for parathyroid tumors or for sentinel nodes in cancer patients (usually breast and melanoma). A parenthetical note has been added to clarify that code 38792 may be used for the interstitial injection preceding surgery, during which a gamma probe may be used for localization of a sentinel node.

Clinical Example (78808)

A 57-year-old male presents with a history of tumor. The patient now presents for surgical resection, and the referring surgeon requests injection of radiopharmaceutical so that the lesion can be intraoperatively localized with a gamma probe.

Description of Procedure (78808)

The physician provides supervision of radioisotope handling, ie, the preparation and injection of the radiopharmaceutical. The interpretation and report of the examination is available.

78816 Positron emission tomography (PET) with concurrently acquired computed tomography (CT) for attenuation correction and anatomical localization imaging; whole body

(Report 78811-78816 only once per imaging session)

(Computed tomography [CT] performed for other than attenuation correction an anatomical localization is reported using the appropriate site-specific CT code with modifier 59)

▶(78890, 78891 have been deleted)◀

Rationale

Nuclear medicine codes 78890 and 78891 and the related cross-reference have been deleted. Codes 78890 and 78891 previously described the components of computer processing required for nuclear medicine procedures. As technology has progressed, the components of computer processing required for nuclear medicine procedures have been included directly in the 78000 series of codes. As such, these services are no longer separately reported. To instruct users, a parenthetical note has been added in the Nuclear Medicine subsection to indicate that computer processing codes 78890 and 78891 have been deleted.

Pathology and Laboratory

Most notable of the revisions of the Pathology and Laboratory section for this year is a new subsection and three new codes for in-vivo point-of-care tests.

Other new codes have been added to report detection of non-viral enzymatic activity, coagulation, and des-gamma-carboxy-prothrombin. The molecular diagnostic testing codes have been revised to specify intent for frequency or quantity when reporting.

Pathology and Laboratory

Organ or Disease-Oriented Panels

▲ **80048**   Basic metabolic panel (Calcium, total)

This panel must include the following:

Calcium▶, total◀ (82310)

Carbon dioxide (82374)

Chloride (82435)

Creatinine (82565)

Glucose (82947)

Potassium (84132)

Sodium (84295)

Urea nitrogen (BUN) (84520)

▲ **80053**   Comprehensive metabolic panel

This panel must include the following:

Albumin (82040)

Bilirubin, total (82247)

Calcium▶, total◀ (82310)

Carbon dioxide (bicarbonate) (82374)

Chloride (82435)

Creatinine (82565)

Glucose (82947)

Phosphatase, alkaline (84075)

Potassium (84132)

Protein, total (84155)

Sodium (84295)

Transferase, alanine amino (ALT) (SGPT) (84460)

Transferase, aspartate amino (AST) (SGOT) (84450)

Urea nitrogen (BUN) (84520)

▲ **80069**   Renal function panel

This panel must include the following:

Albumin (82040)

Calcium▶, total◀ (82310)

Carbon dioxide (bicarbonate) (82374)

Chloride (82435)

Creatinine (82565)

Glucose (82947)

Phosphorus inorganic (phosphate) (84100)

Potassium (84132)

Sodium (84295)

Urea nitrogen (BUN) (84520)

 Rationale

Codes 80048, 80053, 80069 have been revised to specify "Calcium, total" for Organ or Disease-Oriented Panels. This revision will clarify that total calcium, in contrast to ionized calcium, is required when the user reports 80048, 80083, 80069.

Evocative/Suppression Testing

The following test panels involve the administration of evocative or suppressive agents, and the baseline and subsequent measurement of their effects on chemical constituents. These codes are to be used for the reporting of the laboratory component of the overall testing protocol. For the physician's administration of the evocative or suppressive agents, see ▶96360, 96361, 96372-96374, 96375◀; for the supplies and drugs, see 99070. To report physician attendance and monitoring during the testing, use the appropriate evaluation and management code, including the prolonged physician care codes if required. Prolonged physician care codes are not separately reported when evocative/suppression testing involves prolonged infusions reported with ▶96360, 96361◀. In the code descriptors where reference is made to a particular analyte (eg, Cortisol: 82533 x 2) the "x 2" refers to the number of times the test for that particular analyte is performed.

80400 ACTH stimulation panel; for adrenal insufficiency This panel must include the following: Cortisol (82533 x 2)

 Rationale

In support of the deletion and renumbering of codes 90760-90799, the Evocative/Suppression Testing guidelines have been revised to reflect the appropriate codes to report for infusion services.

Chemistry

The material for examination may be from any source unless otherwise specified in the code descriptor. When an analyte is measured in multiple specimens from different sources, or in specimens that are obtained at different times, the analyte is reported separately for each source and for each specimen. The examination is quantitative unless specified. To report an organ or disease oriented panel, see codes 80048-80076.

▲ 82040   Albumin; serum▶, plasma or whole blood◀

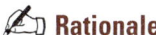

Rationale

Code 82040 was editorially revised by adding "plasma or whole blood" to the descriptor to broaden the list of specimen types appropriately reported with this code.

▲ 82375   ▶Carboxyhemoglobin◀; quantitative

▲ 82376   qualitative

▶(For transcutaneous measurement of carboxyhemoglobin, use 88740)◀

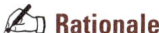

Rationale

Code 82375 was revised to delete the term "carbon monoxide" and replace it with "quantitative carboxyhemoglobin" as a parent code.

A cross-reference was added following code 82376 to direct the user to report 88740 for transcutaneous carboxyhemoglobin determination.

82955   Glucose-6-phosphate dehydrogenase (G6PDP); quantitative

82960   screen

(For glucose tolerance test with medication, use ▶96374◀ in addition)

Rationale

In support of the deletion and renumbering of codes 90760-90799, the cross-reference following code 82960 has been revised to reflect the appropriate codes to report for infusion services.

83026   Hemoglobin; by copper sulfate method, non-automated

83050   methemoglobin, quantitative

▶(For transcutaneous quantitative methemoglobin determination, use 88741)◀

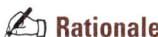

Rationale

An instructional parenthetical note was added following code 83050 to direct users to report code 88742 for transcutaneous quantitative methemoglobin determination.

● **83876** Myeloperoxidase (MPO)

Rationale

Myeloperoxidase (MPO) is a biomarker that can identify troponin-negative patients at risk for myocardial infarction. Code 83876 was established to report quantitative determination of myeloperoxidase assay (analyte specific) as a means to track patients with cardiac markers for ischemic heart disease and as an indicator for risk and prognosis of patients with cardiovascular disease. Myeloperoxidase can be used as an early predictor of cardiac risks in patients who present within as little as 4 hours of the onset of chest pain.

Myeloperoxidase testing can be used in conjunction with clinical history, electrocardiogram (ECG), and cardiac biomarkers to evaluate patients at risk for major adverse cardiac events.

Myeloperoxidase measurement provides independent information separate from B-type natriuretic peptide (BNP) and troponin. Myeloperoxidase is released when plaque is unstable or in the event of ruptured plaque and cell injury. Myeloperoxidase can identify patients with chest pain who are at risk of myocardial infarction but do not have a positive troponin or ECG changes.

Clinical Example (83876)

A 69-year-old man without a prior history of coronary artery disease presents to the emergency department 90 minutes after experiencing 20 minutes of substernal chest pressure.

Description of Procedure (83876)

Upon presentation, the patient has an ECG performed that is interpreted as normal. Aspirin is administered, continuous ECG monitoring is initiated, and venous blood is obtained, including a tube containing lithium heparin. The laboratory tests ordered include a complete blood count, troponin T, creatinine kinase (CK), MB fraction of creatinine kinase (CK-MB), and myeloperoxidase (cardio-MPO).

Blood test results show no evidence of myocardial infarction (normal troponin T, CK, and CK-MB). The repeat ECG is normal. The cardio-MPO is high (>2500 pmol/L). Heparin therapy is initiated and the patient is admitted to the hospital with a greater than 50% risk of requiring coronary revascularization. Serial troponin T and CK/CK-MB are all normal.

The next day, the patient undergoes coronary angiography that reveals a hazy 80% stenosis of the mid–left anterior descending coronary artery. Percutaneous coronary intervention is performed and the patient is discharged home the following day.

83880   Natriuretic peptide

Codes 83890-83914 are intended for use . . .

Codes 83890-83914 are coded by procedure . . .

Code separately for each procedure used . . .

When molecular diagnostic procedures are performed . . .

▶Each nucleic acid preparation may include a digestate, undigested nucleic acid, or other uniquely modified nucleic acid sample (eg, newly synthesized oligonucleotide).◀

▲ 83890 Molecular diagnostics; molecular isolation or extraction▶, each nucleic acid type (ie, DNA or RNA)◀

▲ 83891 isolation or extraction of highly purified nucleic acid▶, each nucleic acid type (ie, DNA or RNA)◀

▲ 83892 enzymatic digestion▶, each enzyme treatment◀

▲ 83893 dot/slot blot production▶, each nucleic acid preparation◀

▲ 83894 separation by gel electrophoresis (eg, agarose, polyacrylamide)▶, each nucleic acid preparation◀

▲ 83896 nucleic acid probe, each

▲ 83897 nucleic acid transfer (eg, Southern, Northern)▶, each nucleic acid preparation◀

83900 amplification, target, multiplex, first 2 nucleic acid sequences

83903 mutation scanning, by physical properties (eg, single strand conformational polymorphisms [SSCP], heteroduplex, denaturing gradient gel electrophoresis [DGGE], RNA'ase A), single segment, each

▲ 83907 lysis of cells prior to nucleic acid extraction (eg, stool specimens, paraffin embedded tissue)▶, each specimen◀

▲ 83909 separation and identification by high resolution technique (eg, capillary electrophoresis)▶, each nucleic acid preparation◀

Rationale

In CPT 2009, there has been a conscious effort to more clearly define the unit of service for the molecular pathology codes. In tandem with these efforts, following code 83887, a paragraph was added to the guidelines to inform users that each nucleic acid preparation may include a digestate, undigested nucleic acid, or other uniquely modified nucleic acid sample (eg, newly synthesized oligonucleotide).

Additionally, many editorial revisions were made to the molecular diagnostic codes to better clarify the original intent of these codes.

Codes 83890 and 83891 were revised to add "each nucleic acid type (ie, DNA or RNA)." Code 83892 was revised to add "each enzyme treatment." Codes 83893, 89894, 83897, and 83909 were revised to add "each nucleic acid preparation." Code 83907 was revised to add "each specimen."

▲ 83925 Opiate▶(s), drug and metabolites, each procedure◀

Rationale

Code 83925 was revised by changing "opiates" to "opiate(s)." The parenthetical note "(eg, morphine, meperidine)" was deleted and the phrase "drug and metabolites, each procedure" was added to the descriptor. This revision was made to clarify that if multiple assays are being performed to identify different opiates and/or metabolites, the user should report each procedure.

▲ **83950**   Oncoprotein▶;◀ HER-2/neu

(For tissue, see 88342, 88365)

● **83951**   des-gamma-carboxy-prothrombin (DCP)

 Rationale

Code 83950 was revised by replacing the comma with a semicolon, making it a parent code for oncoproteins, to accommodate the addition of code 83951.

Code 83951 was established to report des-gamma-carboxy-prothrombin (DCP) oncoprotein and follows code 83950 as a child (indented) code.

The DCP test is intended for the follow-up of patients with chronic liver disease who are at risk for the development of hepatocellular carcinoma (HCC). The DCP values have been demonstrated to be associated with a 4.8-fold increase in the risk of developing HCC within the next 21 months.

Des-gamma-carboxy-prothrombin is an independent oncoprotein biomarker for HCC.

 Clinical Example (83951)

The patient is a 59-year-old woman with a history of chronic hepatitis C infection. The patient has been diagnosed with cirrhosis of the liver. Since she is at increased risk for the development of HCC, her hepatologist follows her twice annually with ultrasound and serum oncoprotein DCP.

Description of Procedure (83951)

The laboratory analysis of DCP involves technology with two distinct analytical steps: (1) exposure of the sample to two labeled antibodies and (2) chromatographic separation of the immunochemically marked DCP. One antibody is an anion-conjugated monoclonal antibody specific for prothrombin; the other is a horseradish peroxidase–conjugated monoclonal antibody specific for oncoprotein DCP. Anion exchange chromatography is used to purify the DCP bound to the two antibody conjugates away from prothrombin and from free enzyme-conjugated antibody. Chromatography is central to the assay because it is necessary to separate the oncoprotein DCP away from the vast excess of native prothrombin and away from the unbound enzyme-labeled monoclonal antibody. The peroxidase enzyme activity is measured in the eluted complex by the generation of a fluorescent product. By the use of calibrators, the concentration of DCP is calculated. The results are reported in nanograms of DCP per milliliter.

Because the DCP results for this patient were less than 7.5 ng/mL, the physician was able to reassure the patient that there are no indications of HCC, and a follow-up visit is made for 6 months hence.

▲ 84132   Potassium; serum▶, plasma or whole blood◀

▲ 84155   Protein, total, except by refractometry; serum▶, plasma or whole blood◀

▲ 84295   Sodium; serum▶, plasma or whole blood◀

Rationale

Codes 84132, 84155, and 84295 were editorially revised by adding "plasma or whole blood" to the descriptors to broaden the list of specimen types appropriately reported with these codes.

Hematology and Coagulation

●85397   Coagulation and fibrinolysis, functional activity, not otherwise specified (eg, ADAMTS-13), each analyte

Rationale

Code 85397 was established to report coagulation and fibrinolysis, functional activity, not otherwise specified for each analyte. Prior to 2009, there was no coagulation assay code for a functional assay of either coagulation or fibrinolysis except for several specific analyte assays. The establishment of code 85397 appropriately fills this void; therefore, providing a code for assays such as a disintegrin and metalloproteinase with a thrombospondin type 1 motif, member 13 (ADAMTS13).

A disintegrin and metalloproteinase with a thrombospondin type 1 motif, member 13 (ADAMTS-13), is a von Willebrand factor cleaving protease and is used as a measurement of activity for proteases. It is a congenital or an acquired deficiency and is associated with thrombotic thrombocytopenic purpura (TTP) and more rarely with the hemolytic uremic syndrome.

The ADAMTS-13 is an example of an assay that is used to diagnose TTP. Code 85397 could be used to report performance of other functional assays that currently are not specifically codifiable due to the lack of a generic functional assay code for other proteins participating in coagulation and fibrinolysis.

Clinical Example (85397)

A 42-year-old woman presents with acute renal failure, generalized petechia, and confusion. A complete blood count is ordered and shows an increased white blood cell count and a decreased platelet count. A blood culture is ordered. The culture contains schistocytes. The physician is concerned about the possibility of TTP. The physician then orders an ADAMTS-13 assay and consultation for therapeutic plasmapheresis.

Immunology

Tissue Typing

86805 Lymphocytotoxicity assay, visual crossmatch; with titration

86806 without titration

86807 Serum screening for cytotoxic percent reactive antibody (PRA); standard method

86822 lymphocyte culture, primed (PLC)

▶(For HLA typing by molecular pathology techniques, see 83890-83914 with appropriate genetic testing modifiers 4A-4G)◀

🖉 Rationale

The instructional parenthetical note following the subheading, Tissue Typing, preceding code 86805, was deleted because the word "appropriate" is nonfunctional for this parenthetical note.

A parenthetical note was added following code 86822 to direct users to codes 83890-83914 with appropriate genetic testing modifiers 4A-4G for human lymphocyte antigen (HLA) typing by molecular pathology techniques to clarify the distinction between genotyping and HLA typing tests. With the advent of genetic testing modifiers, the use of molecular pathology codes with corresponding genetic testing modifiers is more granular than the use of tissue typing codes.

Microbiology

These codes are intended for primary source only. For similar studies on culture material, refer to codes 87140-87158. Infectious agents by antigen detection, immunofluorescence microscopy, or nucleic acid probe techniques should be reported as precisely as possible. The most specific code possible should be reported. If there is no specific agent code, the general methodology code (eg, 87299, 87449, 87450, 87797, 87798, 87799, 87899) should be used. For identification of antibodies to many of the listed infectious agents, see 86602-86804. When separate results are reported for different species or strain of organisms, each result should be coded separately.
▶Use modifier 59 when separate results are reported for different species or strains that are described by the same code.◀

87260 Infectious agent antigen detection by immunofluorescent technique; adenovirus

🖉 Rationale

A sentence was added to the end of the primary source infectious agent detection guidelines following code 87255 to instruct the users to report modifier 59 when separate results are reported for different species or strains that are described by the same CPT® code.

87802	Infectious agent antigen detection by immunoassay with direct optical observation; Streptococcus, group B	
87803	Clostridium difficile toxin A	
87804	Influenza	
87807	respiratory syncytial virus	
87808	Trichomonas vaginalis	
87809	adenovirus	
▲87810	►Chlamydia trachomatis◄	

Rationale

Code 87810 was converted from a parent code (appears with semicolon) to a child (indented) code to be included in the series of codes 87802-87899.

●87905 Infectious agent enzymatic activity other than virus (eg, sialidase activity in vaginal fluid)

►(For virus isolation including identification by nonimmunologic method, other than by cytopathic effect, use 87255)◄

Rationale

Code 87905 was established to report rapid testing utilizing an infectious agent enzymatic activity other than a virus. This code was placed in the Microbiology section of the CPT codebook.

Vaginal fluid sialidase enzyme tests for bacterial vaginosis are performed directly from vaginal swab samples, provide a test result in approximately 10 minutes, and have a reported sensitivity of approximately 90%.

A parenthetical note was added following code 87905 to instruct users to report virus isolation including identification by nonimmunologic method, other than by cytopathic effect, with code 87255.

Clinical Example (87905)

A 24-year-old woman complains to her physician of vaginal itching and/or burning sensation. A pelvic examination reveals a frothy, yellow-green vaginal discharge with odor. Inflammation of the vaginal wall is also observed.

►(88400 has been deleted. To report, use 88720)◄

Rationale

In support of the addition of a new subsection and codes to report in vivo (eg, transcutaneous) tests, code 88400 has been deleted and renumbered to the new subsection.

▶In Vivo (eg, Transcutaneous) Laboratory Procedures◀

● **88720** Bilirubin, total, transcutaneous

▶(For transdermal oxygen saturation, see 94760-94762)◀

● **88740** Hemoglobin, quantitative, transcutaneous, per day; carboxyhemoglobin

▶(For in vitro carboxyhemoglobin measurement, use 82375)◀

● **88741** methemoglobin

▶(For in vitro quantitative methemoglobin determination, use 83050)◀

Rationale

The subheading following code 88399, Transcutaneous Procedures, has been deleted and replaced with a new subheading, In Vivo (eg, Transcutaneous) Laboratory Procedures, for better characterization of these in vivo, transcutaneous procedure codes.

A parenthetical note following the new subheading, In Vivo (eg, Transcutaneous) Laboratory Procedures, has been added to direct users to codes 94760-94762 to report transdermal oxygen saturation.

In tandem with the new subheading, code 88400 has been deleted and renumbered to appear under the new subheading as code 88720. A cross-reference has been added to direct users to report code 88720 for total bilirubin, transcutaneous.

Code 88741 was established to report transcutaneous quantitative carboxyhemoglobin per day. A parenthetical note was added to direct users to code 82375 to report in vitro carboxyhemoglobin measurement.

Code 88742 was established to report transcutaneous quantitative methemoglobin. A parenthetical note was added to direct users to report in vitro quantitative methemoglobin determination with code 83050.

Clinical Example (88740)

A 35-year-old woman with somnolence, headache, and nausea is brought to the hospital emergency department by ambulance. The patient was removed from a fire at her residence. The emergency department physician orders a transcutaneous quantitative carboxyhemoglobin measurement to determine whether the victim suffers from carbon monoxide poisoning.

Clinical Example (88741)

A 65-year-old male undergoing bronchoscopy receives local anesthesia in the form of benzocaine spray. During and after the procedure, the patient complains of shortness of breath. The patient continues to have somnolence, nausea, and headache. The pulmonologist orders a transcutaneous, quantitative methemoglobin measurement to determine whether the patient is suffering from methemoglobinemia.

Medicine

A large number of the revisions for the *CPT® 2009* codebook took place in this section. These revisions include deletion and renumbering of entire code sections, including the therapeutic and hydration infusion codes and the hemodialysis codes. The hemodialysis section now includes many new codes for home and outpatient hemodialysis.

The Cardiovascular subsection also includes large changes, including extensive guideline and code additions and revisions of the Echocardiography section. Extensive revisions have also been applied to the Cardiology section, with revision to most of the codes, and addition of a new subsection with extensive guidelines and many codes to report cardiac device monitoring.

Medicine

Immune Globulins

Codes 90281-90399 identify the immune globulin product only and are reported in addition to the administration codes ▶96365-96368, 96372, 96374, 96375◀ as appropriate. Modifier 51 should not be reported with the immune globulin codes when performed with another procedure. Immune globulin products listed here include broad-spectrum and anti-infective immune globulins, antitoxins, and various iso-antibodies.

90281 Immune globulin (Ig), human, for intramuscular use

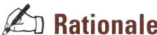 Rationale

The code numbers referenced for reporting administration of immune globulins have been updated to correspond to the relocated and renumbered therapeutic, prophylactic, and diagnostic injections and infusions codes 96365-96368 and 96372-96375.

Immunization Administration for Vaccines/Toxoids

(For therapeutic or diagnostic injections, see ▶96372-96379◀)

90465 Immunization administration younger than 8 years of age (includes percutaneous, intradermal, subcutaneous, or intramuscular injections) when the physician counsels the patient/family; first injection (single or combination vaccine/toxoid), per day

90471 Immunization administration (includes percutaneous, intradermal, subcutaneous, or intramuscular injections); one vaccine (single or combination vaccine/toxoid)

(Do not report 90471 in conjunction with 90473)

+90472 each additional vaccine (single or combination vaccine/toxoid) (List separately in addition to code for primary procedure)

(For administration of immune globulins, see 90281-90399, ▶96360, 96361, 96365-96368, 96374◀)

Vaccines, Toxoids

The "age" descriptions included in . . .

(For immune globulins, see codes 90281-90399, ▶96365-96368, 96372-96375◀ for administration of immune globulins)

90476 Adenovirus vaccine, type 4, live, for oral use

●90650 Human Papilloma virus (HPV) vaccine, types 16, 18, bivalent, 3 dose schedule, for intramuscular use

●90681 Rotavirus vaccine, human, attenuated, 2 dose schedule, live, for oral use

▲=Revised Code ●=New Code ▶◀=New or Revised Text O=Reinstated Code

- ●90696　Diphtheria, tetanus toxoids, acellular pertussis vaccine and poliovirus vaccine, inactivated (DTaP-IPV), when administered to children 4 through 6 years of age, for intramuscular use
- ▲90698　Diphtheria, tetanus toxoids, acellular pertussis vaccine, haemophilus influenza Type B, and poliovirus vaccine, inactivated (DTaP - Hib - IPV), for intramuscular use
- ⟋●90738　Japanese encephalitis virus vaccine, inactivated, for intramuscular use

Rationale

Code 90650 has been established to report a human papilloma virus (HPV) vaccine. This new vaccine will contain an adjuvant formulation and is intended to protect against infection of oncogenic types of cervical cancer (types 16 and 18). The existing HPV vaccine, code 90649, targets both oncogenic (types 16 and 18) and non-oncogenic (types 6 and 11) types of cervical cancer but does not contain the adjuvant. The vaccine adjuvant system is intended to provide a more sustained immune response and may contribute to the cross-protective benefit of the vaccine against other oncogenic HPV types.

The dosing schedules to these HPV vaccines also differ. The administration schedule for the product reported with code 90649 is 0, 2, 6 months for the current product, while the product reported with code 90650 is administered at 0, 1, 6 months for the new vaccine. Code 90650 will appear in the CPT® codebook with the Federal Drug Administration (FDA) approval pending symbol. Updates on the FDA status of these codes are provided on the AMA CPT Web site under Category I Vaccine Codes (www.ama-assn.org/ama/pub/category/10902.html) and in subsequent CPT publications.

Code 90681 has been established to report an attenuated human rotavirus (HRV) vaccine intended to protect against rotavirus gastroenteritis. Rotavirus is the leading recognized cause of diarrhea-related illness, hospitalization, and in some parts of the world death among infants and young children. Rotarix is a liquid for oral administration and is recommended for use in infants in a two-dose schedule. The existing vaccine product for rotavirus reported with code 90680 is administered on a three-dose schedule.

Code 90696 has been established to report a combination vaccine to protect against pertussis, diphtheria, tetanus, and poliomyelitis in a single injection. Previously, administration of each antigen was only possible under separate codes. This vaccine is intended to be administered as a booster dose to healthy children 4 to 6 years of age who completed the recommended immunization schedule for DTaP and poliovirus during their infancy.

The FDA approval pending indicator (⟋) was removed from code 90698 following notification of receipt of FDA approval.

Code 90738 has been established to report an inactivated Japanese encephalitis virus vaccine for intramuscular use. The existing code, 90735, also used to report an inactivated Japanese encephalitis virus vaccine, is administered subcutaneously and is primarily used by the military. In the civilian sector, it is offered to individuals who are traveling to endemic areas in Asia or to persons whose activities place them at a high risk of infection (eg, US expatriates/military personnel) or who plan to reside in areas where Japanese encephalitis is endemic.

Japanese encephalitis is the leading cause of viral encephalitis in Asia. Although it rarely occurs in US civilians and military personnel traveling to and living in Asia, outbreaks have occurred in US territories in the Western Pacific and in Australia. The outcomes for patients who acquire symptomatic Japanese encephalitis may be severe, and survivors may develop serious, permanent neuropsychiatric sequelae.

The currently licensed inactivated vaccine (90735) is produced from infected suckling mouse brains, which are no longer being supplied by the manufacturer. Thus, this particular vaccine will not be available once its supply runs out. The new vaccine will eventually replace the older vaccine (90735) and will be produced from Vero cell cultures administered in a two-dose schedule without thiomersal (mercury).

Code 90738 will appear in the CPT codebook with the FDA approval pending symbol. This symbol was added to CPT in 2006 to identify vaccine or toxoid products that have not yet received, at the time of their code assignment, FDA approval. Updates on the FDA status of these codes are provided on the AMA CPT Web site under Category I Vaccine Codes (www.ama-assn.org/ama/pub/category/10902.html) and in subsequent CPT publications.

The guidelines for the section have also been revised by updating the code numbers referenced for reporting administration of immune globulins to correspond to the relocated and renumbered therapeutic, prophylactic, and diagnostic injections and infusions codes 96365-96368 and 96372-96375.

▶(90760 has been deleted. To report, use 96360)◀

▶(90761 has been deleted. To report, use 96361)◀

▶(90765 has been deleted. To report, use 96365)◀

▶(90766 has been deleted. To report, use 96366)◀

▶(90767 has been deleted. To report, use 96367)◀

▶(90768 has been deleted. To report, use 96368)◀

▶(90769 has been deleted. To report, use 96369)◀

▶(90770 has been deleted. To report, use 96370)◀

▶(90771 has been deleted. To report, use 96371)◀

▶(90772 has been deleted. To report, use 96372)◀

▶(90773 has been deleted. To report, use 96373)◀

▶(90774 has been deleted. To report, use 96374)◀

▶(90775 has been deleted. To report, use 96375)◀

▶(90776 has been deleted. To report, use 96376)◀

▶(90779 has been deleted. To report, use 96379)◀

Rationale

In order to assist users in comparison and use of the infusion services procedures, codes 90760-90779 have been deleted and renumbered for proximity to the chemotherapy and other complex infusion services reported with codes 96401-96549. In addition to deletion and renumbering of these services, movement of the codes allowed condensation of the guidelines with revisions to reflect overarching principles between each of the code series.

Biofeedback

90911 Biofeedback training, perineal muscles, anorectal or urethral sphincter, including EMG and/or manometry

(For incontinence treatment by pulsed magnetic neuromodulation, use ▶53899◀)

Rationale

In support of the deletion of Category III code 0029T, a parenthetical note has been added following code 90911 to direct users to the appropriate code to report for incontinence treatment by pulsed magnetic neuromodulation.

Dialysis

▶(90918, 90922 have been deleted. To report ESRD-related services for patients younger than 2 years of age, see 90953, 90963, 90967)◀

▶(90919, 90923 have been deleted. To report ESRD-related services for patients between 2 and 11 years of age, see 90954-90956, 90964, 90968)◀

▶(90920, 90924 have been deleted. To report ESRD-related services for patients between 12 and 19 years of age, see 90957-90959, 90965, 90969)◀

▶(90921, 90925 have been deleted. To report ESRD-related services for patients 20 years of age and older, see 90960-90962, 90966, 90970)◀

Hemodialysis

90935 Hemodialysis procedure with single physician evaluation

Miscellaneous Dialysis Procedures

90947 Dialysis procedure other than hemodialysis (eg, peritoneal dialysis, hemofiltration, or other continuous renal replacement therapies), requiring repeated physician evaluations, with or without substantial revision of dialysis prescription

▶End-Stage Renal Disease Services◀

Codes 90951-90962 are reported **once** per month to distinguish age-specific services related to the patient's end-stage renal disease (ESRD) performed in an outpatient setting with three levels of service based on the number of face-to-face visits. ESRD-related physician services include establishment of a dialyzing cycle, outpatient evaluation and management of the dialysis visits, telephone calls, and patient management during the dialysis provided during a full month. In the circumstances where the patient has had a complete assessment visit during the month and services are provided over a period of less than a month, 90951-90962 may be used according to the number of visits performed.

Codes 90963-90966 are reported once per month for a full month of service to distinguish age-specific services for end-stage renal disease (ESRD) services for home dialysis patients.

For ESRD and non-ESRD dialysis services performed in an inpatient setting, and for non-ESRD dialysis services performed in an outpatient setting, see 90935-90937 and 90945-90947.

Evaluation and Management services unrelated to ESRD services that cannot be performed during the dialysis session may be reported separately.

Codes 90967-90970 are reported to distinguish age-specific services for end-stage renal disease (ESRD) services for less than a full month of service, per day, for services provided under the following circumstances: home dialysis patients less than a full month, transient patients, partial month where there was one or more face-to-face visits without the complete assessment, the patient was hospitalized before a complete assessment was furnished, dialysis was stopped due to recovery or death, or the patient received a kidney transplant. For reporting purposes, each month is considered 30 days.

Examples

ESRD-related services:

ESRD-related services are initiated on July 1 for a 57-year-old male. On July 11, he is admitted to the hospital as an inpatient and is discharged on July 27. He has had a complete assessment, and the physician has performed two face-to-face visits prior to admission. Another face-to-face visit occurs after discharge during the month.

In this example, 90961 is reported for the three face-to-face outpatient visits. Report inpatient E/M services as appropriate. Dialysis procedures rendered during the hospitalization (July 11-27) should be reported as appropriate (90935-90937, 90945-90947).

If the patient did not have a complete assessment during the month or was a transient or dialysis was stopped due to recovery or death, 90970 would be used to report each day outside the inpatient hospitalization as described in the home dialysis example below.

ESRD-related services for the home dialysis patient:

Home ESRD-related services are initiated on July 1 for a 57-year-old male. On July 11, he is admitted to the hospital as an inpatient and is discharged on July 27.

In this example, 90970 should be reported for each day outside of the inpatient hospitalization (30 days/month less 17 days/hospitalization = 13 days). Report inpatient E/M services as appropriate. Dialysis procedures rendered during the hospitalization (July 11-27) should be reported as appropriate (90935-90937, 90945-90947).

●**90951** End-stage renal disease (ESRD) related services monthly, for patients younger than 2 years of age to include monitoring for the adequacy of nutrition, assessment of growth and development, and counseling of parents; with 4 or more face-to-face physician visits per month

●**90952** with 2-3 face-to-face physician visits per month

●**90953** with 1 face-to-face physician visit per month

●**90954** End-stage renal disease (ESRD) related services monthly, for patients 2-11 years of age to include monitoring for the adequacy of nutrition, assessment of growth and development, and counseling of parents; with 4 or more face-to-face physician visits per month

●**90955** with 2-3 face-to-face physician visits per month

●**90956** with 1 face-to-face physician visit per month

●**90957** End-stage renal disease (ESRD) related services monthly, for patients 12-19 years of age to include monitoring for the adequacy of nutrition, assessment of growth and development, and counseling of parents; with 4 or more face-to-face physician visits per month

●**90958** with 2-3 face-to-face physician visits per month

●**90959** with 1 face-to-face physician visit per month

●**90960** End-stage renal disease (ESRD) related services monthly, for patients 20 years of age and older; with 4 or more face-to-face physician visits per month

●**90961** with 2-3 face-to-face physician visits per month

●**90962** with 1 face-to-face physician visit per month

●**90963** End-stage renal disease (ESRD) related services for home dialysis per full month, for patients younger than 2 years of age to include monitoring for the adequacy of nutrition, assessment of growth and development, and counseling of parents

●**90964** End-stage renal disease (ESRD) related services for home dialysis per full month, for patients 2-11 years of age to include monitoring for the adequacy of nutrition, assessment of growth and development, and counseling of parents

●**90965** End-stage renal disease (ESRD) related services for home dialysis per full month, for patients 12-19 years of age to include monitoring for the adequacy of nutrition, assessment of growth and development, and counseling of parents

●**90966** End-stage renal disease (ESRD) related services for home dialysis per full month, for patients 20 years of age and older

●**90967**   End-stage renal disease (ESRD) related services for dialysis less than a full month of service, per day; for patients younger than 2 years of age

●**90968**   for patients 2-11 years of age

●**90969**   for patients 12-19 years of age

●**90970**   for patients 20 years of age and older

▶Other Dialysis Procedures◀

90989   Dialysis training, patient, including helper where applicable, any mode, completed course

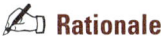
Rationale

In 2008, the Centers for Medicare and Medicaid Services (CMS) established 20 Healthcare Common Procedure Coding System (HCPCS) Level II "G" codes to describe end-stage renal disease (ESRD)-related services based on the age of the patient and the number of face-to-face physician visits that occurred per month. In order to provide consistency between the "G" codes and CPT codes, the ESRD-related CPT codes were restructured for the CPT codebook for 2009. The restructuring of these CPT codes consisted of the deletion of codes 90918-90925 and the establishment of 20 new codes, with three levels of service based on the number of face-to-face visits. The new codes also differentiate provision of hemodialysis services in the outpatient setting (90951-90962) from home dialysis services (90963-90970). The ESRD-related services guidelines have been revised in accordance with the restructured codes.

Codes 90951-90953 were established to report ESRD-related services for patients younger than 2 years of age. The codes include monitoring for the adequacy of nutrition, assessment of growth and development, and counseling of parents. Code 90951 is reported when four or more physician visits occurred during the month. Code 90952 is reported when two to three physician visits occurred during the month. Code 90953 is reported when one physician visit occurred during the month. In addition, codes 90954-90956 and 90957-90959, which were established to report ESRD-related services, are based on the same reporting structure and include the same services. However, codes 90954-90956 are reported for patients between 2 and 11 years of age, and codes 90957-90959 are reported for patients between 12 and 19 years of age. Codes 90951-90959 are reported once per month.

Codes 90960-90962 were established to report ESRD-related services for patients 20 years of age or older. These codes do not include the services that are included for younger patients (ie, monitoring for the adequacy of nutrition, assessment of growth and development, and counseling of parents). As with codes 90951-90959, code selection is based on the number of face-to-face physician visits that occurred during the month.

Codes 90963-90965 were established to report a full month of ESRD-related services for home dialysis for patients younger than 20 years of age. As with codes 90951-90959, they are reported based on patient age and include monitoring for the adequacy of nutrition, assessment of growth and development, and counseling of parents. Code 90966 describes a full month of ESRD-related services for home dialysis for patients 20 years of age and older and does not include monitoring for the adequacy of nutrition, assessment of growth and development, and counseling of parents. Codes 90963-90966 are reported once per month.

Codes 90967-90970 were established to report ESRD-related services for dialysis with less than a full month of service, per day. These codes are reported based on the patient's age and should be reported for each day of ESRD-related services for dialysis. The example in the guidelines shown previously provides an illustration of how to report these codes.

Clinical Example (90951)

A 7-month-old boy with renal dysplasia, end-stage renal disease from birth, and failed peritoneal dialysis undergoes chronic hemodialysis at a pediatric facility. His disease burden includes catheter access problems, renal osteodystrophy, anemia, acidosis, growth failure, developmental delay, anorexia and feeding problems, family dysfunction related to a technologically dependent infant, modified childhood immunizations, and polypharmacy (more than seven medications).

Description of Procedure (90951)

The patient's pediatric nephrologist will manage his condition over the entire month by providing the following services: scheduled examinations for management of known and anticipated problems; episodic examinations for intercurrent changes in his general condition; evaluation of the integrity and functionality of his dialysis access; episodic changes in his dialysis prescription; frequent adjustment of target weight for growth and fluid intake; scheduled review of routinely collected laboratory data, including frequent hemoglobin assessment for blood loss in the dialyzer; episodic adjustment of intravenous erythropoietin stimulating agents, iron, and vitamin D metabolites given during the dialysis treatment and of home medications including oral iron supplements, vitamin D metabolites or surrogates, potassium supplements or exchange resins, calcium supplements, phosphate supplements or binders, and growth hormone injections; growth and nutritional monitoring with frequent adjustments of gastrostomy or nasogastric tube feedings of a special infant formula with added protein, carbohydrate, and/or oil for adequate caloric intake for growth; monitoring of developmental progress and initiation and coordination of intervention for delayed milestones; coordination and appropriate dosing of childhood immunizations; establishing and modifying short- and long-term care plans in cooperation with social services, nutritional support services, child life specialists, transplantation centers, and other medical specialists; and overall care coordination with regular counseling and support of the parents/caregivers and siblings for the care of a technologically dependent infant with chronic kidney disease. The pediatric nephrologist is likely to have multiple unscheduled telephone and electronic interventions generated by the dialysis center, an emergency room, another physician, or the patient's parents/caregivers and will see the patient during dialysis sessions four or more times during the month in order to accomplish his care and comply with facility-specific quality requirements.

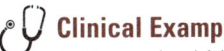

Clinical Example (90952)

A 7-month-old boy with renal dysplasia, end-stage renal disease from birth, and failed peritoneal dialysis undergoes chronic hemodialysis at a pediatric facility. His disease burden includes catheter access problems, renal osteodystrophy, anemia, acidosis, growth failure, developmental delay, anorexia and feeding problems, family dysfunction related to a technologically dependent infant, modified childhood immunizations, and polypharmacy (greater than seven medications).

Description of Procedure (90952)

The patient's pediatric nephrologist will manage his condition over the entire month by providing the following services: scheduled examinations for management of known and anticipated problems; episodic examinations for intercurrent changes in his general condition; evaluation of the integrity and functionality of his dialysis access; episodic changes in his dialysis prescription; frequent adjustment of target weight for growth and fluid intake; scheduled review of routinely collected laboratory data, including frequent hemoglobin assessment for blood loss in the dialyzer; episodic adjustment of intravenous erythropoietin stimulating agents, iron, and vitamin D metabolites given during the dialysis treatment and of home medications including oral iron supplements, vitamin D metabolites or surrogates, potassium supplements or exchange resins, calcium supplements, phosphate supplements or binders, and growth hormone injections; growth and nutritional monitoring with frequent adjustments of gastrostomy or nasogastric tube feedings of a special infant formula with added protein, carbohydrate, and/or oil for adequate caloric intake for growth; monitoring of developmental progress and initiation and coordination of intervention for delayed milestones; coordination and appropriate dosing of childhood immunizations; establishing and modifying short- and long-term care plans in cooperation with social services, nutritional support services, child life specialists, transplantation centers, and other medical specialists; and overall care coordination with regular counseling and support of the parents/caregivers and siblings for the care of a technologically dependent infant with chronic kidney disease. The pediatric nephrologist is likely to have multiple unscheduled telephone and electronic interventions generated by the dialysis center, an emergency room, another physician, or the patient's parents/caregivers and will see the patient during dialysis sessions two to three times during the month in order to accomplish his care and comply with facility-specific quality requirements.

Clinical Example (90953)

A 7-month-old boy with renal dysplasia, end-stage renal disease from birth, and failed peritoneal dialysis undergoes chronic hemodialysis at a pediatric facility. His disease burden includes catheter access problems, renal osteodystrophy, anemia, acidosis, growth failure, developmental delay, anorexia and feeding problems, family dysfunction related to a technologically dependent infant, modified childhood immunizations, and polypharmacy (greater than seven medications).

Description of Procedure (90953)

The patient's pediatric nephrologist will manage his condition over the entire month by providing the following services: scheduled examinations for management of known and anticipated problems; episodic examinations for intercurrent changes in his general condition; evaluation of the integrity and functionality of his dialysis access; episodic changes in his dialysis prescription; frequent adjustment of target weight for growth and fluid intake; scheduled review of routinely collected laboratory data, including frequent hemoglobin assessment for blood loss in the dialyzer; episodic adjustment of intravenous erythropoietin stimulating agents, iron, and vitamin D metabolites given during the dialysis treatment and of home medications including oral iron supplements, vitamin D metabolites or surrogates, potassium supplements or exchange resins, calcium supplements, phosphate supplements or binders, and growth hormone injections; growth and nutritional monitoring with frequent adjustments of gastrostomy or nasogastric tube feedings of a special infant formula with added protein, carbohydrate, and/or oil for adequate caloric intake for growth; monitoring of developmental progress and initiation and coordination of intervention for delayed milestones; coordination and appropriate dosing of childhood immunizations; establishing and modifying short- and long-term care plans in cooperation with social services, nutritional support services, child life specialists, transplantation centers, and other medical specialists; and overall care coordination with regular counseling and support of the parents/caregivers and siblings for the care of a technologically dependent infant with chronic kidney disease. The pediatric nephrologist is likely to have multiple unscheduled telephone and electronic interventions generated by the dialysis center, an emergency room, another physician, or by the patient's parents/caregivers and will see the patient during dialysis sessions once during the month in order to accomplish his care and comply with facility-specific quality requirements.

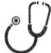 **Clinical Example (90954)**

A 9-year-old girl with end-stage renal disease from congenital renal anomalies and failed renal transplant, who is now anephric, undergoes chronic hemodialysis at a pediatric facility. Her disease burden includes catheter access problems, hypertension, fluid overload, intermittent hyperkalemia, renal osteodystrophy, anemia, acidosis, growth failure, behavior problems, family dysfunction related to a technologically dependent child, and polypharmacy (greater than seven medications).

Description of Procedure (90954)
The patient's pediatric nephrologist will manage her condition over the entire month by providing the following services: scheduled examinations for management of known and anticipated problems; episodic examinations for intercurrent changes in her general condition; evaluation of the integrity and functionality of her dialysis access; episodic changes in her dialysis prescription for growth, weight gain or loss, and fluid overload; scheduled review of routinely collected laboratory data; episodic adjustment of intravenous erythropoietin stimulating agents, iron, and vitamin D metabolites given during the dialysis treatment and of home medications including oral antihypertensives, iron supplements, vitamin D metabolites or surrogates, phosphate binders, potassium exchange resins, anti-constipation drugs, and growth hormone injections; establishing and modifying short- and long-term care plans in cooperation with social services, nutritional support services, child life specialists, school personnel, transplantation centers, and other medical

specialists; and overall care coordination. Growth and nutritional monitoring and intervention plus monitoring of developmental and school progress and intervention will be accomplished along with counseling of the parents/caregivers for patient's behavior problems related to dietary and fluid restriction, medication non-adherence, and coping with a technologically dependent child with chronic kidney disease. The pediatric nephrologist is likely to have multiple unscheduled telephone and electronic interventions generated by the dialysis center, an emergency room, another physician, or by the patient's parents/caregivers and may see the patient during dialysis sessions four or more times during the month in order to accomplish her care and to comply with facility-specific quality requirements.

Clinical Example (90955)

A 9-year-old girl with end-stage renal disease from congenital renal anomalies and failed renal transplant, who is now anephric, undergoes chronic hemodialysis at a pediatric facility. Her disease burden includes catheter access problems, hypertension, fluid overload, intermittent hyperkalemia, renal osteodystrophy, anemia, acidosis, growth failure, behavior problems, family dysfunction related to a technologically dependent child, and polypharmacy (greater than seven medications).

Description of Procedure (90955)

The patient's pediatric nephrologist will manage her condition over the entire month by providing the following services: scheduled examinations for management of known and anticipated problems; episodic examinations for intercurrent changes in her general condition; evaluation of the integrity and functionality of her dialysis access; episodic changes in her dialysis prescription for growth, weight gain or loss, and fluid overload; scheduled review of routinely collected laboratory data; episodic adjustment of intravenous erythropoietin stimulating agents, iron, and vitamin D metabolites given during the dialysis treatment and of home medications including oral antihypertensives, iron supplements, vitamin D metabolites or surrogates, phosphate binders, potassium exchange resins, anti-constipation drugs, and growth hormone injections; establishing and modifying short- and long-term care plans in cooperation with social services, nutritional support services, child life specialists, school personnel, transplantation centers, and other medical specialists; and overall care coordination. Growth and nutritional monitoring and intervention plus monitoring of developmental and school progress and intervention will be accomplished along with counseling of the parents/caregivers for patient's behavior problems related to dietary and fluid restriction, medication non-adherence, and coping with a technologically dependent child with chronic kidney disease. The pediatric nephrologist is likely to have multiple unscheduled telephone and electronic interventions generated by the dialysis center, an emergency room, another physician, or the patient's parents/caregivers and may see the patient during dialysis sessions two to three times during the month in order to accomplish her care and comply with facility-specific quality requirements.

Clinical Example (90956)

A 9-year-old girl with end-stage renal disease from congenital renal anomalies and failed renal transplant, who is now anephric, undergoes chronic hemodialysis at a pediatric facility. Her disease burden includes catheter access problems, hypertension, fluid overload, intermittent hyperkalemia, renal osteodystrophy, anemia, acidosis, growth failure, behavior problems, family dysfunction related to a technologically dependent child, and polypharmacy (greater than seven medications).

Description of Procedure (90956)
The patient's pediatric nephrologist will manage her condition over the entire month by providing the following services: scheduled examinations for management of known and anticipated problems; episodic examinations for intercurrent changes in her general condition; evaluation of the integrity and functionality of her dialysis access; episodic changes in her dialysis prescription for growth, weight gain or loss, and fluid overload; scheduled review of routinely collected laboratory data; episodic adjustment of intravenous erythropoietin stimulating agents, iron, and vitamin D metabolites given during the dialysis treatment and of home medications including oral antihypertensives, iron supplements, vitamin D metabolites or surrogates, phosphate binders, potassium exchange resins, anti-constipation drugs, and growth hormone injections; establishing and modifying short- and long-term care plans in cooperation with social services, nutritional support services, child life specialists, school personnel, transplantation centers, and other medical specialists; and overall care coordination. Growth and nutritional monitoring and intervention plus monitoring of developmental and school progress and intervention will be accomplished along with counseling of the parents/caregivers for patient's behavior problems related to dietary and fluid restriction, medication non-adherence, and coping with a technologically dependent child with chronic kidney disease. The pediatric nephrologist is likely to have multiple unscheduled telephone and electronic interventions generated by the dialysis center, an emergency room, another physician, or the patient's parents/caregivers and may see the patient during dialysis sessions once during the month in order to accomplish her care and comply with facility-specific quality requirements.

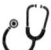

Clinical Example (90957)
A 14-year-old boy with end-stage renal disease from focal segmental glomerulosclerosis undergoes chronic hemodialysis at a dialysis facility. His disease burden includes dialysis access problems, hypertension, fluid overload, hyperkalemia, renal osteodystrophy, anemia, acidosis, anorexia and malnutrition, growth failure, adolescent non-adherent behavior, school problems, family stress, and polypharmacy (greater than seven medications).

Description of Procedure (90957)
The patient's pediatric nephrologist will manage his condition over the entire month by providing the following services: scheduled examinations for management of known and anticipated problems; episodic examinations for intercurrent changes in his general condition; evaluation of the integrity and functionality of his dialysis access; episodic changes in his dialysis prescription for growth, weight gain or loss, and fluid overload; scheduled review of routinely collected laboratory data; episodic adjustment of intravenous erythropoietin stimulating agents, iron, and vitamin D metabolites given during the dialysis treatment and of home medications including oral antihypertensives, iron supplements, vitamin D metabolites

or surrogates, phosphate binders, potassium exchange resins, anti-constipation drugs, and growth hormone injections; establishing and modifying short- and long-term care plans in cooperation with social services, nutritional support services, child life specialists, school personnel, transplantation centers, and other medical specialists; and overall care coordination. Growth and nutritional monitoring and intervention plus the monitoring of pubertal development and school progress will be accomplished along with counseling of the parents/caregivers for malnutrition, need for special renal dietary supplements, delayed puberty and growth failure, behavioral problems related to dietary and fluid restriction, medication non-adherence, and coping with a technologically dependent adolescent with chronic kidney disease. Planning for future transition to adult care will be initiated and progress periodically addressed. The pediatric nephrologist is likely to have multiple unscheduled telephone and electronic interventions generated by the dialysis center, an emergency room, another physician, or the patient's parents/caregivers and will see the patient during dialysis sessions four or more times during the month in order to accomplish his care and comply with facility-specific quality requirements.

Clinical Example (90958)

A 14-year-old boy with end-stage renal disease from focal segmental glomerulosclerosis undergoes chronic hemodialysis at a dialysis facility. His disease burden includes dialysis access problems, hypertension, fluid overload, hyperkalemia, renal osteodystrophy, anemia, acidosis, anorexia and malnutrition, growth failure, adolescent non-adherent behavior, school problems, family dysfunction, and polypharmacy (greater than seven medications).

Description of Procedure (90958)

The patient's pediatric nephrologist will manage his condition over the entire month by providing the following services: scheduled examinations for management of known and anticipated problems; episodic examinations for intercurrent changes in his general condition; evaluation of the integrity and functionality of his dialysis access; episodic changes in his dialysis prescription for growth, weight gain or loss and fluid overload; scheduled review of routinely collected laboratory data; episodic adjustment of intravenous erythropoietin stimulating agents, iron, and vitamin D metabolites given during the dialysis treatment and of home medications including oral antihypertensives, iron supplements, vitamin D metabolites or surrogates, phosphate binders, potassium exchange resins, anti-constipation drugs and growth hormone injections; establishing and modifying short and long term care plans in cooperation with social services, nutritional support services, child life specialists, school personnel, transplantation centers, and other medical specialists; and overall care coordination. Growth and nutritional monitoring and intervention plus the monitoring of pubertal development and school progress will be accomplished along with counseling of the parents/caregivers for malnutrition, need for special renal dietary supplements, delayed puberty and growth failure, behavioral problems related to dietary and fluid restriction, medication non-adherence and coping with an technologically dependent adolescent with chronic kidney disease. Planning for future transition to adult care will be initiated, and progress periodically addressed. The pediatric nephrologist is likely to have multiple unscheduled telephone and electronic interventions generated by the dialysis center, an emergency room, another physician, or the patient's parents/caregivers, and will see the patient during dialysis sessions two to three times during the month in order to accomplish his care and comply with facility specific quality requirements.

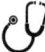

Clinical Example (90959)

A 14-year-old boy with end-stage renal disease from focal segmental glomerulosclerosis undergoes chronic hemodialysis at a dialysis facility. His disease burden includes dialysis access problems, hypertension, fluid overload, hyperkalemia, renal osteodystrophy, anemia, acidosis, anorexia and malnutrition, growth failure, adolescent non-adherent behavior, school problems, family stress, and polypharmacy (greater than seven medications)

Description of Procedure (90959)

The patient's pediatric nephrologist will manage his condition over the entire month by providing the following services: scheduled examinations for management of known and anticipated problems; episodic examinations for intercurrent changes in his general condition; evaluation of the integrity and functionality of his dialysis access; episodic changes in his dialysis prescription for growth, weight gain or loss and fluid overload; scheduled review of routinely collected laboratory data; episodic adjustment of intravenous erythropoietin stimulating agents, iron and vitamin D metabolites given during the dialysis treatment and of home medications including oral antihypertensives, iron supplements, vitamin D metabolites or surrogates, phosphate binders, potassium exchange resins, anti-constipation drugs, and growth hormone injections; establishing and modifying short- and long-term care plans in cooperation with social services, nutritional support services, child life specialists, school personnel, transplantation centers, and other medical specialists; and overall care coordination. Growth and nutritional monitoring and intervention plus the monitoring of pubertal development and school progress will be accomplished along with counseling of the parents/caregivers for malnutrition, need for special renal dietary supplements, delayed puberty and growth failure, behavioral problems related to dietary and fluid restriction, medication non-adherence, and coping with a technologically dependent adolescent with chronic kidney disease. Planning for future transition to adult care will be initiated and progress periodically addressed. The pediatric nephrologist is likely to have multiple unscheduled telephone and electronic interventions generated by the dialysis center, an emergency room, another physician, or the patient's parents/caregivers and will see the patient during dialysis sessions once during the month in order to accomplish his care and comply with facility-specific quality requirements.

Clinical Example (90960)

A 65-year-old man receives hemodialysis at a dialysis facility. His disease burden includes Type II diabetes mellitus, vascular disease, multiple access problems, hypertension, secondary hyperparathyroidism, anemia, and polypharmacy (greater than seven medications).

Description of Procedure (90960)

His nephrologist will manage his condition over the entire month by providing the following services: scheduled examinations for management of known and anticipated problems; episodic examinations for intercurrent changes in his general condition including post-hospitalization (the typical patient has 2.0 admissions per year or 14 hospitalization days per year); evaluation of the integrity and functionality of his dialysis access; episodic changes in his dialysis prescription; scheduled review of routinely collected laboratory data including intravenous erythropoietin stimulating agents, iron, and vitamin D or its surrogates; episodic adjustments of home medications including antihypertensives and phosphate binders; establishing and modifying short- and long-term care plans in cooperation with social services, nutritional support services, transplantation centers, and other medical specialists; and overall care coordination. The nephrologist is likely to have multiple unscheduled telephone and electronic interventions generated by the dialysis center, an emergency room, another physician, or the patient or his caregiver. He will see the patient during dialysis sessions four or more times during the month in order to accomplish his care and comply with facility-specific quality requirements.

Clinical Example (90961)

A 65-year-old man receives hemodialysis at a dialysis facility. His disease burden includes Type II diabetes mellitus, vascular disease, multiple access problems, hypertension, secondary hyperparathyroidism, anemia, and polypharmacy (greater than seven medications).

Description of Procedure (90961)

His nephrologist will manage his condition over the entire month by providing the following services: scheduled examinations for management of known and anticipated problems; episodic examinations for intercurrent changes in his general condition including post-hospitalization (the typical patient has 2.0 admissions per year or 14 hospitalization days per year); evaluation of the integrity and functionality of his dialysis access; episodic changes in his dialysis prescription; scheduled review of routinely collected laboratory data including intravenous erythropoietin stimulating agents, iron, and vitamin D or its surrogates; episodic adjustments of home medications including antihypertensives and phosphate binders; establishing and modifying short- and long-term care plans in cooperation with social services, nutritional support services, transplantation centers, and other medical specialists; and overall care coordination. The nephrologist is likely to have multiple unscheduled telephone and electronic interventions generated by the dialysis center, an emergency room, another physician, or the patient or his caregiver. He will see the patient during dialysis sessions two to three times during the month in order to accomplish his care and comply with facility-specific quality requirements.

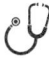

Clinical Example (90962)

A 65-year-old man receives hemodialysis at a dialysis facility. His disease burden includes Type II diabetes mellitus, vascular disease, multiple access problems, hypertension, secondary hyperparathyroidism, anemia, and polypharmacy (greater than seven medications).

Description of Procedure (90962)

His nephrologist will manage his condition over the entire month by providing the following services: scheduled examinations for management of known and anticipated problems; episodic examinations for intercurrent changes in his general condition including post-hospitalization (the typical patient has 2.0 admissions per year or 14 hospitalization days per year); evaluation of the integrity and functionality of his dialysis access; episodic changes in his dialysis prescription; scheduled review of routinely collected laboratory data including intravenous erythropoietin stimulating agents, iron, and vitamin D or its surrogates; episodic adjustments of home medications including antihypertensives and phosphate binders; establishing and modifying short- and long-term care plans in cooperation with social services, nutritional support services, transplantation centers, and other medical specialists; and overall care coordination. The nephrologist is likely to have multiple unscheduled telephone and electronic interventions generated by the dialysis center, an emergency room, another physician, or the patient or his caregiver. He will see the patient during dialysis sessions once during the month in order to accomplish his care and comply with facility-specific quality requirements.

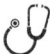

Clinical Example (90963)

A 10-month-old boy with end-stage renal disease from prune belly syndrome with renal dysplasia receives nightly home continuous cycling peritoneal dialysis by parent caregivers. His disease burden includes catheter access problems, renal osteodystrophy, anemia, acidosis, growth failure, developmental delay, anorexia and feeding problems, family dysfunction related to a technologically dependent infant, modified childhood immunizations, and polypharmacy (greater than seven medications).

Description of Procedure (90963)

The patient's pediatric nephrologist will manage his condition over the entire month by providing the following services: scheduled examinations for management of known and anticipated problems; episodic examinations for intercurrent changes in his general condition; evaluation of the integrity and functionality of his dialysis access; episodic changes in his dialysis prescription; frequent adjustment of target weight for growth and fluid intake; scheduled review of routinely collected laboratory data; episodic adjustment of home medications including oral iron supplements, vitamin D metabolites or surrogates, potassium supplements or exchange resins, calcium supplements, phosphate supplements or binders, erythropoietin stimulating agents, and growth hormone injections; growth and nutritional monitoring with frequent adjustments of gastrostomy or nasogastric tube feedings of a special infant formula with added protein, carbohydrate, and/or oil for adequate caloric intake for growth; monitoring of developmental progress and initiation and coordination of intervention for delayed milestones; coordination and appropriate dosing of childhood immunizations; establishing and modifying short- and long-term care plans in cooperation with social services, nutritional support services, child life specialists, transplantation centers, and other medical specialists; and overall care coordination with regular counseling and support of the parents/caregivers and siblings for the care of a technologically dependent infant with chronic kidney disease using high-tech home therapy. The pediatric nephrologist is likely to have multiple unscheduled telephone and electronic interventions generated by the dialysis center, an emergency room, another physician, or the patient's parents/caregivers. He will see the patient one or more times during the month in order to accomplish his care and comply with facility-specific quality requirements.

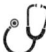

Clinical Example (90964)

A 6-year-old boy with posterior urethral valves and obstructive uropathy receives home continuous cycling peritoneal dialysis by parent caregivers. His disease burden includes catheter access problems, renal osteodystrophy, anemia, acidosis, growth failure, behavior problems, family stress related to a technologically dependent child, and polypharmacy (greater than seven medications).

Description of Procedure (90964)

The patient's pediatric nephrologist will manage his condition over the entire month by providing the following services: scheduled examinations for management of known and anticipated problems; episodic examinations for intercurrent changes in his general condition; evaluation of the integrity and functionality of his dialysis access; episodic changes in his dialysis prescription; frequent adjustment of target weight for growth and fluid intake; scheduled review of routinely collected laboratory data; episodic adjustment of home medications including oral iron supplements, vitamin D metabolites or surrogates, potassium supplements or exchange resins, calcium supplements, phosphate supplements or binders, erythropoietin stimulating agent, and growth hormone injections; establishing and modifying short- and long-term care plans in cooperation with social services, nutritional support services, child life specialists, transplantation centers, and other medical specialists; and overall care coordination. Growth and nutritional monitoring and intervention with special renal supplemental formula plus monitoring of developmental, behavioral, and school problems and initiation of intervention will be accomplished along with counseling of the parents or caregivers for coping with a technologically dependent child with chronic kidney disease receiving high-tech home therapy. The pediatric nephrologist is likely to have multiple unscheduled telephone interventions generated by the dialysis center, an emergency room, another physician, or the patient's parents/caregivers and may see the patient one or more times during the month in order to accomplish his care and comply with facility-specific quality requirements.

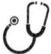

Clinical Example (90965)

A 16-year-old anuric girl with IgA nephropathy and failed renal transplant does her own home continuous cycling peritoneal dialysis treatments with back-up supervision from her parents. Her disease burden includes dialysis access problems, hypertension, fluid overload, renal osteodystrophy, anemia, acidosis, anorexia and malnutrition, growth failure, adolescent non-adherent behavior, school problems, and polypharmacy (greater than seven medications).

Description of Procedure (90965)

The patient's pediatric nephrologist will manage her condition over the entire month by providing the following services: scheduled examinations for management of known and anticipated problems; episodic examinations for intercurrent changes in her general condition; evaluation of the integrity and functionality of her dialysis access; episodic changes in her dialysis prescription for growth, weight gain or loss, and fluid overload; scheduled review of routinely collected laboratory data; episodic adjustment of home medications including oral antihypertensives, iron supplements, vitamin D metabolites or surrogates, phosphate binders, potassium exchange resins, anti-constipation drugs, erythropoietin stimulating agents, and growth hormone injections; establishing and modifying short- and long-term care plans in cooperation with social services, nutritional support services, child life specialists, school personnel, transplantation centers, and other medical specialists; and overall care coordination. Growth and nutritional monitoring and intervention plus the monitoring of pubertal development and school progress will be accomplished along with counseling of the parents/caregivers for malnutrition, need for special renal dietary supplements, delayed puberty and growth failure, behavioral problems related to dietary and fluid restriction, medication non-adherence, and coping with a technologically dependent adolescent with chronic kidney disease. Planning for future transition to adult care will be initiated and progress periodically addressed. The pediatric nephrologist is likely to have multiple unscheduled telephone and electronic interventions generated by the dialysis center, an emergency room, another physician, or the patient/parents/caregivers and may see the patient one or more times during the month in order to accomplish her care and comply with facility-specific quality requirements.

Clinical Example (90966)

A 59-year-old chronic peritoneal dialysis patient dialyzes at home. His disease burden includes Type II diabetes mellitus, vascular disease, hypertension, secondary hyperparathyroidism, anemia, and polypharmacy (greater than seven medications).

Description of Procedure (90966)

His nephrologist will manage his condition over the entire month by providing the following services: scheduled examinations for management of known and anticipated problems; episodic examinations for intercurrent changes in his general condition including post-hospitalization; evaluation of the integrity and functionality of his dialysis access; episodic changes in his dialysis prescription; scheduled review of routinely collected laboratory data; episodic administration of IV iron or other medications in the dialysis center; episodic adjustments of home medications including antihypertensives and phosphate binders; establishing and modifying short- and long-term care plans in cooperation with social services, nutritional support services, transplantation centers, and other medical specialists; and overall care coordination. The nephrologist is likely to have multiple unscheduled telephone and electronic interventions generated by the dialysis center, an emergency room, another physician, or the patient or his caregiver.

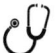
Clinical Example (90967)

A 10-month-old boy with end-stage renal disease from prune belly syndrome with renal dysplasia receives nightly home continuous cycling peritoneal dialysis by parent caregivers. His disease burden includes catheter access problems, renal osteodystrophy, anemia, acidosis, growth failure, developmental delay, anorexia and feeding problems, family stress related to a technologically dependent infant, modified childhood immunizations, and polypharmacy (greater than seven medications).

Description of Procedure (90967)

The patient's pediatric nephrologist will manage his condition over the day by providing the following services: scheduled examinations for management of known and anticipated problems; episodic examinations for intercurrent changes in his general condition; evaluation of the integrity and functionality of his dialysis access; episodic changes in his dialysis prescription; frequent adjustment of target weight for growth and fluid intake; scheduled review of routinely collected laboratory data; episodic adjustment of home medications including oral iron supplements, vitamin D metabolites or surrogates, potassium supplements or exchange resins, calcium supplements, phosphate supplements or binders, erythropoietin stimulating agent, and growth hormone injections; growth and nutritional monitoring with frequent adjustments of gastrostomy or nasogastric tube feedings of a special infant formula with added protein, carbohydrate, and/or oil for adequate caloric intake for growth; monitoring of developmental progress and initiation and coordination of intervention for delayed milestones; coordination and appropriate dosing of childhood immunizations; establishing and modifying short- and long-term care plans in cooperation with social services, nutritional support services, child life specialists, transplantation centers, and other medical specialists; and overall care coordination with regular counseling and support of the parents/caregivers and siblings for the care of a technologically dependent infant with chronic kidney disease using high-tech home therapy. The pediatric nephrologist is likely to have multiple unscheduled telephone and electronic interventions generated by the dialysis center, an emergency room, another physician, or the patient's parents/caregivers. He will see the patient one or more times during the month in order to accomplish his care and comply with facility-specific quality requirements.

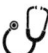
Clinical Example (90968)

A 6-year-old boy with posterior urethral valves and obstructive uropathy receives home continuous cycling peritoneal dialysis by parent caregivers. His disease burden includes catheter access problems, renal osteodystrophy, anemia, acidosis, growth failure, behavior problems, family stress related to a technologically dependent child, and polypharmacy (greater than seven medications).

Description of Procedure (90968)

The patient's pediatric nephrologist will manage his condition over the day by providing the following services: scheduled examinations for management of known and anticipated problems; episodic examinations for intercurrent changes in his general condition; evaluation of the integrity and functionality of his dialysis access; episodic changes in his dialysis prescription; frequent adjustment of target weight for growth and fluid intake; scheduled review of routinely collected laboratory data; episodic adjustment of home medications including oral iron supplements, vitamin D metabolites or surrogates, potassium supplements or exchange resins, calcium supplements, phosphate supplements or binders, erythropoietin stimulating agents, and growth hormone injections; establishing and modifying short- and long-term care plans in cooperation with social services, nutritional support services, child life specialists, transplantation centers, and other medical specialists; and overall care coordination. Growth and nutritional monitoring and intervention with special renal supplemental formula plus monitoring of developmental, behavioral, and school problems and initiation of intervention will be accomplished along with counseling of the parents or caregivers for coping with a technologically dependent child with chronic kidney disease receiving high-tech home therapy. The pediatric nephrologist is likely have multiple unscheduled telephone interventions generated by the dialysis center, an emergency room, another physician, or the patient's parents/caregivers and may see the patient one or more times during the month in order to accomplish his care and comply with facility-specific quality requirements.

Clinical Example (90969)
A 16-year-old anuric girl with IgA nephropathy and failed renal transplant does her own home continuous cycling peritoneal dialysis treatments with back-up supervision from her parents. Her disease burden includes hypertension, fluid overload, renal osteodystrophy, anemia, acidosis, anorexia and malnutrition, growth failure, adolescent non-adherent behavior, school problems, and polypharmacy (greater than seven medications).

Description of Procedure (90969)
The patient's pediatric nephrologist will manage her condition over the day by providing the following services: scheduled examinations for management of known and anticipated problems; episodic examinations for intercurrent changes in her general condition; evaluation of the integrity and functionality of her dialysis access; episodic changes in her dialysis prescription for growth, weight gain or loss, and fluid overload; scheduled review of routinely collected laboratory data; episodic adjustment of home medications including oral antihypertensives, iron supplements, vitamin D metabolites or surrogates, phosphate binders, potassium exchange resins, anti-constipation drugs, erythropoietin stimulating agents, and growth hormone injections; establishing and modifying short- and long-term care plans in cooperation with social services, nutritional support services, child life specialists, school personnel, transplantation centers, and other medical specialists; and overall care coordination. Growth and nutritional monitoring and intervention plus the monitoring of pubertal development and school progress will be accomplished along with counseling of the parents/caregivers for malnutrition, need for special renal dietary supplements, delayed puberty and growth failure, behavioral problems related to dietary and fluid restriction, medication non-adherence, and coping with a technologically dependent adolescent with chronic kidney disease. Planning for future transition to adult care will be initiated and progress periodically addressed. The pediatric nephrologist is likely to have multiple

unscheduled telephone and electronic interventions generated by the dialysis center, an emergency room, another physician, or the patient/parents/caregivers and may see the patient one or more times during the month in order to accomplish her care and comply with facility-specific quality requirements.

Clinical Example (90970)

A 59-year-old chronic peritoneal dialysis patient dialyzes for less than a full month. His disease burden includes Type II diabetes mellitus, vascular disease, hypertension, secondary hyperparathyroidism, anemia, and polypharmacy (greater than seven medications).

Description of Procedure (90970)

His nephrologist will manage his condition over the day by providing the following services: scheduled examinations for management of known and anticipated problems; episodic examinations for intercurrent changes in his general condition including post-hospitalization; evaluation of the integrity and functionality of his dialysis access; episodic changes in his dialysis prescription; scheduled review of routinely collected laboratory data; episodic administration of IV iron or other medications in the dialysis center; episodic adjustments of home medications including antihypertensives and phosphate binders; establishing and modifying short- and long-term care plans in cooperation with social services, nutritional support services, transplantation centers, and other medical specialists; and overall care coordination. The nephrologist is likely have multiple unscheduled telephone and electronic interventions generated by the dialysis center, an emergency room, another physician, or the patient or his caregiver.

Gastroenterology

▶(91100 has been deleted)◀

▶(To report placement of an esophageal tamponade tube for management of variceal bleeding, use 43460. To report placement of a long intestinal Miller-Abbott tube, use 44500)◀

Rationale

Code 91100 has been deleted as therapeutic and diagnostic developments for the evaluation of gastrointestinal tract bleeding over the past 20 years have made this procedure obsolete. To direct users to the appropriate codes to report placement of an esophageal tamponade tube for management of variceal bleeding and placement of a long intestinal Miller-Abbott tube, an instructional parenthetical note has been added to direct users to codes 43460 and 44500, respectively.

Ophthalmology

Special Ophthalmological Services

92025 Computerized corneal topography, unilateral or bilateral, with interpretation and report

(Do not report 92025 in conjunction with 65710-▶65771◀)

✎ Rationale
The list of codes included in the exclusionary parenthetical instruction currently following code 92025 for computerized corneal topography has been expanded to encompass not only codes 65710-65755 but also codes 65760-65771.

Special Otorhinolaryngologic Services

Diagnostic or treatment procedures ▶that are reported as evaluation and management services (eg, otoscopy, anterior rhinoscopy, tuning fork test, removal of non-impacted cerumen) are not reported separately.◀

Special otorhinolaryngologic services are those diagnostic and treatment services not included in ▶an Evaluation and Management service◀. These services are reported separately using codes 92502-92700.

92506 Evaluation of speech, language, voice, communication, and/or auditory processing

▶Vestibular Function Tests, Without Electrical Recording◀

92531 Spontaneous nystagmus, including gaze

92532 Positional nystagmus test

▶(Do not report 92531, 92532 with evaluation and management services)◀

▶Vestibular Function Tests, With Recording (eg, ENG)◀

92541 Spontaneous nystagmus test, including gaze and fixation nystagmus, with recording

▶Audiologic Function Tests◀

The audiometric tests listed below require the use of calibrated electronic equipment, ▶recording of results and a report with interpretation◀. ▶H◀earing tests (such as whispered voice, tuning fork) ▶that◀ are otorhinolaryngologic ▶Evaluation and Management◀ services are not reported separately. All services include testing of both ears. Use modifier 52 if a test is applied to one ear instead of two ears. All codes (except 92559) apply to testing of individuals. For testing of groups, use 92559 and specify test(s) used.

(For evaluation of speech, language and/or hearing problems through observation and assessment of performance, use 92506)

92551   Screening test, pure tone, air only

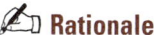
Rationale
The introductory language and subheading titles within the Special Otorhinolaryngologic Services section (92502-92700) of the CPT codebook were revised to remove references to and prevent misinterpretation of the use of the vestibular and audiologic function test codes in conjunction with evaluation and management (E/M) services. The tests included in this section are typically not provided by physicians, thus all references that infer that physician observation, evaluation, or medical diagnostic evaluations are included in this series of codes have been eliminated. Additional clarification to indicate that special otorhinolaryngologic services are not part of E/M services performed on the same date of service in which these tests have been provided, with the exception of codes 92531 and 92532, which include E/M, is included in a new parenthetical note. Additionally, the acronym PENG (photoelectronystagmography) was omitted from the Vestibular Function Tests, with Recording subheading, because it is an outdated term.

Cardiovascular

Therapeutic Services and Procedures

(For nonsurgical septal reduction therapy [eg, alcohol ablation], use ▶93799◀)

92950   Cardiopulmonary resuscitation (eg, in cardiac arrest)

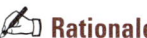
Rationale
In support of the deletion of Category III code 0024T, the cross-reference following the Therapeutic Services and Procedures subheading has been revised to direct users to code 93799 for nonsurgical septal reduction therapy.

92960   Cardioversion, elective, electrical conversion of arrhythmia; external

92961   internal (separate procedure)

(Do not report 92961 in addition to codes 93282, 93283, 93289, 93292, 93295, 93662, 93618-93624, 93631, 93640-93642, 93650-93652)

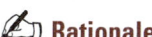
Rationale
In support of the changes to the cardiac device monitoring section, the instructional note following code 92961 has been revised to reflect the appropriate codes.

Cardiography

▶Cardiovascular monitoring services are diagnostic medical procedures using in-person and remote technology to assess cardiovascular rhythm (ECG) data.◀

▶*Attended surveillance* is the immediate availability of a remote technician to respond to rhythm or device alert transmissions from a patient, either from an implanted or wearable monitoring or therapy device, as they are generated and transmitted to the remote surveillance location or center.◀

▶*Mobile cardiovascular telemetry (MCT)* continuously records the electrocardiographic rhythm from external electrodes placed on the patient's body. Segments of the ECG data are automatically (without patient intervention) transmitted to a remote surveillance location by cellular or landline telephone signal. The segments of the rhythm, selected for transmission, are triggered automatically (MCT device algorithm) by rapid and slow heart rates or by the patient during a symptomatic episode. There is continuous real time data analysis by preprogrammed algorithms in the device and attended surveillance of the transmitted rhythm segments by a surveillance center technician to evaluate any arrhythmias and to determine signal quality. The surveillance center technician reviews the data and notifies the physician depending on the prescribed criteria.◀

▶ECG rhythm derived elements are distinct from physiologic data, even when the same device is capable of producing both. Implantable cardiovascular monitor (ICM) device services are always separately reported from Implantable cardioverter-defibrillator (ICD) service.◀

▶For other services related to a wearable defibrillator, see 93745.◀

▶(For echocardiography, see 93303-93350)◀

▶(For electrocardiogram, 64 leads or greater, with graphic presentation and analysis, see 0178T-0180T)◀

93000 Electrocardiogram, routine ECG with at least 12 leads; with interpretation and report

93014 physician review with interpretation and report only

▶(Do not report 93014 in conjunction with 93228, 93229)◀

93040 Rhythm ECG, 1-3 leads; with interpretation and report

▲**93224** Wearable electrocardiographic rhythm derived monitoring for 24 hours by continuous original waveform recording and storage, with visual superimposition scanning; includes recording, scanning analysis with report, physician review and interpretation

▲**93225** recording (includes connection, recording, and disconnection)

▲**93226** scanning analysis with report

▲**93227** physician review and interpretation

●**93228** Wearable mobile cardiovascular telemetry with electrocardiographic recording, concurrent computerized real time data analysis and greater than 24 hours of accessible ECG data storage (retrievable with query) with ECG triggered and patient selected events transmitted to a remote attended surveillance center for up to 30 days; physician review and interpretation with report

▶(Report 93228 only once per 30 days)◀

▶(Do not report 93228 in conjunction with 93014)◀

● **93229** technical support for connection and patient instructions for use, attended surveillance, analysis and physician prescribed transmission of daily and emergent data reports

▶(Report 93229 only once per 30 days)◀

▶(Do no report 93229 in conjunction with 93014)◀

▶(For wearable cardiovascular monitors that do not perform automatic ECG triggered transmissions to an attended surveillance center, see 93224-93227, 93230-93272)◀

▲ **93230** Wearable electrocardiographic rhythm derived monitoring for 24 hours by continuous original waveform recording and storage without superimposition scanning utilizing a device capable of producing a full miniaturized printout; includes recording, microprocessor-based analysis with report, physician review and interpretation

▲ **93231** recording (includes connection, recording, and disconnection)

▲ **93232** microprocessor-based analysis with report

▲ **93233** physician review and interpretation

▲ **93235** Wearable electrocardiographic rhythm derived monitoring for 24 hours by continuous computerized monitoring and non-continuous recording, and real-time data analysis utilizing a device capable of producing intermittent full-sized waveform tracings, possibly patient activated; includes monitoring and real-time data analysis with report, physician review and interpretation

▲ **93236** monitoring and real-time data analysis with report

▲ **93237** physician review and interpretation

▶(For wearable mobile telemetry with ECG triggered transmissions to an attended surveillance center, see 93228, 93229)◀

▲ **93268** Wearable patient activated electrocardiographic rhythm derived event recording with presymptom memory loop, 24-hour attended monitoring, per 30 day period of time; includes transmission, physician review and interpretation

▲ **93270** recording (includes connection, recording, and disconnection)

▲ **93271** monitoring, receipt of transmissions, and analysis

▲ **93272** physician review and interpretation

(For postsymptom recording, see 93012, 93014)

(For implanted patient activated cardiac event recording, see 33282, ▶93285, 93291, 93298◀)

93278 Signal-averaged electrocardiography (SAECG), with or without ECG

(For interpretation and report only, use 93278 with modifier 26)

(For unlisted cardiographic procedure, use 93799)

▶Cardiovascular Device Monitoring—Implantable and Wearable Devices◀

▶Cardiovascular monitoring services are diagnostic medical procedures using in-person and remote technology to assess device therapy and cardiovascular physiologic data. Codes 93279-93299 describe this technology and technical/professional physician and service center practice. Codes 93279-93292 are reported per procedure. Codes 93293-93296 are reported no more than **once** every 90 days. Do not report 93293-93296 if the monitoring period is less than 30 days. Codes 93297, 93298 are reported no more than **once** up to every 30 days. Do not report 93297-93299 if the monitoring period is less than 10 days.◀

▶A service center may report 93296 or 93299 during a period in which a physician performs an in-person interrogation device evaluation. A physician may not report an in-person and remote interrogation of the same device during the same period. Report only remote services when an in-person interrogation device evaluation is performed during a period of remote interrogation device evaluation. A period is established by the initiation of the remote monitoring or the 91st day of a pacemaker or implantable cardioverter-defibrillator (ICD) monitoring or the 31st day of an implantable loop recorder (ILR) or implantable cardiovascular monitor (ICM) monitoring and extends for the subsequent 30 or 90 days, respectively, for which remote monitoring is occurring. Programming device evaluations and in-person interrogation device evaluations may not be reported on the same date by the same physician. Programming device evaluations and remote interrogation device evaluations may both be reported during the remote interrogation device evaluation period.◀

▶ECG rhythm derived elements are distinct from physiologic data, even when the same device is capable of producing both. ICM device services are always separately reported from ICD services. When ILR data is derived from an ICD or pacemaker, do not report ILR services with pacemaker or ICD services.◀

▶For monitoring by wearable devices, see 93224-93272, 93228, 93229.◀

▶For other services related to a wearable defibrillator, use 93745.◀

▶Do not report 93012, 93014 when performing 93279-93289, 93291-93296 or 93298-93299. Do not report 93040-93042 when performing 93279-93289, 93291-93296, or 93298-93299.◀

▶The pacemaker and ICD interrogation device evaluations, peri-procedural device evaluations and programming, and programming device evaluations may not be reported in conjunction with pacemaker or ICD device and/or lead insertion or revision services by the same physician.◀

▶The following definitions and instructions apply to codes 93279-93299:◀

▶*Attended surveillance:* the immediate availability of a remote technician to respond to rhythm or device alert transmissions from a patient, either from an implanted or wearable monitoring or therapy device, as they are generated and transmitted to the remote surveillance location or center.◀

▶*Device, single lead:* a pacemaker or implantable cardioverter-defibrillator with pacing and sensing function in only one chamber of the heart.◀

▶*Device, dual lead:* a pacemaker or implantable cardioverter-defibrillator with pacing and sensing function in only two chambers of the heart.◀

▶*Device, multiple lead:* a pacemaker or implantable cardioverter-defibrillator with pacing and sensing function in three or more chambers of the heart.◀

▶*Electrocardiographic rhythm derived:* data analysis derived from recordings of the electrical activation of the heart including, but not limited to, heart rhythm, rate, ST analysis, heart rate variability, T-wave alternans.◀

▶*Implantable cardiovascular monitor (ICM):* an implantable cardiovascular device used to assist the physician in the management of non-rhythm related cardiac conditions such as heart failure. The device collects longitudinal physiologic cardiovascular data elements from one or more internal sensors (such as right ventricular pressure, left atrial pressure or an index of lung water) and/or external sensors (such as blood pressure or body weight) for patient assessment and management. The data are stored and transmitted to the physician by either local telemetry or remotely to an Internet based file server or surveillance technician. The function of the ICM may be an additional function of an implantable cardiac device (eg, implantable cardioverter-defibrillator) or a function of a stand-alone device. When ICM functionality is included in an ICD device, the ICM data and the ICD heart rhythm data such as sensing, pacing, and tachycardia detection therapy are distinct and, therefore, the monitoring processes are distinct.◀

▶*Implantable cardioverter-defibrillator (ICD):* an implantable device that provides high-energy and low-energy stimulation to one or more chambers of the heart to terminate rapid heart rhythms called tachycardia or fibrillation. ICDs also have pacemaker functions to treat slow heart rhythms called bradycardia. In addition to the tachycardia and bradycardia functions, the ICD may or may not include the functionality of an implantable cardiovascular monitor or an implantable loop recorder.◀

▶*Implantable loop recorder (ILR):* an implantable device that continuously records the electrocardiographic rhythm triggered automatically by rapid and slow heart rates or by the patient during a symptomatic episode. The ILR function may be the only function of the device or it may be part of a pacemaker or implantable cardioverter- defibrillator device. The data are stored and transmitted to the physician by either local telemetry or remotely to an Internet based file server or surveillance technician.◀

▶*Interrogation device evaluation (in person):* a face-to-face evaluation of an implantable device such as a cardiac pacemaker, implantable cardioverter-defibrillator, implantable cardiovascular monitor, or implantable loop recorder. Using an office, hospital, or emergency room instrument, stored and measured information about the lead(s) when present, sensor(s) when present, battery and the implanted pulse generator function as well as data collected about the patient's heart rhythm and heart rate is retrieved. The retrieved information is evaluated to determine the current programming of the device and to evaluate certain aspects of the device function such as battery voltage, lead impedance, tachycardia detection settings, and rhythm treatment settings.◀

▶The components that must be evaluated for the various types of implantable cardiac devices are listed below. (The required components for both remote and in-person interrogations are the same.)◀

▶*Pacemaker:* Programmed parameters, lead(s), battery, capture and sensing function and heart rhythm.◀

▶*Implantable cardioverter-defibrillator:* Programmed parameters, lead(s), battery, capture and sensing function, presence or absence of therapy for ventricular tachyarrhythmias and underlying heart rhythm.◀

▶*Implantable cardiovascular monitor:* Programmed parameters and analysis of at least one recorded physiologic cardiovascular data element from either internal or external sensors.◀

▶ *Implantable loop recorder:* Programmed parameters and the heart rate and rhythm during recorded episodes from both patient initiated and device algorithm detected events, when present. ◀

▶ *Pacemaker* is an implantable device that provides low energy localized stimulation to one or more chambers of the heart to initiate contraction in that chamber. ◀

▶ *Peri-procedural device evaluation and programming:* an evaluation of an implantable device system (either a pacemaker or implantable cardioverter defibrillator) to adjust the device to settings appropriate for the patient prior to a surgery, procedure, or test. The device system data are interrogated to evaluate the lead(s), sensor(s), and battery in addition to review of stored information, including patient and system measurements. The device is programmed to settings appropriate for the surgery, procedure, or test, as required. A second evaluation and programming are performed after the surgery, procedure, or test to provide settings appropriate to the postprocedural situation, as required. If one provider performs both the pre- and post-evaluation and programming service, the appropriate code, either 93286 or 93287, would be reported two times. If one provider performs the pre-surgical service and a separate provider performs the post-surgical service, each reports either 93286 or 93287 only one time. ◀

▶ *Physiologic cardiovascular data elements:* data elements from one or more internal sensors (such as right ventricular pressure, left atrial pressure or an index of lung water) and/or external sensors (such as blood pressure or body weight) for patient assessement and management. It does not include ECG rhythm derived data elements. ◀

▶ *Programming device evaluation:* a procedure performed for patients with a pacemaker, implantable cardioverter-defibrillator, or implantable loop recorder. All device functions, including the battery, programmable settings and lead(s), when present, are evaluated. To assess capture thresholds, iterative adjustments (eg, progressive changes in pacing output of a pacing lead) of the programmable parameters are conducted. The iterative adjustments provide information that permits the operator to assess and select the most appropriate final program parameters to provide for consistent delivery of the appropriate therapy and to verify the function of the device. The final program parameters may or may not change after evaluation. ◀

▶ The programming device evaluation includes all of the components of the interrogation device evaluation (remote) or the interrogation device evaluation (in person), and it includes the selection of patient specific programmed parameters depending on the type of device. ◀

▶ The components that must be evaluated for the various types of programming device evaluations are listed below. (See also required interrogation device evaluation [remote and in person] components above.) ◀

▶ *Pacemaker:* Programmed parameters, lead(s), battery, capture and sensing function, and heart rhythm. Often, but not always, the sensor rate response, lower and upper heart rates, AV intervals, pacing voltage and pulse duration, sensing value, and diagnostics will be adjusted during a programming evaluation. ◀

▶ *Implantable cardioverter-defibrillator:* Programmed parameters, lead(s), battery, capture and sensing function, presence or absence of therapy for ventricular tachyarrhythmias and underlying heart rhythm. Often, but not always, the sensor rate response, lower and upper heart rates, AV intervals, pacing voltage and pulse duration, sensing value, and diagnostics will be adjusted during a programming evaluation. In addition, ventricular tachycardia detection and therapies are sometimes altered depending on the interrogated data, patient's rhythm, symptoms, and condition. ◀

▶*Implantable loop recorder:* Programmed parameters and the heart rhythm during recorded episodes from both patient initiated and device algorithm detected events. Often, but not always, the tachycardia and bradycardia detection criteria will be adjusted during a programming evaluation.◄

▶*Transtelephonic rhythm strip pacemaker evaluation:* service of transmission of an electrocardiographic rhythm strip over the telephone by the patient using a transmitter and recorded by a receiving location using a receiver/recorder (also commonly known as transtelephonic pacemaker monitoring). The electrocardiographic rhythm strip is recorded both with and without a magnet applied over the pacemaker. The rhythm strip is evaluated for heart rate and rhythm, atrial and ventricular capture (if observed) and atrial and ventricular sensing (if observed). In addition, the battery status of the pacemaker is determined by measurement of the paced rate on the electrocardiographic rhythm strip recorded with the magnet applied.◄

●**93279**   Programming device evaluation with iterative adjustment of the implantable device to test the function of the device and select optimal permanent programmed values with physician analysis, review and report; single lead pacemaker system

▶(Do not report 93279 in conjunction with 93286, 93288)◄

●**93280**   dual lead pacemaker system

▶(Do not report 93280 in conjunction with 93286, 93288)◄

●**93281**   multiple lead pacemaker system

▶(Do not report 93281 in conjunction with 93286, 93288)◄

●**93282**   single lead implantable cardioverter-defibrillator system

▶(Do not report 93282 in conjunction with 93287, 93289, 93745)◄

●**93283**   dual lead implantable cardioverter-defibrillator system

▶(Do not report 93283 in conjunction with 93287, 93289)◄

●**93284**   multiple lead implantable cardioverter-defibrillator system

▶(Do not report 93284 in conjunction with 93287-93289)◄

●**93285**   implantable loop recorder system

▶(Do not report 93285 in conjunction with 33282, 93279, 93284, 93291)◄

●**93286**   Peri-procedural device evaluation and programming of device system parameters before or after a surgery, procedure, or test with physician analysis, review and report; single, dual, or multiple lead pacemaker system

▶(Report 93286 once before and once after surgery, procedure, or test, when device evaluation and programming is performed before and after surgery, procedure, or test)◄

▶(Do not report 93286 in conjunction with 93279-93281, 93288)◄

●**93287**   single, dual, or multiple lead implantable cardioverter-defibrillator system

▶(Report 93287 once before and once after surgery, procedure, or test, when device evaluation and programming is performed before and after surgery, procedure, or test)◄

▶(Do not report 93287 in conjunction with 93282-93284, 93289)◄

●**93288** Interrogation device evaluation (in person) with physician analysis, review and report, includes connection, recording and disconnection per patient encounter; single, dual, or multiple lead pacemaker system

▶(Do not report 93288 in conjunction with 93279-93281, 93286, 93294, 93296)◀

●**93289** single, dual, or multiple lead implantable cardioverter-defibrillator system, including analysis of heart rhythm derived data elements

▶(For monitoring physiologic cardiovascular data elements derived from an ICD, use 93290)◀

▶(Do not report 93289 in conjunction with 93282-93284, 93287, 93295, 93296)◀

●**93290** implantable cardiovascular monitor system, including analysis of 1 or more recorded physiologic cardiovascular data elements from all internal and external sensors

▶(For heart rhythm derived data elements, use 93289)◀

▶(Do not report 93290 in conjunction with 93297, 93299)◀

●**93291** implantable loop recorder system, including heart rhythm derived data analysis

▶(Do not report 93291 in conjunction with 33282, 93288-93290, 93298, 93299)◀

●**93292** wearable defibrillator system

▶(Do not report 93292 in conjunction with 93745)◀

●**93293** Transtelephonic rhythm strip pacemaker evaluation(s) single, dual, or multiple lead pacemaker system, includes recording with and without magnet application with physician analysis, review and report(s), up to 90 days

▶(Do not report 93293 in conjunction with 93294)◀

▶(For in person evaluation, see 93040, 93041, 93042)◀

▶(Report 93293 only once per 90 days)◀

●**93294** Interrogation device evaluation(s) (remote), up to 90 days; single, dual, or multiple lead pacemaker system with interim physician analysis, review(s) and report(s)

▶(Do not report 93294 in conjunction with 93288, 93293)◀

▶(Report 93294 only once per 90 days)◀

●**93295** single, dual, or multiple lead implantable cardioverter-defibrillator system with interim physician analysis, review(s) and report(s)

▶(For remote monitoring of physiologic cardiovascular data elements derived from an ICD, use 93297)◀

▶(Do not report 93295 in conjunction with 93289)◀

▶(Report 93295 only once per 90 days)◀

●**93296** single, dual, or multiple lead pacemaker system or implantable cardioverter-defibrillator system, remote data acquisition(s), receipt of transmissions and technician review, technical support and distribution of results

▶(Do not report 93296 in conjunction with 93288, 93289, 93299)◀

▶(Report 93296 only once per 90 days)◀

●**93297** Interrogation device evaluation(s), (remote) up to 30 days; implantable cardiovascular monitor system, including analysis of 1 or more recorded physiologic cardiovascular data elements from all internal and external sensors, physician analysis, review(s) and report(s)

▶(For heart rhythm derived data elements, use 93295)◀

▶(Do not report 93297 in conjunction with 93290, 93298)◀

▶(Report 93297 only once per 30 days)◀

●**93298** implantable loop recorder system, including analysis of recorded heart rhythm data, physician analysis, review(s) and report(s)

▶(Do not report 93298 in conjunction with 33282, 93291, 93297)◀

▶(Report 93298 only once per 30 days)◀

●**93299** implantable cardiovascular monitor system or implantable loop recorder system, remote data acquisition(s), receipt of transmissions and technician review, technical support and distribution of results

▶(Do not report 93299 in conjunction with 93290, 93291, 93296)◀

▶(Report 93299 only once per 30 days)◀

Rationale

In an effort to bring the CPT codebook up to date with current cardiac device monitoring practices, two sections in the Medicine/Cardiovascular section were updated for 2009. In the first section, Cardiography, new guidelines and two new codes were established, and 15 codes were revised. The second section, Noninvasive Physiologic Studies and Procedures, was restructured with the addition of a new subheading and guidelines, deletion of 11 codes, and establishment of 21 codes.

In the Cardiography section, the new guidelines define cardiovascular monitoring services, attended surveillance, and mobile cardiovascular telemetry (MCT). The guidelines also explain that ECG rhythm-derived elements are distinct from physiologic data, even if the same device is capable of producing both types of data. This is stressed in the new guidelines because implantable cardiovascular monitor (ICM) devices are to be reported separately from implantable cardioverter defibrillator (ICD) services. The guidelines also direct users to code 93745 for other services related to a wearable defibrillator. Modifier 51 should not be used in conjunction with codes 93000-93229, which is also noted in the guidelines.

In the Cardiography section, codes 93228 and 93229 were established to report wearable rhythm-derived cardiovascular telemetry. Code 93228 describes the physician review and interpretation with report. Two parenthetical notes were added following code 93228. One note instructs users that code 93228 is only reported once per 30 days. The second parenthetical note directs users not to report code 93228 in conjunction with code 93014. Code 93229 describes the technical support for connection and patient instructions for use, attended surveillance, analysis and physician's prescribed transmission of daily and emergent data reports. Three new parenthetical notes follow code 93229. The first note instructs users that code 93229 is only reported once per 30 days. The second note indicates that 93229 should not be reported with code 93014. The third note indicates that codes 93224-93272 should be reported for wearable cardiovascular monitors that do not perform automatic ECG triggered transmissions sent to attended surveillance centers.

Codes 93224-93237 and 93268-93272 were revised to specify wearable electrocardiography rhythm-derived monitoring. A parenthetical note was added following code 93237 referring users to codes 93228 and 93229 for wearable mobile telemetry with ECG-triggered transmissions to an attended surveillance center.

In the Noninvasive Physiologic Studies and Procedures section, codes 93727-93736 and 93741-93744 were deleted and replaced with 21 new codes. The new codes provide a mechanism that more accurately reflects current cardiac device monitoring practices. Throughout the section, parenthetical notes have been added to inform users of which codes should not be reported in conjunction with these new codes. Each code family is based upon the type of service performed and the type of device involved (eg, single lead pacemaker system, implantable cardioverter-defibrillator system, etc).

These new codes were placed within a new subsection of the Noninvasive Physiologic Studies and Procedures section, titled Cardiovascular Device Monitoring-Implantable and Wearable Devices. New guidelines were added to this subsection, which define cardiovascular device monitoring services and provide instructions on the proper reporting of the new cardiac device monitoring codes. The guidelines also provide education on the terminology used in the descriptors of the new codes.

Codes 93279-93285 describe programming device evaluation with iterative adjustment of the device to test the function of the device and select optimal permanent programmed values and includes physician analysis, review, and report.

> **NOTE:** The parenthetical note following code 93285 includes codes 93279-93284. This is a corrected version of the note as shown in the 2009 CPT codebook, which indicates 93279 AND 93284, rather than 93279 through 93284. This correction will be posted to the CPT Web site errata document and will be clarified in the *CPT® Assistant* newsletter.

Codes 93286 and 93287 describe peri-procedural evaluation and programming of the device parameters before or after a surgery, procedure, or test. These codes include physician analysis, review, and report. A parenthetical note has been added following each code instructing users to report the service once before and once after the surgery, procedure, or test when the device evaluation and programming are performed before and after the surgery, procedure, or test.

Codes 93288-93292 describe in-person interrogation device evaluation. These codes include physician analysis, review and report, connection, recording, and disconnection. Codes 93288-93292 are reported per patient encounter.

A parenthetical note following code 93288 instructs users not to report this code with codes 93279-93281, 93286, 93294, or 93296. A parenthetical note following code 93289 refers users to code 93290 for monitoring of physiologic cardiovascular data elements derived from an ICD. A second note following code 93289 instructs users not to report this code with codes 93282-93284, 93287, 93295, or 93296. A parenthetical note following code 93290 refers users to code 93289 for heart rhythm-derived data elements.

Code 93293 was established to report transtelephonic rhythm strip pacemaker evaluation of a single, dual, or multiple lead pacemaker system and includes the recording with and without magnet application, physician analysis, review, and report(s). Code 93293 is reported once per every 90 days. A parenthetical note was added following code 93293 to indicate this. A second note was added to instruct users not to report code 93293 with code 93294. Finally, a third note was added to refer users to codes 93040-93042 for in-person evaluations.

Codes 93294-93296 were established to report remote interrogation device evaluation(s). These codes are reported once per 90 days of interrogation evaluation. Code 93296 describes nonphysician technical services, for example provided in an independent testing facility (IDTF). Parenthetical notes were added following each of these codes indicating this. A parenthetical note was added following code 93294 instructing users not to report this code with codes 93288 or 93293. A parenthetical note was added following code 93295 referring users to code 93297 for remote monitoring of physiologic cardiovascular data elements derived from an ICD.

Codes 93297-93299 are similar to codes 93294-93296, except that they reflect up to 30 days of interrogation evaluation. As such, they are reported once per 30 days, and parenthetical notes were added following each code to indicate this. Code 93299 describes nonphysician technical services, for example provided in an IDTF. A cross-reference was added following 93297 directing users to code 93295 for evaluation of heart rhythm-derived data elements. Exclusionary notes were added following each code instructing users as to which codes should not be reported in conjunction with each service.

NOTE: The parenthetical note following code 93298 includes code 33282. This is a corrected version of the note as shown in the 2009 CPT codebook, which erroneously excludes code 33282 from the note. This correction will be posted to the CPT Web site errata document and will be clarified in the *CPT® Assistant* newsletter.

Clinical Example (93228)

A 52-year-old patient receives a mobile cardiovascular telemetry monitor to investigate severe near syncopal episodes that occur once or twice a month. Electrocardiographic rhythm strips are transmitted to the physician for review, demonstrating atrial fibrillation with a rapid ventricular heart rate and with a 4-second pause correlating with a near syncopal symptom.

This is for all evaluations received for up to a 30-day period.

Description of Procedure (93228)
The information from the mobile cardiovascular telemetry is interrogated by telemetric communication and either printed for review or reviewed on the programmer or computer monitor. Critical review of the interrogated data along with the assessment of the appropriateness of the function of the wearable device and appropriateness of the current programmed parameters, is performed.

Data that are reviewed may include, but are not limited to, electrograms, stored episodes of data, alerts generated from electronic devices, battery voltage and impedance, pacing and shocking lead impedance, sensed electrogram voltage amplitude, histogram, and/or counters of paced and sensed events from each chamber.

Additionally, stored episodes of data are reviewed to assess the history and trends identified by any of the collected data.

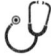 **Clinical Example (93279)**
A 65-year-old woman with chronic atrial fibrillation and complete heart block had a single-chamber, rate-adaptive, ventricular pacemaker implanted 2 years ago. The patient contacted her internist because she had "passed out." The physician has the patient come in for a symptom assessment and a programming device evaluation.

Description of Procedure (93279)
After verbal consent is obtained from the patient to proceed, the patient is connected to a single- or multi-lead free-running electrocardiogram monitor. A communication link is obtained between the pacemaker and the programmer. The current rhythm is assessed and recorded. The magnet mode response is assessed and recorded. An attempt to obtain and record the patient's underlying rhythm is performed. The appropriate safety techniques are given to the patient who is pacemaker-dependent.

A full interrogation of the stored pacemaker data is obtained and reviewed for alert conditions. The current interrogated measurements are compared to the extensive stored and trended data. These data are reviewed for device alerts in regard to battery and lead function including voltage, impedance, and current. Additional measurements are made when necessary to assess the status of the insulation and conductors of the leads. The appropriate lead polarity for sensing and capture parameters are identified. Stored summary and recorded rhythm information are reviewed for evidence of atrial fibrillation, premature ventricular contractions, and nonsustained and sustained ventricular tachycardia. The appropriate rhythm alerts and recording parameters are identified. The pacing capture threshold is measured in a single chamber by varying the voltage output and pulse width in a step-wise fashion to determine the appropriate safety margin for final device parameters and to optimize pacemaker device longevity. The appropriate voltage and pulse width parameters are identified.

The sensing threshold is measured by recording the signal from a single lead and chamber and by iterative (step-wise) adjustment of pacemaker sensing value to determine the appropriate sensing safety margin. The appropriate mode and threshold for sensing is identified. Heart rate adaptation to exercise or physiologic stress data is reviewed and adjusted in an iterative (step-wise) technique. Data considered to select the appropriate final programmed values include multiple heart rate histograms and trended activity levels. When necessary, in-office assessment is completed through the patient's exercise activity to establish adequate heart rate response to exercise. The appropriate rate response parameters are identified.

After detailed analysis of each of the above parameters, a decision is made about the adequacy of the initial programmed pacemaker parameters and any identified changes that need to be made to optimize the device performance relative to the patient's clinical condition. These device programming changes are made, and any additional recommendations for further cardiac evaluation or treatment are given.

Clinical Example (93280)

A 70-year-old male with acquired complete heart block had a dual-chamber pacemaker implanted 5 years ago. The patient calls his general cardiologist concerned about increasing "shortness of breath" and some "palpitations." The cardiologist orders a programming device evaluation.

Description of Procedure (93280)

After obtaining verbal consent from the patient to proceed, the patient is connected to a single- or multi-lead free-running electrocardiogram monitor. A communication link is obtained between the pacemaker and the programmer. The current rhythm is assessed and recorded. The magnet mode response is assessed and recorded. An attempt to obtain and record the patient's underlying rhythm is performed with appropriate safety considerations given to the patient who is pacemaker dependent.

A full interrogation of the stored pacemaker data is obtained and reviewed for alert conditions. Current interrogated measurements are compared to the extensive stored data. Trended data is reviewed for device alerts in regard to battery and lead function, including voltage, impedance, and current. Additional measurements are made when necessary to assess the status of the insulation and conductors of the leads. The appropriate lead polarity for sensing and capture parameters are identified. Stored summary and recorded rhythm information is reviewed for evidence of atrial fibrillation, premature ventricular contractions, and nonsustained and sustained ventricular tachycardia. The appropriate rhythm alerts and recording parameters are identified.

The pacing capture threshold is measured in a single chamber by varying the voltage output and pulse width in a step-wise fashion to determine the appropriate safety margin for final device parameters and to optimize pacemaker device longevity. The appropriate voltage and pulse width parameters are identified. The sensing threshold is measured by recording the signal from a single lead and chamber and by iterative (step-wise) adjustment of pacemaker sensing value to determine the appropriate sensing safety margin. The appropriate mode and threshold for sensing is identified. Heart rate adaptation to exercise or physiologic stress data is reviewed and adjusted in an iterative (step-wise) technique. Data considered to select the appropriate final programmed values include multiple heart rate histograms and trended activity levels. When necessary, in-office assessment is completed through patient exercise activity to establish adequate heart rate response to exercise. The appropriate rate response parameters are identified.

After the detailed analysis of each of the above parameters, a decision is made about the adequacy of the initial programmed pacemaker parameters and any identified changes which need to be made to optimize the device performance relative to the patient's clinical condition. These device programming changes are made and any additional recommendations for further cardiac evaluation or treatment are given.

Clinical Example (93281)

A 75-year-old male with nonischemic cardiomyopathy, left ventricular ejection fraction of 35%, sinus rhythm, and QRS duration of 160 ms had a biventricular pacemaker implanted for treatment of moderately severe heart failure symptoms. The patient returns for a programming device evaluation of his pacemaker and lead function 1 year after his last programming device evaluation.

Description of Procedure (93281)

After verbal consent is obtained from the patient to proceed, the patient is connected to a single- or multi-lead free-running electrocardiogram monitor. A communication link is obtained between the pacemaker and the programmer. The current rhythm is assessed and recorded. The magnet mode response is assessed and recorded. An attempt to obtain and record the patient's underlying rhythm is performed with appropriate safety considerations given to the patient who is pacemaker dependent.

A full interrogation of the stored pacemaker data is obtained and results are reviewed for alert conditions. The current interrogated measurements are compared to the extensive stored data. Trended data are reviewed for device alerts with regard to battery and lead function, including voltage, impedance, and current. Additional measurements are made when necessary to assess the status of the insulation and lead conductors. The appropriate lead polarity for sensing and capture parameters are identified. Appropriate sensing of chamber-specific electrical activity and adjustment of pacemaker device parameters to accommodate for interim changes in the patient's status are performed. Stored summary and recorded rhythm information is reviewed for evidence of atrial fibrillation, premature ventricular contractions, and nonsustained and sustained ventricular tachycardia. The appropriate rhythm alerts and recording parameters are identified.

The pacing capture threshold is measured separately in three or more chambers (usually right atrium, right ventricle, and left ventricle) by varying the voltage output and pulse width in a step-wise fashion to determine the appropriate safety margin for final device parameters and to optimize pacemaker device longevity. Care is taken to appropriately identify the capture of the ventricular chamber of interest (right, left, or both) to avoid incorrect conclusions about capture safety margins. The appropriate voltage and pulse width parameters are identified. The sensing threshold is measured separately in both chambers (usually right atrium and right ventricle) by recording the signal from each lead and chamber and by iterative (step-wise) adjustment of the pacemaker sensing value to determine the appropriate sensing safety margin. The appropriate mode and threshold for sensing are identified. Influence of the stimulation of one chamber on the sensing and activation of the other chamber is evaluated for atrial to right and left ventricular, ventricular to atrial, right ventricle to left ventricle, and left ventricle to right ventricle conduction; cross-talk sensing between the chambers; and far-field electrogram detection. The potential influence of these issues for permanent programming is identified.

Anodal right ventricular stimulation during left ventricular pacing is assessed, and the presence or absence of phrenic nerve (diaphragmatic) stimulation in regard to pacing output and pacing polarity configuration is identified for permanent programming. Iterative (step-wise) programming of arteriovenous interval timing, whether fixed or dynamic, and determination of its influence on the percentage of ventricular pacing and hemodynamics or limitation of heart rate response are completed. Heart rate adaptation to exercise or physiologic stress data are reviewed and adjusted using an iterative (step-wise) technique. Data considered to select the appropriate final programmed values include multiple heart rate histograms and trended activity levels. When necessary, in-office assessment is completed through patient's exercise activity to establish adequate heart rate response to exercise. The appropriate rate response parameters are identified.

After detailed analysis of each of the above parameters, a decision is made about the adequacy of the initial programmed pacemaker parameters and any identified changes that need to be made to optimize the device performance relative to the patient's clinical condition. These device programming changes are made, and any additional recommendations for further cardiac evaluation or treatment are given.

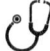

Clinical Example (93282)
A 65-year-old woman with sinus rhythm and an ischemic cardiomyopathy with a left ventricular ejection fraction of 30% had a single-chamber implantable cardioverter-defibrillator (VVI ICD) implanted. The patient tells her cardiologist that she "fainted" without palpitations, warning, or feeling a shock. The cardiologist requests a programming device evaluation.

Description of Procedure (93282)
After verbal consent from the patient is obtained, the patient is connected to a single- or multi-lead electrocardiogram recording system. A communication link is established between the device and the programmer.

A full interrogation of the stored device parameters is obtained. The current rhythm is assessed and recorded. The stored pacing and tachyarrhythmia episode data are retrieved, and detailed physician analysis of these data are performed.

The stored summary and recorded rhythm data are reviewed. Pacing capture threshold data and lead impedance are measured within the ventricular chamber. Based on this information, the physician identifies any pacing or integrity issues with the existing lead and determines the appropriate pacing output settings. Sensing threshold data are obtained by recording the signal from the ventricular chamber and utilizing iterative (step-wise) adjustment of ICD sensing level. Based on this information, the physician identifies the appropriate ICD sensing settings. Ventricular stimulation and the presence or absence of phrenic nerve (diaphragmatic) stimulation are assessed in regard to pacing output and pacing polarity configuration is made.

After detailed analysis of the data, a decision is made regarding the appropriateness of the initial programmed pacing and anti-tachycardia parameters and therapies relative to the patient's clinical status. If indicated, the device's programming is altered at this time.

Clinical Example (93283)

A 70-year-old male with intermittent complete heart block had an implantable defibrillator with dual-chamber pacemaker capacity (DDD ICD) implanted. The patient had an interrogation device evaluation (remote) that noted a marked elevation of shocking impedance. The ICD clinic contacted the patient to assess his current symptoms and to urge him to come to the ICD clinic for a programming device evaluation.

Description of Procedure (93283)

After verbal consent from the patient to proceed is obtained, the patient is connected to a single- or multi-lead electrocardiogram recording system. A communication link is established between the device and the programmer.

A full interrogation of the stored device parameters is obtained. The current rhythm is assessed and recorded to include the differentiation between the presence of an underlying native rhythm (if present). Stored pacing and tachyarrhythmia episode data are retrieved, and detailed physician analysis of these data is performed. The stored summary and recorded rhythm data are reviewed for evidence of interval arrhythmias. The pacing capture threshold data and lead impedance are measured separately in both chambers (usually the right atrium and ventricle). Based on this information, the physician identifies any pacing or integrity issues within the existing leads and determines the appropriate pacing output settings (voltage, pulse width duration) individually for each chamber. The sensing threshold data are obtained in each chamber by recording the signal from the atrial and the ventricular chambers individually. Influence of the stimulation of one chamber on the sensing and activation of the other chambers (cross talk) is evaluated. Atrial and ventricular stimulation individually in each chamber is assessed to confirm the presence or absence of phrenic nerve (diaphragmatic) stimulation.

Iterative programming of the arteriovenous interval timing, whether fixed or dynamic, is completed. The heart rate adaptation to exercise or physiologic stress data are reviewed and adjustments are made in an iterative fashion. Based on this information, the physician identifies the appropriate ICD sensing settings to allow for appropriate sensing safety margins.

After a detailed analysis of the data, a decision is made regarding the appropriateness of the initial programmed pacing and anti-tachycardia parameters. The therapies relative to the patient's clinical status are evaluated, and, if indicated, alteration in the device's programming is performed at this time.

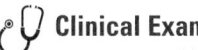 **Clinical Example (93284)**

A 68-year-old male with an ischemic cardiomyopathy, left ventricular ejection fraction of 35%, NYHA FC III heart failure symptoms, and a complete left bundle branch block had an implantable cardioverter-defibrillator (ICD) with biventricular pacemaker stimulation implanted. The patient returns to the ICD clinic for a programming device evaluation 6 months later because, although the patient initially improved, he is now feeling more "short of breath."

Description of Procedure (93284)

After the patient provides verbal consent to proceed, he is connected to a single- or multi-lead electrocardiogram recording system. A communication link is established between the device and the programmer.

A full interrogation of the stored device parameters is obtained and reviewed. The current rhythm is assessed and recorded to include the differentiation between the presence of an underlying native rhythm (if present) in each chamber. Stored pacing and tachyarrhythmia episode data are retrieved. Detailed physician analysis of these data is performed. The stored summary and recorded rhythm data are reviewed for evidence of interval arrhythmias. Pacing capture threshold data and lead impedance are measured separately in all chambers (usually the right atrium and ventricle and the left ventricle).

Based on this information, the physician identifies any pacing or integrity issues within the existing leads and determines the appropriate pacing output settings (voltage, pulse width duration) individually for each chamber.

The sensing threshold data are obtained in each chamber by recording the signal from atrial (sensed P waves) and ventricular (sensed R waves) activity, if present. Influence of the stimulation of one chamber on the sensing and activation of the other chambers (cross talk) is evaluated.

Atrial and ventricular stimulation individually in each chamber is assessed to confirm the presence or absence of phrenic nerve (diaphragmatic) stimulation in regard to pacing output and pacing polarity configuration. Iterative programming of the arteriovenous interval timing, whether fixed or dynamic, and its influence on the percentage of ventricular pacing and hemodynamics or limitation of heart rate response is completed. Heart rate adaptation to exercise or physiologic stress data are reviewed and adjusted in an iterative fashion.

After detailed analysis of the data, a decision is made regarding the appropriateness of the initial programmed pacing and anti-tachycardia parameters. The therapies relative to the patient's clinical status are evaluated, and, if indicated, alteration in the device's programming is performed at this time.

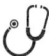 **Clinical Example (93285)**

A 52-year-old male with coronary artery disease and diabetes who received an implantable loop recorder (ILR) implant 2 months ago presents for in-office device evaluation of near syncope and palpitations and adjustment of his rhythm detection parameters with a programming device evaluation.

Description of Procedure (93285)

After verbal consent from the patient is obtained, a communication link is created between the ILR and the programmer. Programmed parameters are obtained. Stored ILR data are obtained and downloaded for physician review.

A full interrogation of the stored ILR data is obtained and reviewed for alert conditions. The current interrogated measurements are compared to the extensive stored and trended data and reviewed for device alerts with regard to battery function, including voltage and impedance. The underlying signal strength is assessed. The sensing threshold is measured by recording the signal from the ILR and by iterative (step-wise) adjustment of the sensing value to determine the appropriate sensing safety margin. The appropriate threshold for sensing is identified. The sensing and gain parameters are programmed as appropriate to ensure optimal device sensing.

The patient-activated recorded rhythm episodes are reviewed for evidence of tachycardia, bradycardia, and cardiac rhythm pauses. Specific rhythm waveforms are downloaded and reviewed for atrial fibrillation, premature atrial contractions (PACs), supraventricular tachycardia (SVT), premature ventricular contractions (PVCs), nonsustained ventricular tachycardia, sustained ventricular tachycardia, sinus pauses, evidence of cardiac arteriovenous (AV) block, and recording system artifact. The appropriate rhythm alerts and recording parameters are identified.

The automatically recorded rhythm episodes (based on previously programmed detection parameters) are reviewed for evidence of tachycardia, bradycardia, and cardiac rhythm pauses. Specific rhythm waveforms are downloaded and reviewed for atrial fibrillation, PACs, SVT, PVCs, nonsustained ventricular tachycardia, sustained ventricular tachycardia, sinus pauses, evidence of cardiac AV block, and recording system artifact. The appropriate rhythm alerts and recording parameters are identified. Parameters describing the criteria for automatic rhythm detection are reviewed for appropriateness and programmed for optimal rhythm detection. Parameters describing the device memory capacity as well as the recording capacity of the number of patient-activated and automatically detected episodes are reviewed. The amount of pre- and post-detection electrocardiographic recording time is assessed. Programmed changes to these values are made as appropriate to optimize ILR recording function.

After detailed analysis of each of the above parameters, a decision is made about the adequacy of the initial programmed ILR parameters and any identified changes that need to be made to optimize the device performance relative to the patient's clinical condition. These device programming changes are made, and any additional recommendations for further cardiac evaluation or treatment are given.

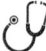

Clinical Example (93286)

A 65-year-old woman with chronic atrial fibrillation and complete heart block had a single-chamber, rate-adaptive, ventricular pacemaker implanted. The patient requires a contralateral breast mastectomy with electrosurgical cautery. To avoid pacemaker-induced heart rate increases or inhibition during the surgery, the surgeon requests evaluation and programming of the pacemaker sensor and settings to prepare the patient for the surgery. After the surgery, the surgeon requests a reevaluation of the pacemaker system with appropriate adjustment of the device to permit full activity of the patient.

Description of Procedure (93286)
After obtaining verbal consent from the patient to proceed, a communication link is obtained between the pacemaker and the programmer. The doctor-specified parameter(s) is changed and device reinterrogation completed to confirm programming. The patient's stability is assessed after the pre-procedural (test, surgery) programming. The patient is informed about temporary changes that have been made and the expected timing of post-procedure (test, surgery) restoration to baseline settings. An initial note is placed in the patient's chart documenting the temporary changes.

After intervention (test, surgery), an interim history is obtained and the appropriateness of returning the pacemaker to the original programmed settings is determined. After obtaining verbal consent from the patient to proceed, a communication link is obtained between the pacemaker and the programmer. The doctor-specified parameter(s) is changed and device reinterrogation completed to confirm programming. The patient's stability is assessed after the post-procedural (test, surgery) programming. The patient is informed about the permanent changes (restoration of programming) that have been made and the expected timing of their next pacemaker evaluation. A second note is placed in the patient's chart documenting the changes.

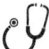

Clinical Example (93287)
A 67-year-old woman with chronic atrial fibrillation and complete heart block had a single-chamber implantable cardioverter-defibrillator (ICD) with rate adaptive ventricular pacemaker function (VVIR ICD) implanted. The patient requires an abdominal aortic aneurysm surgery. To avoid ICD shocks during the surgery related to electrosurgical cautery and manipulation, the surgeon requests evaluation and programming of the ICD to prepare the patient for the surgery. After the surgery, the surgeon requests a reevaluation of the ICD system in the intensive care unit with appropriate adjustment of the device to permit full protection of the patient from bradycardia and tachycardia events.

The reevaluation is reported separately from the initial evaluation.

Description of Procedure (93287)
After verbal consent from the patient to proceed is obtained, a communication link is established between the device and the programmer. The doctor-specified changes in the device's programmed pacing are made, anti-tachycardia parameters based upon the pre-procedural evaluation are performed, and the device reinterrogated to confirm programming changes. The changes made to the device, including expected timing of post-procedure restoration or reprogramming of settings, are explained to the patient. An initial report documenting the device issues and the changes made prior to the procedure is placed in the patient's chart.

After intervention (test, surgery), stability of the patient is assessed. An interim history is obtained, and the appropriateness of returning the device to its original settings is determined. After verbal consent is obtained from the patient to proceed, a communication link is established between the ICD and the programmer. Physician-specified changes in the device programming are made and the device is interrogated to confirm programming. Stability of the patient is assessed. The patient is informed of any changes or restoration of the original programmed settings. A second report is placed in the patient's chart.

Clinical Example (93288)

A 74-year-old patient with a pacemaker for sick sinus syndrome and congestive heart failure is followed with interrogation device evaluations (in person) for lightheadedness and dyspnea.

Description of Procedure (93288)

The information from the pacemaker is interrogated by telemetric communication and either printed for review or reviewed on the programmer or computer monitor. Critical review of the interrogated data with assessment of normal pacemaker function and safety of the current programmed parameters are completed.

Data from an electrogram for appropriateness or presence of arrhythmia and appropriate sensing and capture are reviewed. The stored episodes of data are reviewed for appropriate sensing, capture, magnet reversion, and noise reversions.

Alerts generated from the pacemaker device are reviewed, if required. Battery voltage and impedance, pacing lead impedance, and sensed electrogram voltage amplitude for each lead are reviewed. Counts of paced and sensed events from each chamber for which there are leads located are provided for review. The stored episodes of sensed events including arrhythmias, ectopic beats, nonsustained and sustained atrial and ventricular arrhythmias, and, when appropriate, mode switch episodes are evaluated. The frequency, rate, and duration are noted for heart rate response during activities, rate histograms, and indicators of patient activity level.

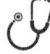

Clinical Example (93289)

A 74-year-old patient with a pacemaker for sick sinus syndrome and congestive heart failure is followed with interrogation device evaluations (in person) for lightheadedness and dyspnea.

Description of Procedure (93289)

The information from the pacemaker is interrogated by telemetric communication and either printed for review or reviewed on the programmer or computer monitor. The interrogated data are critically reviewed in order to assess the appropriateness of the pacemaker's function and the safety of the current programmed parameters and to determine if device function is normal.

The data reviewed includes the presenting electrogram for appropriateness or presence of arrhythmia and appropriate sensing and capture; stored episodes of data for appropriate sensing, capture, magnet reversion, and noise reversions; alerts generated from the pacemaker device; battery voltage and impedance, pacing lead impedance, and sensed electrogram voltage amplitude for each lead; counters of paced and sensed events from each chamber for which there are leads located; stored episodes of sensed events including arrhythmias, ectopic beats, nonsustained and sustained atrial and ventricular arrhythmias, and, when appropriate, mode switch episodes, with the frequency, rate, and duration noted; and the heart rate response during activities, rate histograms, and indicators of patient activity level.

Clinical Example (93290)

A 58-year-old patient with prior myocardial infarction, ventricular tachycardia, and congestive heart failure had an implantable cardioverter-defibrillator system that monitors physiologic cardiovascular data in addition to the heart rhythm implanted. The patient has ongoing dyspnea, orthopnea, and peripheral edema and is evaluated in the heart failure clinic with interrogation device evaluations (in person).

Description of Procedure (93290)
The information from the implantable cardiovascular monitor (ICM) is interrogated by telemetric communication and either printed for review or reviewed on the programmer or computer monitor. The interrogated data, with assessment of the appropriateness of the function of the ICM and appropriateness of the current programmed parameters, are critically reviewed.

Data reviewed may include, but are not limited to, (1) weight; (2) systemic blood pressure; (3) right atrial, right ventricular, left atrial, left ventricular, pulmonary arterial pressures; (4) intra-thoracic impedance measurements; and (5) other measures of physiologic parameters.

Additionally, stored episodes of data are reviewed to assess the history and trends identified by any of the collected data. Further, alerts generated from the ICM are reviewed along with battery voltage and sensor information to validate the integrity of the ICM system.

Clinical Example (93291)

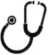

A 41-year-old patient receives an implantable loop recorder (ILR) for recurrent syncopal spells. The patient has a syncopal episode resulting in a laceration to the head. The patient comes in for an interrogation device evaluation (in person).

Description of Procedure (93291)
Verbal consent from the patient to proceed is obtained. A communication link is created between the ILR and the programmer. Programmed parameters are obtained. Stored ILR data are obtained and downloaded for physician review.

A full interrogation of the stored ILR data is obtained and reviewed for alert conditions. The current interrogated measurements are compared to the extensive stored and trended data and reviewed for device alerts with regard to battery function, including voltage and impedance. The underlying signal strength is assessed. If sensing is inadequate, instructions are given to the patient for further follow-up and potential reprogramming. Patient-activated recorded rhythm episodes are reviewed for evidence of tachycardia, bradycardia, and cardiac rhythm pauses. Specific rhythm waveforms are downloaded and reviewed for atrial fibrillation, premature atrial contractions (PACs), supraventricular tachycardia (SVT), premature ventricular contractions (PVCs), nonsustained ventricular tachycardia, sustained ventricular tachycardia, sinus pauses, evidence of cardiac arteriovenous (AV) block, and recording system artifact. The appropriate rhythm alerts and recording parameters are identified. Automatically recorded rhythm episodes (based on previously programmed detection parameters) are reviewed for evidence of tachycardia, bradycardia, and cardiac rhythm pauses. Specific rhythm waveforms are downloaded and reviewed for atrial fibrillation, PACs, SVT, PVCs, nonsustained ventricular tachycardia, sustained ventricular tachycardia, sinus pauses, evidence of cardiac AV block, and recording system artifact. The appropriate rhythm alerts and recording parameters are identified. Parameters describing the criteria for automatic rhythm detect are reviewed for appropriateness. Parameters describing the device memory capacity and the recording capacity of the number of patient-activated and automatically detected episodes are reviewed. The amount of pre- and post-detection electrocardiographic recording time is assessed.

After detailed physician analysis of each of the above parameters, recommendations for further cardiac evaluation or treatment are given.

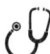

Clinical Example (93292)

A 66-year-old patient with a history of sustained ventricular tachycardia treated with an implantable cardioverter-defibrillator (ICD) requires ICD and lead extraction and intravenous antibiotics for 3 months because of a bacterial infection with intracardiac vegetations before an ICD can be reimplanted. The patient returns 1 month later with her wearable cardioverter-defibrillator for interrogation device evaluation (in person).

Description of Procedure (93292)

The information from the wearable device is interrogated by telemetric communication and either printed for review or reviewed on the programmer or computer monitor. The interrogated data, with assessment of the appropriateness of the wearable device's function and appropriateness of the current programmed parameters, are critically reviewed.

The data reviewed may include, but are not limited to, presenting electrograms; stored episodes of data; alerts generated from the device; battery voltage and impedance; pacing and shocking lead impedance and sensed electrogram voltage amplitude; and histogram and/or counters of paced and sensed events from each chamber. Stored episodes of sensed arrhythmia events including the type, frequency, rate, and duration are noted.

Heart rate response during activities, rate histograms, and indicators of patient activity level are evaluated. A rhythm strip is recorded for 30 seconds and evaluated for heart rate and capture, sensing of each lead, and for atrial or ventricular arrhythmias. A second rhythm strip may be recorded, with a magnet located over the device, and evaluated for capture and sensing of each lead for atrial or ventricular arrhythmias, and the magnet response including paced rate. Physician review of these data produces an assessment of the adequacy of each lead's sensing and capture and of battery function. Additionally, stored episodes of data are reviewed to assess the history and trends identified by any of the collected data.

Clinical Example (93293)

A 69-year-old patient with complete heart block has a 6-year-old dual-chamber pacemaker that is being monitored for battery depletion with transtelephonic rhythm strip pacemaker evaluations.

Description of Procedure (93293)

A TA rhythm strip is recorded for 30 seconds and evaluated for heart rate and capture, sensing of each lead, and for atrial or ventricular arrhythmias. A second rhythm strip is recorded, with a magnet located over the pacemaker, and evaluated for capture and sensing of each lead, for atrial or ventricular arrhythmias, and for the magnet response including paced rate. Physician review of these data produces an assessment of the adequacy of each lead's sensing and capture and of battery function.

The technician receives the rhythm strip data with a second rhythm strip after application of a magnet to the pacemaker. The technician reviews the rhythm strips for sensing, capture, and intrinsic and paced heart rates. The parameters are reviewed and analyzed by the technician.

If presented to the technician, he/she documents any patient symptoms that are patient-reported during the interrogation. The technician reports to the physician on any parameters that are designated by the physician. The technician enters findings into the monitoring center or local independent diagnostic testing facility's database. The technician validates function by assessing if the lead data and arrhythmia events are normal or abnormal. After the data are entered and evaluated, the technician generates a comprehensive report of all evaluated parameters, which is then delivered to the physician. The physician reviews the data and confirms the function of each lead, the battery, capture, and sensing. An assessment is made of the adequacy of the function and the time interval to the next analysis as well as the type of device evaluation that should be done at that time.

Clinical Example (93294)

A 74-year-old patient with a pacemaker for sick sinus syndrome and congestive heart failure is followed with interrogation device evaluations (remote) of the pacemaker from the patient's home. The patient has intermittent brief palpitations and light-headedness.

Description of Procedure (93294)

The information from the pacemaker is interrogated by telemetric communication and either printed for review or reviewed on the programmer or computer monitor. The interrogated data are critically reviewed to with assessment of the appropriateness of the pacemaker's function and safety of the current programmed parameters and to assess if the device function is normal.

The data reviewed include the presenting electrogram for appropriateness or presence of arrhythmia and appropriate sensing and capture; stored episodes of data for appropriate sensing, capture, appropriate magnet reversion, and noise reversions; alerts generated from the pacemaker device; battery voltage and impedance, pacing lead impedance, and sensed electrogram voltage amplitude for each lead; and counters of paced and sensed events from each chamber for which there are leads located. Stored episodes of sensed events including arrhythmias, ectopic beats, nonsustained and sustained atrial and ventricular arrhythmias, and, when appropriate, mode switch episodes, frequency, rate, and duration are noted. Heart rate response during activities, rate histograms, and indicators of patient activity level are evaluated.

Clinical Example (93295)

A 66-year-old patient with a history of sustained ventricular tachycardia treated with an implantable cardioverter-defibrillator (ICD) is followed with interrogation device evaluations (remote) of the ICD from the patient's home. The patient has dyspnea on exertion and intermittent palpitations with light-headedness.

Description of Procedure (93295)

The information from the ICD is interrogated by telemetric communication and either printed for review or reviewed on the programmer or computer monitor. The interrogated data, with assessment of the appropriateness of the function of ICD, safety of the current programmed pacing, and anti-tachycardia parameters and assessment of device function, is critically assessed.

The data reviewed include the presenting electrograms for appropriateness of pacing and sensing; stored episodes of data; alerts generated from the device; battery voltage and impedance; pacing and shocking lead impedance; and sensed electrogram voltage amplitude for each lead. Histogram and/or counters of paced and sensed events from each chamber and stored episodes of sensed arrhythmia events including the type, frequency, rate, and duration are noted. Adequacy of heart rate response is evaluated.

Clinical Example (93296)

A 66-year-old patient with a history of sustained ventricular tachycardia treated with an implantable cardioverter-defibrillator (ICD) is followed with interrogation device evaluations (remote) of the ICD from the patient's home. The patient has dyspnea on exertion and intermittent palpitations with light-headedness.

This is for all evaluations received within a 90-day period.

Description of Procedure (93296)

Remote ICD device evaluation includes monitoring of all programmed parameters, leads, battery, capture and sensing function, presence or absence of therapy for ventricular tachyarrhythmias and underlying heart rhythm. Based on the physician's order, a patient with an ICD is registered for remote interrogation at a monitoring facility. The monitoring facility delivers the equipment to the patient with instructions for connection to the telephone system. The provider provides additional telephone support to help the patient complete the connections. The provider establishes a schedule for device interrogations based on the physician's order.

The interrogated data is assembled and sent to the provider by an electrodiagnostic technician. It is then reviewed by the nurse for device alerts and is compared to the physician-directed parameters for communication to the patient's physician. The interrogated data are both scheduled and triggered by the patient and/or device alarm-initiated episodes.

The technician receives data through the device information system and inputs that data into the provider's database. The technician then reviews all of the data generated from the system (20-65 pages, depending on the number of episodes). The data is then incorporated into the provider's system. The parameters are reviewed and analyzed by the technician and, if present, patient symptoms are documented. The technician reports to the physician if any parameters designated by the physician are exceeded. The technician enters findings into the provider's database and validates function by assessing if the lead data and arrhythmia events are normal or abnormal. After data is entered and evaluated, the technician generates a comprehensive report of all evaluated parameters, which is then delivered to the physician.

There is an average of 1.25 events per patient per quarter.

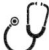

Clinical Example (93297)

A 58-year-old patient with prior myocardial infarction, ventricular tachycardia, and congestive heart failure has an implantable cardioverter-defibrillator system that monitors physiologic cardiovascular data in addition to the heart rhythm. The patient is followed with interrogation device evaluations (remote). The patient has NYHA FC III heart failure symptoms. The physiologic cardiovascular data are transmitted from the patient's home to the remote surveillance database.

This is for all evaluations received within a 30-day period.

Description of Procedure (93297)

The information from the implantable cardiovascular monitor (ICM) is interrogated by telemetric communication and either printed for review or reviewed on the programmer or computer monitor. The interrogated data, with assessment of the appropriateness of the function of the ICM and appropriateness of the current programmed parameters, is critically reviewed.

Data reviewed may include, but are not limited to, (1) weight; (2) systemic blood pressure; (3) right atrial, right ventricular, left atrial, left ventricular, pulmonary arterial pressures; (4) intra-thoracic impedance measurements; and (5) other measures of physiologic parameters.

Additionally, stored episodes of data are reviewed to assess the history and trends identified by any of the collected data. Further, alerts generated from the ICM are reviewed along with battery voltage and sensor information to validate the integrity of the ICM system.

Clinical Example (93298)

A 41-year-old patient receives an implantable loop recorder (ILR) for recurrent syncopal spells. The patient is followed with interrogation device evaluations (remote) for light-headed but non-syncopal episodes.

This is for all evaluations received within a 30-day period.

Description of Procedure (93298)

Verbal consent from the patient to proceed is obtained. A communication link is created between the ILR and the programmer. Programmed parameters are obtained. Stored ILR data are obtained and downloaded for physician review.

A full interrogation of the stored ILR data is obtained and reviewed for alert conditions. The current interrogated measurements are compared to the extensive stored and trended data and reviewed for device alerts with regard to battery function, including voltage and impedance. The underlying signal strength is assessed. Sensing threshold is measured by recording the signal from the ILR and by iterative (step-wise) adjustment of the sensing value to determine the appropriate sensing safety margin. The appropriate threshold for sensing is identified. The sensing and gain parameters are programmed as appropriate to ensure optimal device sensing. Patient-activated recorded rhythm episodes are reviewed for evidence of tachycardia, bradycardia, and cardiac rhythm pauses. Specific rhythm waveforms are downloaded and reviewed for atrial fibrillation, premature atrial contractions (PACs), supraventricular tachycardia (SVT), premature ventricular contractions (PVCs), non-sustained ventricular tachycardia, sustained ventricular tachycardia, sinus pauses, evidence of cardiac arteriovenous (AV) block, and recording system artifact. The appropriate rhythm alerts and recording parameters are identified. Automatically recorded rhythm episodes (based on previously programmed detection parameters) are reviewed for evidence of tachycardia, bradycardia, and cardiac rhythm pauses. Specific rhythm waveforms are downloaded and reviewed for atrial fibrillation, PACs, SVT, PVCs, non-sustained ventricular tachycardia, sustained ventricular tachycardia, sinus pauses, evidence of cardiac AV block, and recording system artifact. The appropriate rhythm alerts and recording parameters are identified. Parameters describing the criteria for automatic rhythm detection are reviewed for appropriateness and programmed for optimal rhythm detection. Parameters describing the device memory capacity and the recording capacity of the number of patient-activated and automatically detected episodes are reviewed. The amount of pre- and post-detection electrocardiographic recording time is assessed. Programmed changes to these values are made as appropriate to optimize ILR recording function.

After the physician performs a detailed analysis of each parameter, a decision is made about the adequacy of the initial programmed ILR parameters and any identified changes that need to be made to optimize the device performance relative to the patient's clinical condition. These device programming changes are made and any additional recommendations for further cardiac evaluation or treatment are given.

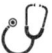 **Clinical Example (93299)**

A 58-year-old patient with prior myocardial infarction, ventricular tachycardia, and congestive heart failure has an implantable cardioverter-defibrillator system that monitors physiologic cardiovascular data in addition to the heart rhythm. The patient is followed with interrogation device evaluations (remote). The patient has NYHA FC III heart failure symptoms. The physiologic cardiovascular data are transmitted from the patient's home to the remote surveillance database.

This is for all evaluations received within a 30-day period.

Description of Procedure (93299)

An implantable loop recorder (ILR) is an implantable device that continuously records ECG rhythm triggered automatically by rapid and slow heart rates or by the patient during a symptomatic episode. It is designed to detect transient symptoms, most significantly syncope, which may not be detected by other types of cardiac monitoring. After implantation, the ECG segments data is automatically stored for those episodes when the R-R interval falls outside of predetermined limits. The patient can also trigger storage, when symptoms are experienced.

A patient with an ILR is referred by the physician to the testing facility for round-the-clock ECG monitoring. The facility enrolls the patient and educates the patient on the use of the service. An assessment of the underlying signal strength is made and if sensing is inadequate, instructions are given to the patient for further follow-up and potential reprogramming. The facility furnishing this service transmits the data via modem. Interrogated ECG data is transmitted to the monitoring center, which includes automatically recorded (trending samples) rhythm episodes (based on previously programmed detection parameters) as well as patient-activated rhythm (symptomatic and asymptomatic transmissions) episodes, are reviewed by the electrodiagnostic technician (a certified cardiographic technician) for device alerts, and compared to physician directed parameters for possible communication to the physician if the criteria is met. The interrogated data is transmitted to the physician for review with the frequency of delivery determined by the physician based upon the patient's condition. An average of 6 trending samples are transmitted each day (ie, every four hours) in addition to an average of 300 asymptomatic transmissions per month and approximately 4 symptomatic transmissions generated by the patient. This data is compiled into a monthly report and distributed to the physician.

Echocardiography

Echocardiography includes obtaining ultrasonic signals from the heart and great ▶vessels, with real time◀ image and/or Doppler ultrasonic signal documentation, ▶with◀ interpretation and report. When interpretation is performed separately, use modifier 26.

A complete transthoracic echocardiogram ▶without spectral or color flow Doppler◀ (93307) is a comprehensive procedure that includes 2-dimensional and selected M-mode examination of the left and right atria, left and right ventricles, the aortic, mitral, and tricuspid valves, the pericardium, and adjacent portions of the aorta. ▶Multiple views are required to obtain a complete functional and anatomic evaluation, and appropriate measurements are obtained and recorded.◀ Despite significant effort, identification and measurement of some structures may not always be possible. In such instances, the reason that an element could not be visualized must be documented. Additional structures that may be visualized (eg, pulmonary veins, pulmonary artery, pulmonic valve, inferior vena cava) would be included as part of the service.

▶A complete transthoracic echocardiogram with spectral and color flow Doppler (93306) is a comprehensive procedure that includes spectral Doppler and color flow Doppler in addition to the

2-dimensional and selected M-mode examinations. Spectral Doppler (93320, 93321) and color flow Doppler (93325) provide information regarding intracardiac blood flow and hemodynamics.◄

A follow-up or limited echocardiographic study (93308) is an examination that does not evaluate or document the attempt to evaluate all the structures that comprise the complete echocardiographic exam. This is typically ►limited to or◄ performed in follow-up of a focused clinical concern.

►In stress echocardiography, echocardiographic images are recorded from multiple cardiac windows before, after, and in some protocols, during stress. The stress is achieved by (1) walking on a treadmill; (2) using a bicycle (supine or upright); or (3) the administration of pharmacological agents that either simulate exercise (by increasing heart rate, blood pressure, or myocardial contractility) or alter coronary flow (vasodilation). The patient's ECG, heart rate, and blood pressure are monitored at baseline, throughout the procedure and during recovery. Reports are prepared to evaluate (1) the duration of stress, the reason for stopping, and the hemodynamic response to stress; and (2) the electrocardiographic response to stress.◄

►When a stress echocardiogram is performed◄ with a complete cardiovascular stress test (continuous electrocardiographic monitoring, physician supervision, interpretation and report), use 93351. ►Code 93350 is used to report the performance and interpretation of a stress echocardiogram only, with the components of the cardiovascular stress test reported separately using the appropriate codes (93016–93018).◄

►When left ventricular endocardial borders cannot be adequately identified by standard echocardiographic imaging, echocardiographic contrast may be infused intravenously both at rest and with stress to achieve that purpose. Code 93352 is used to report the administration of echocardiographic contrast agent in conjunction with the stress echocardiography codes (93350 or 93351). Supply of contrast agent and/or drugs used for pharmacological stress are reported separately in addition to the procedure code.◄

Report of an echocardiographic study, whether . . .

Use of ultrasound, without thorough evaluation . . .

(For fetal echocardiography, see 76825-76828)

93303	Transthoracic echocardiography for congenital cardiac anomalies; complete
93304	follow-up or limited study
●**93306**	Echocardiography, transthoracic, real-time with image documentation (2D), includes M-mode recording, when performed, complete, with spectral Doppler echocardiography, and with color flow Doppler echocardiography

►(For transthoracic echocardiography without spectral and color Doppler, use 93307)◄

▲**93307**	Echocardiography, transthoracic, real-time with image documentation (2D), includes M-mode recording, when performed, complete, without spectral or color Doppler echocardiography

►(Do not report 93307 in conjunction with 93320, 93321, 93325)◄

▲**93308**	Echocardiography, transthoracic, real-time with image documentation (2D), includes M-mode recording, when performed, follow-up or limited study
⊙**93312**	Echocardiography, transesophageal, real-time with image documentation (2D) (with or without M-mode recording); including probe placement, image acquisition, interpretation and report

+ 93320   Doppler echocardiography, pulsed wave and/or continuous wave with spectral display (List separately in addition to codes for echocardiographic imaging); complete

(Use 93320 in conjunction with 93303, 93304, 93312, 93314, 93315, 93317, 93350, ▶93351◀)

+ 93321   follow-up or limited study (List separately in addition to codes for echocardiographic imaging)

(Use 93321 in conjunction with 93303, 93304, 93308, 93312, 93314, 93315, 93317, 93350, ▶93351◀)

+ 93325   Doppler echocardiography color flow velocity mapping (List separately in addition to codes for echocardiography)

(Use 93325 in conjunction with 76825, 76826, 76827, 76828, 93303, 93304, 93308, 93312, 93314, 93315, 93317, 93350, ▶93351◀)

▲ 93350   Echocardiography, transthoracic, real-time with image documentation (2D), includes M-mode recording, when performed, during rest and cardiovascular stress test using treadmill, bicycle exercise and/or pharmacologically induced stress, with interpretation and report;

(The appropriate stress testing code(s) from the ▶93016◀-93018 series should be reported in addition to 93350 to capture the exercise stress portion of the study)

● 93351   including performance of continuous electrocardiographic monitoring, with physician supervision

▶(Do not report 93351 in conjunction with 93015-93018, 93350)◀

+ ● 93352   Use of echocardiographic contrast agent during stress echocardiography (List separately in addition to code for primary procedure)

▶(Do not report 93352 more than once per stress echocardiogram)◀

▶(Use 93352 in conjunction with 93350, 93351)◀

Rationale

To address changes in clinical practice and allow the performance and interpretation of contrast enhanced echocardiography before and during stress to be reported, the Echocardiography subsection of the CPT codebook has been updated.

The role of stress echocardiography in the detection of ischemia and infarction, cardiac risk stratification, and assessment of myocardial viability is well documented. The efficacy of intravenous contrast agents for left ventricular (LV) opacification to improve endocardial border visualization is well documented in patients with more than one LV wall segment. When used with stress (as well as resting) echocardiography, opacification of the LV cavity with contrast increases the number of interpretable LV wall segments, improves the qualitative assessment of LV ejection fraction, and improves quantitative assessment of LV volume and systolic function. A contrast agent is considered medically necessary when it is used to improve the delineation of the left ventricular endocardial borders in a patient whose non-contrast study is inadequate or suboptimal and for whom the LV function information is essential to the management of the patient.

Because the current stress echo code (93350) only reflects performance and interpretation of a baseline resting echocardiogram and the subsequent images acquired during and/or post exercise/stress, codes 93306, 93351, and add-on code 93352 have been established to describe a complete transthoracic echocardiogram (93306), a stress echocardiogram combined with a complete cardiovascular stress test (93351), and administration of an echocardiographic contrast agent in conjunction with stress echocardiography (93352).

The Echocardiography subsection guidelines have been revised to instruct the appropriate reporting for codes 93306-93308, 93016-93018, 93320-93321, 93325, 93350-93352. In addition, the guidelines were revised to clarify that pharmaceuticals or drugs should be reported separately.

Parenthetical notes have been added to accompany revisions and additions in the Echocardiography subsection. A parenthetical note following code 93306 was added to direct users to report code 93307 for transthoracic echocardiograpy without color flow or velocity. An exclusionary parenthetical note was added following code 93307 to indicate that it should not be used in conjunction with codes 93320, 93321, or 93325. Also, an exclusionary parenthetical note was added following code 93351 to indicate that it should not be used in conjunction with codes 93015-93018, 93350. A parenthetical note following code 93352 was added to indicate that code 93350 or 93351 should be reported in conjunction with code 93352.

The instructional parenthetical notes following codes 93320-93325 have been revised by deleting codes 93307, 93308, and 93320, 93321 from the respective parentheticals. Although the Echocardiography guidelines have been revised, existing codes 93016-93018, 93320, 93321, and 93325 are reported according to their original intent.

Code 93306 was established to report a complete transthoracic echoardiogram with spectral and color flow Doppler in addition to the 2-dimensional and selected M-mode examinations.

Code 93307 was revised for standardization of nomenclature to describe a complete transthoracic echocardiogram without spectral and color flow Doppler and includes 2-dimensional and selected M-mode examinations and to clarify the lack of Doppler echocardiography in this test.

Code 93308 was revised to clarify that this is intended to report only a follow-up or limited echocardiographic study.

Previously, code 93350 was a stand-alone code. Code 93350 has been revised to support the establishment of a child (indented) code 93351. Code 93350 is used to report the performance and interpretation of a stress echocardiogram only.

Code 93351 was established to report a stress echocardiogram combined with a complete cardiovascular stress test.

Code 93352 was established to report the administration of echocardiographic contrast agent in conjunction with the stress echocardiography codes 93350 or 93351.

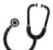 **Clinical Example (93306)**
A 67-year-old man with a history of coronary artery disease and hypertension presents with exertional shortness of breath and progressive exercise intolerance. On clinical evaluation, blood pressure is 140/90 mmHg, heart rate is regular at

90 bpm, and respirations are elevated at 20 per minute. Examination is notable for rales in the lung fields, and a systolic murmur is heard. Cardiomegaly and pulmonary congestion are noted on chest X ray, and left ventricular hypertrophy is noted on electrocardiogram.

Description of Procedure (93306)

A sequence of real-time tomographic images of cardiac structure and dynamics is obtained from multiple views and recorded on videotape or digitally. Selected M-mode (time-motion) recordings may be made to facilitate dimensional measurement. Using color Doppler flow imaging, blood flow velocity patterns are viewed and recorded across the cardiac valves and along the atrial and ventricular septae as well as in the great arteries and veins. When abnormal findings indicate valvular regurgitation or an intracardiac or extracardiac shunt, additional views are recorded. Using spectral Doppler (by means of pulsed and/or continuous wave techniques), flow velocities are recorded across the cardiac valves, and abnormal flow signals (such as with stenotic or regurgitant valves) are recorded usually from multiple transducer positions and orientations. The interpreting physician may verify the suitability of the images and Doppler flow data prior to completion of the study and may obtain additional views, if necessary. The interpreting physician reviews videotaped or digitally recorded views of the heart and analyzes and measures the structure and dynamics of the heart chambers, valves, and great vessels. In the context of the anatomic and dynamic findings, the presence of any abnormalities of the flow stream in the heart and great vessels is noted and, where appropriate, measures of jet width, jet area, proximal flow convergence, and flow propagation velocity are made to help quantitate the severity of abnormalities noted. The interpreting physician also reviews spectral Doppler velocity recordings and makes or verifies quantitative measures. Doppler velocities are used for hemodynamic assessment of systolic and diastolic left ventricular function as well as pressures in the right atrium, right ventricle, pulmonary artery, and left atrium. When appropriate, calculations include pressure gradients and valve orifice areas in patients with stenotic valves and regurgitant volumes, regurgitant fractions, and effective regurgitant orifice areas in patients with pathologic valvular regurgitation. From these anatomic and hemodynamic data, a complete interpretation is developed. Quantitative anatomic and functional measures such as left ventricular size, wall thickness, mass, ejection fraction, and regional wall motion are made, and the sizes of the left atrium, aorta, and right heart chambers are documented. Final interpretation typically also involves review of relevant tomographic views and hemodynamic data in comparison to previous study findings in order to determine if qualitative and quantitative changes have occurred.

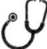 **Clinical Example (93351)**

A 40-year-old woman with non-diagnostic chest pain concerned about a family history of coronary artery disease presents to the office for a stress echocardiogram.

Description of Procedure (93351)

The sonographer hooks up a three-lead electrocardiogram (ECG) for gating, places the patient in left lateral decubitus position, and obtains a baseline echocardiogram at rest, including assessment of ventricular function, chamber sizes, wall thicknesses, wall motion, aortic root, and valves. Images are acquired from multiple cardiac windows, including the parasternal long axis, parasternal short axis, and apical four-chamber and two-chamber views.

The physician reviews the resting echocardiographic images to be sure there is adequate visualization of all left ventricle (LV) segments.

The nurse initiates the stress protocol by having the patient begin exercise on the treadmill. The heart rate, blood pressure, and ECG are continuously monitored. A staged stress protocol is followed with blood pressure, pulse, and ECG recordings made at the end of each stage. The patient's response to stress is watched for the appearance of any indicators requiring cessation of the stress test; eg, (1) severe symptoms, (2) significant ventricular arrhythmia, (3) hypotension, or (4) echocardiographic evidence of new regional LV wall motion abnormality. If no such indicators appear, stress continues until exercise cannot be continued or target heart rate is achieved during a pharmacologic stress test. The patient is monitored until all symptoms have resolved.

The sonographer records echocardiographic images for assessment of left ventricular wall motion immediately after exercise ends. In the case of treadmill exercise, the patient must be moved onto the examination table and placed in the left decubitus position. The sonographer organizes acquired selected images in a side-by-side format for review and interpretation by the physician.

The physician reviews the sequence of tomographic images, recorded both at baseline and again immediately following completion of treadmill exercise. Global and regional ventricular performance is evaluated carefully. Other cardiac causes of chest pain are also assessed. Where appropriate, measurements of cardiac structure and function are made. When available, prior studies are retrieved and reviewed side-by-side with the current images. A diagnostic interpretation is developed. The physician also reviews and analyzes the stress electrocardiogram, which includes starting and ending hemodynamics, arrhythmias, symptoms (especially chest pain), ST segment changes, functional capacity, and any other elements that are relevant to the interpretation of a stress electrocardiogram examination.

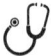 **Clinical Example (93352)**
An overweight 60-year-old man with non-diagnostic chest pain presents for a stress echocardiogram. Resting images of the left ventricle are inadequate to fully assess wall motion and contractility. Preparations for contrast administration are made; contrast is then administered at rest and again during stress to provide adequate left ventricular images.

Description of Procedure (93352)
The physician oversees and directs the prescribed dose of contrast that is administered intravenously. The physician is available to answer questions for the sonographer or review components of the study. The physician verifies completeness and adequacy of study and may request additional images as necessary.

A nurse injects the echocardiographic contrast agent intravenously. The dose is titrated through an iterative process to achieve adequate left ventricle (LV) opacification. Pre-stress contrast-enhanced echocardiographic images are obtained by the sonographer to provide optimal definition of the LV endocardium. At peak stress or immediately post-stress, the nurse administers a second infusion of the echocardiographic contrast, and the sonographer obtains post-stress images. Dose adjustments may be required. The patient is monitored until the heart rate has returned to baseline, all symptoms have resolved, and 30 minutes have passed since contrast administration. The intravenous catheter is removed and hemostasis achieved.

The physician reviews and interprets the contrast-enhanced echocardiographic images.

Cardiac Catheterization

Modifier 51 should not be appended to ▶93503◀, 93539▶, 93540, 93544◀-93556.

⊙93501   Right heart catheterization

INJECTION PROCEDURES

When injection procedures are performed in conjunction with cardiac catheterization, these services do not include introduction of catheters but do include repositioning of catheters when necessary and use of automatic power injectors. Injection procedures 93539-93545 represent separate identifiable services and may be coded in conjunction with one another when appropriate. The technical details of angiography, supervision of filming and processing, interpretation, and report are not included. To report radiological supervision, interpretation, and report for 93542 or 93543, use 93555. To report radiological supervision, interpretation, and report for 93539, 93540, 93541, 93544, or 93545, use 93556. Modifier 51 should not be appended to 93539▶, 93540, 93544◀-93556.

⊘⊙93539   Injection procedure during cardiac catheterization; for selective opacification of arterial conduits (eg, internal mammary), whether native or used for bypass

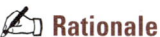 **Rationale**

The instructional note preceding code 93501 was revised to specify that modifier 51 should not be appended to codes 93503, 93539, 93540, and 93544-93556.

The instructions in the Injection Procedures subsection have been revised to specify that modifier 51 should not be appended to codes 93539, 93540, and 93544-93556.

Intracardiac Electrophysiological Procedures/Studies

Modifier 51 should not be appended to 93600-93603, 93610, 93612, 93615-93618, and 93631.

⊘93600   Bundle of His recording

⊘93631   Intra-operative epicardial and endocardial pacing and mapping to localize the site of tachycardia or zone of slow conduction for surgical correction

▶(For operative ablation of an arrhythmogenic focus or pathway by a separate provider, see 33250-33261)◀

Rationale

The instructional note preceding code 93600 has been revised to indicate that modifier 51 should not be appended to codes 93600-93603, 93610, 93612, 93615-93618, and 93631.

A cross-reference has been added following code 93631 to instruct and assist users in locating the appropriate codes for intraoperative pacing and mapping versus operative ablation of an arrythmogenic focus or pathway. These revisions are intended to assist in differentiating and reporting the services provided by a cardiac electrophysiologist versus those of a surgeon. It is not appropriate for both codes to be reported by a single provider for pacing/mapping and ablation for the same arrythmogenic focus, because ablation of the focus by the same provider is included and not separately reported.

Noninvasive Physiologic Studies and Procedures

▶(93727 has been deleted. For programming of implantable loop recorder, use 93285. For interrogation of implantable loop recorder, see 93291, 93298)◀

▶(93731, 93732 have been deleted. For interrogation of dual lead pacemaker, see 93288, 93294. For programming of dual chamber pacemaker, use 93280)◀

▶(93733 has been deleted. For transtelephonic rhythm strip pacemaker, single and dual, or multiple lead pacemaker evaluation, use 93293)◀

▶(93734, 93735 have been deleted. For interrogation of single lead pacemaker, see 93288, 93294. For programming of single lead pacemaker, use 93279)◀

▶(93736 has been deleted. For transtelephonic rhythm strip pacemaker, single and dual, or multiple lead pacemaker evaluation, use 93293)◀

93740 Temperature gradient studies

▶(93741, 93742 have been deleted. For interrogation of single implantable cardioverter-defibrillator [ICD], see 93289, 93295. For programming of single ICD, use 93282. For interrogation of wearable cardioverter-defibrillator, use 93292)◀

▶(93743, 93744 have been deleted. For interrogation of dual implantable cardioverter-defibrillator [ICD], see 93289, 93295. For programming of dual ICD, use 93283)◀

93745 Initial set-up and programming by a physician of wearable cardioverter-defibrillator includes initial programming of system, establishing baseline electronic ECG, transmission of data to data repository, patient instruction in wearing system and patient reporting of problems or events

(Do not report 93745 in conjunction with ▶93282, 93292◀)

▶(93760, 93762 have been deleted)◀

Rationale

In the Noninvasive Physiologic Studies and Procedures section, codes 93727-93736 and 93741-93744 were deleted and replaced with 21 new codes listed in the Cardiovascular Device Monitoring—Implantable and Wearable Devices section. The new codes provide a mechanism that more accurately reflects current cardiac device monitoring practices. Throughout the section, parenthetical notes have been added to inform users of which codes should not be reported in conjunction with these new codes. Each code family is based upon the type of service performed and the type of device involved (eg, single-lead pacemaker system, implantable cardioverter-defibrillator system, etc).

In support of the changes to the Cardiac Device Monitoring subsection, the instructional note following code 93745 has been revised to direct the user to the appropriate codes.

A parenthetical instruction has been added to indicate that the thermography studies codes 93760 and 93762 have been deleted.

Pulmonary

Other Procedures

94760   Noninvasive ear or pulse oximetry for oxygen saturation; single determination

(For blood gases, see 82803-82810)

94762   by continuous overnight monitoring (separate procedure)

▶(For other in vivo laboratory procedures, see 88720-88741)◀

Rationale

In tandem with the addition of the new subheading, In Vivo (eg, Transcutaneous) Laboratory Procedures, and the establishment of codes 88720, 88740, and 88741, a parenthetical note was added following code 94762 to direct users to codes 88720-88741 to report other in vivo laboratory procedures.

Allergy and Clinical Immunology

Allergy Testing

(For therapy for severe or intractable allergic disease, see ▶96365-96368, 96372, 96374, 96375◀)

▲**95010**   Percutaneous tests (scratch, puncture, prick) sequential and incremental, with drugs, biologicals, or venoms, immediate type reaction, including test interpretation and report by a physician, specify number of tests

▲**95015**   Intracutaneous (intradermal) tests, sequential and incremental, with drugs, biologicals, or venoms, immediate type reaction, including test interpretation and report by a physician, specify number of tests

Rationale

In support of the deletion and relocation of codes 90765-90768, 90772, 90774, and 90775, the cross-reference following the Allergy Testing subheading has been revised to indicate the appropriate codes to report therapy for severe or intractable allergic disease.

Codes 95010 and 95015 were revised to be consistent with the intent reflected in other allergy skin testing codes (eg, 95004, 95024, and 95027) to include the physician's interpretation of the test as well as the report. As indicated in the introductory language preceding the allergy testing codes, Evaluation and Management (E/M) services should not be reported for test interpretation and report, because these services, as stated in the descriptors for these particular codes, are inclusive of allergy testing. However, if a significant, separately identifiable E/M service is performed, the appropriate E/M service code should be reported using modifier 25.

Endocrinology

▲ **95250** Ambulatory continuous glucose monitoring of interstitial tissue fluid via a subcutaneous sensor for a minimum of 72 hours; sensor placement, hook-up, calibration of monitor, patient training, removal of sensor, and printout of recording

►(Do not report 95250 more than once per month)◄

(Do not report 95250 in conjunction with 99091)

▲ **95251** interpretation and report

►(Do not report 95251 more than once per month)◄

(Do not report ►95251◄ in conjunction with 99091)

Rationale

Codes 95250 and 95251 have been revised to reflect ambulatory continuous glucose monitoring of interstitial tissue fluid for a minimum of up to 72 hours. Prior to 2009, code 95250 specified monitoring of up to 72 hours. This change is more reflective of current practice. Code 95251 has been revised by removing the specification of interpretation and report performed by a physician, because the interpretation and report may be performed by a health care professional other than a physician. Codes 95250 and 95251 may not be reported more than once per month, and instructional notes have been added following each code to indicate this. Another instructional note was added following code 95251 indicating that this code may not be reported in conjunction with the collection and interpretation of physiologic data code 99091.

Neurology and Neuromuscular Procedures

Sleep Testing

●**95803**   Actigraphy testing, recording, analysis, interpretation, and report (minimum of 72 hours to 14 consecutive days of recording)

▶(Do not report 95803 more than once in any 14 day period)◀

▶(Do not report 95803 in conjunction with 95806-95811)◀

Rationale

Code 95803 was established with the conversion of Category III code 0089T to Category I status to report actigraphy sleep assessment. Actigraphy provides objective long-term data on circadian rhythm and sleep patterns. Unlike attended polysomnography, actigraphy provides days or weeks of data that can be used to assess the stability of sleep wake patterns and circadian rhythms and provide a good estimate of sleep time. Actigraphy data are collected via a small device, downloaded to a computer at the end of the recording period, and analyzed by a physician trained in sleep medicine. It provides data on rest and activity, which has been shown to be a reliable estimate of sleep and wakefulness.

Code 95803 is intended to be reported for a minimum of 72 hours to a maximum of 14 consecutive days of recording. It is not appropriate to report code 95803 more than once in any 14-day period. An exclusionary parenthetical note was added instructing that code 95803 should not be reported in conjunction with code 95806 to reflect the overlapping services described in these codes.

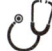

Clinical Example (95803)

A 29-year-old male complained of excessive sleepiness, including difficulty maintaining wakefulness while driving. There was no history of snoring, abnormal breathing while sleeping, cataplexy, hypnagogic hallucinations, sleep paralysis, unusual behaviors during sleep, drug abuse, or psychiatric illness. He reported difficulty falling asleep until late at night and struggling to get out of bed most mornings. Actigraphy monitoring is performed.

Description of Procedure (95803)

The technician reviews the printout and raw data to determine if the test was conducted in an overall valid manner. The technician edits the raw data for sections that need to be excluded, adjusts lights out and lights on times to stated times according to sleep diary data, and correlates the objective data from the printout with the subjective data of the sleep diary provided by patient and initial history from the patient record.

The sleep diary consists of a standardized form covering a week at a time, with separate entries for each 24-hour segment. It is an integral part of the test. The diary consists of patient's recording of lights out and lights on times; awakenings including when they were experienced during the sleep period and their estimated duration; perception of the total sleep time, sleep episodes, and their estimated durations during the regular wake period; and perception of alertness throughout the day. This allows objective correlation with the patient's subjective report of such essential elements as total sleep time, awakening numbers, naps, etc. The final technical data report, consisting of a graphic activity plot, epoch by epoch data printout classified as wake or sleep, and summary data table of sleep latency, total, sleep time, etc, is created. An interpretation of the data is completed and diagnosis established.

►Electromyography◄

Needle electromyographic procedures include the interpretation . . .

95860 Needle electromyography; one extremity with or without related paraspinal areas

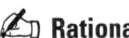
Rationale
To accommodate the addition of new headings, the heading preceding the peripheral nervous system testing codes 95860-95904 has been revised to more distinctly describe the hierarchy of these tests and to limit this heading to codes 95860-95872. A new heading has been added to immediately precede the nerve conduction testing codes 95900-95903.

►Guidance for Chemodenervation and Ischemic Muscle Testing◄

+95873 Electrical stimulation for guidance in conjunction with chemodenervation (List separately in addition to code for primary procedure)

+95874 Needle electromyography for guidance in conjunction with chemodenervation (List separately in addition to code for primary procedure)

(Use 95873, 95874 in conjunction with 64612-64614)

(Do not report 95874 in conjunction with 95873)

(Do not report 95873, 95874 in conjunction with 95860-95870)

95875 Ischemic limb exercise test with serial specimen(s) acquisition for muscle(s) metabolite(s)

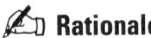
Rationale
A new heading has been added to immediately precede code 95873 to more accurately group codes 95873-95875 into a set of codes used to report chemodenervation guidance and ischemic muscle testing.

►Nerve Conduction Tests◄

⊘95900 Nerve conduction, amplitude and latency/velocity study, each nerve; motor, without F-wave study

⊘95903 motor, with F-wave study

⊘95904   sensory

(Report 95900, 95903, and/or 95904 only once when multiple sites on the same nerve are stimulated or recorded)

▶(For preconfigured electrode array nerve testing, use 95999)◀

 Rationale

A new heading has been added to immediately precede the nerve conduction testing codes 95900-95903. A cross-reference has been added following code 95904 directing users to code 95999 for reporting preconfigured electrode array nerve testing.

Neurostimulators, Analysis-Programming

Code 95980 describes intraoperative electronic analysis of an implanted gastric neurostimulator pulse generator system, with programming; code 95981 describes subsequent analysis of the device; code 95982 describes subsequent analysis and reprogramming. For electronic analysis and reprogramming of gastric neurostimulator, lesser curvature, ▶see 95980-95982.◀

 Rationale

In support of the deletion of Category III code 0162T, the guidelines in the Neurostimulators, Analysis-Programming subsection have been revised to direct users to codes 95980-95982 for electronic analysis and reprogramming of a gastric neurostimulator in the lesser curvature.

Other Procedures

⊘●95992   Canalith repositioning procedure(s) (eg, Epley maneuver, Semont maneuver), per day

▶(Do not report 95992 in conjunction with 92531, 92532)◀

 Rationale

Code 95992 was established to report the maneuvers required to accomplish canalith repositioning. Canalith repositioning procedure describes a prescribed series of movements of the patient's body and head. The maneuver is designed to use the force of gravity to redeposit calcium crystal debris that is in the semi-circular canal system (debris causes benign paroxysmal positional vertigo [BPPV]) into a "neutral" part of the end organ where it cannot cause vertigo.

This procedure (ie, BPPV) is unilateral in nature and is typically performed unilaterally. This procedure is commonly performed by a physician on the same day as an Evaluation and Management (E/M) service that would be separately reported with the appropriate E/M code and the modifier 25. Audiologists and physical therapists also perform this service, but these providers do not typically report E/M services. Therefore, it would not be appropriate to append modifier 51 to code 95992. It would also not be appropriate to report code 95992 in conjunction with nystagmus testing codes 92531 and 92532 on the same day.

Clinical Example (95992)

A 65-year-old man reports brief attacks of position-related vertigo. He has been diagnosed as having benign paroxysmal positional vertigo, and the appropriate involved canal has been determined. The decision is made to perform a canalith repositioning procedure.

Description of Procedure (95992)

The physician or other qualified health care provider instructs the patient in the canalith repositioning procedure. He is counseled that during the repositioning maneuver he may experience dizziness and nausea and may vomit, but that dizziness is expected and is not cause for alarm.

Position 1-2: The patient is rapidly moved from the sitting-upright position to the head-hanging-right position. The head is held at about 45 degrees to the right in the supine position with the neck slightly hyperextended. The nystagmus evoked is observed. Once it subsides, the patient is moved to position 3.

Position 3: From the head-hanging-right position, the head is then turned about 90 degrees to the left so that the head is in the head-hanging-left position.

Position 4: The patient rolls over to his/her left side about 90 degrees and turns toward the opposite ear.

Position 5: From this position, the patient is moved in a manner that allows the head to turn nearly facing the floor. The head is held in that position for 1-30 seconds.

Position 6: From position 5, the patient is taken en bloc to a seated position. The patient's head is straightened and the patient remains seated upright for posterior canal debris to settle in the vestibule. The entire process (positions 1-5) is then repeated at least once.

Health and Behavior Assessment/Intervention

Health and behavior assessment procedures are . . .

The focus of the assessment is . . .

Codes 96150-96155 describe services offered to . . .

For patients that require psychiatric services . . .

Evaluation and Management services codes (including ▶Counseling Risk Factor Reduction and Behavior Change Intervention [99401-99412]◀), should not be reported on the same day.

(For health and behavior assessment and/or . . .

96150 Health and behavior assessment (eg, health-focused clinical interview, behavioral observations, psychophysiological monitoring, health-oriented questionnaires), each 15 minutes face-to-face with the patient; initial assessment

✍ Rationale

The Health and Behavior Assessment/Intervention guidelines have been revised to indicate that the Counseling Risk Factor Reduction and Behavior Change Intervention E/M codes (99401-99412) should not be reported on the same day as codes 96150-96155.

►Hydration, Therapeutic, Prophylactic, Diagnostic Injections and Infusions, and Chemotherapy and Other Highly Complex Drug or Highly Complex Biologic Agent Administration◄

►Physician work related to hydration, injection, and infusion services predominantly involves affirmation of treatment plan and direct supervision of staff.◄

►If a significant, separately identifiable Evaluation and Management service is performed, the appropriate E/M service code should be reported using modifier 25 in addition to 96360-96549. For same day E/M service, a different diagnosis is not required.◄

►If performed to facilitate the infusion or injection, the following services are included and are not reported separately:◄

►a. Use of local anesthesia◄

►b. IV start◄

►c. Access to indwelling IV, subcutaneous catheter or port◄

►d. Flush at conclusion of infusion◄

►e. Standard tubing, syringes, and supplies◄

►(For declotting a catheter or port, use 36593)◄

►When multiple drugs are administered, report the service(s) and the specific materials or drugs for each.◄

►When administering multiple infusions, injections or combinations, only one "initial" service code should be reported, unless protocol requires that two separate IV sites must be used. If an injection or infusion is of a subsequent or concurrent nature, even if it is the first such service within that group of services, then a subsequent or concurrent code from the appropriate section should be reported (eg, the first IV push given subsequent to an initial one-hour infusion is reported using a subsequent IV push code).◄

►When these codes are reported by the physician, the "initial" code that best describes the key or primary reason for the encounter should always be reported irrespective of the order in which the infusions or injections occur.◄

►When these codes are reported *by the facility*, the following instructions apply. The initial code should be selected using a hierarchy whereby chemotherapy services are primary to therapeutic, prophylactic, and diagnostic services which are primary to hydration services. Infusions are primary to pushes, which are primary to injections.◄

►When reporting codes for which infusion time is a factor, use the actual time over which the infusion is administered. Intravenous or intra-arterial push is defined as: (a) an injection in which the health care professional who administers the substance/drug is continuously present to administer the injection and observe the patient, or (b) an infusion of 15 minutes or less.◄

►Hydration◄

●96360　Intravenous infusion, hydration; initial, 31 minutes to 1 hour

►Codes 96360-96361 are intended to report a hydration IV infusion to consist of a pre-packaged fluid and electrolytes (eg, normal saline, D5-1/2 normal saline + 30mEq KCl/liter) but are not used to report infusion of drugs or other substances. Hydration IV infusions typically require direct physician supervision for purposes of consent, safety oversight, or intraservice supervision of staff. Typically such infusions require little special handling to prepare or dispose of, and staff that administer these do not typically require advanced practice training. After initial set-up, infusion typically entails little patient risk and thus little monitoring. These codes are not intended to be reported by the physician in the facility setting.◄

►(Do not report 96360 if performed as a concurrent infusion service)◄

►(Do not report intravenous infusion for hydration of 30 minutes or less)◄

+●96361　　each additional hour (List separately in addition to code for primary procedure)

►(Use 96361 in conjunction with 96360)◄

►(Report 96361 for hydration infusion intervals of greater than 30 minutes beyond 1 hour increments)◄

►(Report 96361 to identify hydration if provided as a secondary or subsequent service after a different initial service [96360, 96365, 96374, 96409, 96413] is administered through the same IV access)◄

►Therapeutic, Prophylactic, and Diagnostic Injections and Infusions (Excludes Chemotherapy and Other Highly Complex Drug or Highly Complex Biologic Agent Administration)◄

►A therapeutic, prophylactic, or diagnostic IV infusion or injection (other than hydration) is for the administration of substances/drugs. When fluids are used to administer the drug(s), the administration of the fluid is considered incidental hydration and is not separately reportable. These services typically require direct physician supervision for any or all purposes of patient assessment, provision of consent, safety oversight, and intra-service supervision of staff. Typically, such infusions require special consideration to prepare, dose or dispose of, require practice training and competency for staff who administer the infusions, and require periodic patient assessment with vital sign monitoring during the infusion. These codes are not intended to be reported by the physician in the facility setting.◄

►See codes 96401-96549 for the administration of chemotherapy or other highly complex drug or highly complex biologic agent services. These highly complex services require advanced practice training and competency for staff who provide these services; special considerations for preparation, dosage or disposal; and commonly, these services entail significant patient risk and frequent monitoring. Examples are frequent changes in the infusion rate, prolonged presence of nurse administering the solution for patient monitoring and infusion adjustments, and frequent conferring with the physician about these issues.◄

▶(Do not report 96365-96379 with codes for which IV push or infusion is an inherent part of the procedure [eg, administration of contrast material for a diagnostic imaging study])◄

●**96365** Intravenous infusion, for therapy, prophylaxis, or diagnosis (specify substance or drug); initial, up to 1 hour

+●**96366** each additional hour (List separately in addition to code for primary procedure)

▶(Report 96366 in conjunction with 96365, 96367)◄

▶(Report 96366 for additional hour[s] of sequential infusion)◄

▶(Report 96366 for infusion intervals of greater than 30 minutes beyond 1 hour increments)◄

+●**96367** additional sequential infusion, up to 1 hour (List separately in addition to code for primary procedure)

▶(Report 96367 in conjunction with 96365, 96374, 96409, 96413 if provided as a secondary or subsequent service after a different initial service is administered through the same IV access. Report 96367 only once per sequential infusion of same infusate mix)◄

+●**96368** concurrent infusion (List separately in addition to code for primary procedure)

▶(Report 96368 only once per encounter)◄

▶(Report 96368 in conjunction with 96365, 96366, 96413, 96415, 96416)◄

●**96369** Subcutaneous infusion for therapy or prophylaxis (specify substance or drug); initial, up to 1 hour, including pump set-up and establishment of subcutaneous infusion site(s)

▶(For infusions of 15 minutes or less, use 96372)◄

+●**96370** each additional hour (List separately in addition to code for primary procedure)

▶(Use 96370 in conjunction with 96369)◄

▶(Use 96370 for infusion intervals of greater than 30 minutes beyond 1 hour increments)◄

+●**96371** additional pump set-up with establishment of new subcutaneous infusion site(s) (List separately in addition to code for primary procedure)

▶(Use 96371 in conjunction with 96369)◄

▶(Use 96369, 96371 only once per encounter)◄

●**96372** Therapeutic, prophylactic, or diagnostic injection (specify substance or drug); subcutaneous or intramuscular

▶(For administration of vaccines/toxoids, see 90465, 90466, 90471, 90472)◄

▶(Report 96372 for non-antineoplastic hormonal therapy injections)◄

▶(Report 96401 for anti-neoplastic nonhormonal injection therapy)◄

▶(Report 96402 for anti-neoplastic hormonal injection therapy)◄

▶(Physicians do not report 96372 for injections given without direct physician supervision. To report, use 99211. Hospitals may report 96372 when the physician is not present)◄

▶(96372 does not include injections for allergen immunotherapy. For allergen immunotherapy injections, see 95115-95117)◄

●96373   intra-arterial

●96374   intravenous push, single or initial substance/drug

+ ●96375   each additional sequential intravenous push of a new substance/drug (List separately in addition to code for primary procedure)

▶(Use 96375 in conjunction with 96365, 96374, 96409, 96413)◄

▶(Report 96375 to identify intravenous push of a new substance/drug if provided as a secondary or subsequent service after a different initial service is administered through the same IV access)◄

+ ●96376   each additional sequential intravenous push of the same substance/drug provided in a facility (List separately in addition to code for primary procedure)

▶(Do not report 96376 for a push performed within 30 minutes of a reported push of the same substance or drug)◄

▶(96376 may be reported by facilities only)◄

●96379   Unlisted therapeutic, prophylactic, or diagnostic intravenous or intra-arterial injection or infusion

▶(For allergy immunology, see 95004 et seq)◄

▶Chemotherapy and Other Highly Complex Drug or Highly Complex Biologic Agent Administration◄

▶Chemotherapy administration codes 96401-96549 apply to parenteral administration of non-radionuclide anti-neoplastic drugs; and also to anti-neoplastic agents provided for treatment of noncancer diagnoses (eg, cyclophosphamide for auto-immune conditions) or to substances such as certain monoclonal antibody agents, and other biologic response modifiers. The highly complex infusion of chemotherapy or other drug or biologic agents requires physician work and/or clinical staff monitoring well beyond that of therapeutic drug agents (96360-96379) because the incidence of severe adverse patient reactions are typically greater. These services can be provided by any physician. Chemotherapy services are typically highly complex and require direct physician supervision for any or all purposes of patient assessment, provision of consent, safety oversight, and intraservice supervision of staff. Typically, such chemotherapy services require advanced practice training and competency for staff who provide these services; special considerations for preparation, dosage, or disposal; and commonly, these services entail significant patient risk and frequent monitoring. Examples are frequent changes in the infusion rate, prolonged presence of the nurse administering the solution for patient monitoring and infusion adjustments, and frequent conferring with the physician about these issues. When performed to facilitate the infusion of injection, preparation of chemotherapy agent(s), highly complex agent(s), or other highly complex drugs is included and is not reported separately. To report infusions that do not require this level of complexity, see 96360-96379. Codes 96401-96402, 96409-96425, 96521-96523 are not intended to be reported by the physician in the facility setting.◄

▶The term "chemotherapy" in 96401-96549 includes other highly complex drugs or highly complex biologic agents.◀

▶Report separate codes for each parenteral method of administration employed when chemotherapy is administered by different techniques. The administration of medications (eg, antibiotics, steroidal agents, antiemetics, narcotics, analgesics) administered independently or sequentially as supportive management of chemotherapy administration, should be separately reported using 96360, 96361, 96365, 96379 as appropriate.◀

▶Report both the specific service as well as code(s) for the specific substance(s) or drug(s) provided. The fluid used to administer the drug(s) is considered incidental hydration and is not separately reportable.◀

▶INJECTION AND INTRAVENOUS INFUSION CHEMOTHERAPY AND OTHER HIGHLY COMPLEX DRUG OR HIGHLY COMPLEX BIOLOGIC AGENT ADMINISTRATION◀

96413 Chemotherapy administration, intravenous infusion technique; up to 1 hour, single or initial substance/drug

(Report ▶96361◀ to identify hydration if administered as a secondary or subsequent service in association with 96413 through the same IV access)

(Report ▶96366, 96367, 96375◀ to identify therapeutic, prophylactic, or diagnostic drug infusion or injection, if administered as a secondary or subsequent service in association with 96413 through the same IV access)

INTRA-ARTERIAL CHEMOTHERAPY ▶AND OTHER HIGHLY COMPLEX DRUG OR HIGHLY COMPLEX◀ BIOLOGIC AGENT ADMINISTRATION

96420 Chemotherapy administration, intra-arterial; push technique

96422   infusion technique, up to 1 hour

OTHER ▶INJECTION AND INFUSION SERVICES◀

Code 96523 does not . . .

🖉 Rationale

In order to assist users in more convenient comparison and use of the infusion services procedures, codes 90760-90779 have been deleted and renumbered for proximity to the chemotherapy and other complex infusion services reported with codes 96401-96549. With the deletion and renumbering of codes 90760-90779 to codes 96360-96379, the overarching guidelines that previously appeared before these codes have been relocated and revised to reflect the application of the overarching principles to the entire set of infusion codes, through codes 96401-96542. To reflect this change in focus, the subheading has also been revised to reflect the applicability of the guidelines for chemotherapy and other complex infusions, in addition to hydration and therapeutic infusion services, and to include these codes in the major subsection. The subsection titles and guidelines for the hydration and therapeutic infusion codes have also been editorially revised to differentiate the use of codes 96401-96549 for complex infusions from codes 93665-93679 for less complex infusions.

The guidelines now refer the user to the complex infusion codes when the services required meet the defined required level of service (advanced practice training and competency for staff; entail significant patient risk and frequent monitoring, including frequent changes in the infusion rate; prolonged presence of nurse administering the solution for patient monitoring and infusion adjustments; and frequent conferring with the physician). The overarching guidelines that precede codes 96360-96379 have also been revised by inclusion of text that was previously only included in parenthetical instructions. These guidelines apply to the entire series of codes 96360-96549. An example of this type of revision is the inclusion of the push injection definition. Additional instructions have been added to address the use and interpretation of the hierarchy of the injections to assist the user in determining the instructions that are most applicable when a coding situation is addressed by the guidelines and parenthetical instructions.

In order to reflect current use of the infusion codes, the instructions related to use of some codes in the facility setting have been revised. As an example of this revision, the last sentence of the first paragraph in the complex injections section has been revised to specify that codes 96401, 96402, 96409-96425, 96521-96523 should not be reported for physician services in the facility setting. The gaps in these series include codes 96405, 96406, 96440, 96445, and 96450, which describe services that may require reporting in the facility setting.

Category II Codes

This section continues to be the fastest growing section of the CPT® codebook, with the addition of 143 codes for quality improvement measures, 12 new clinical conditions, and 14 revised clinical conditions.

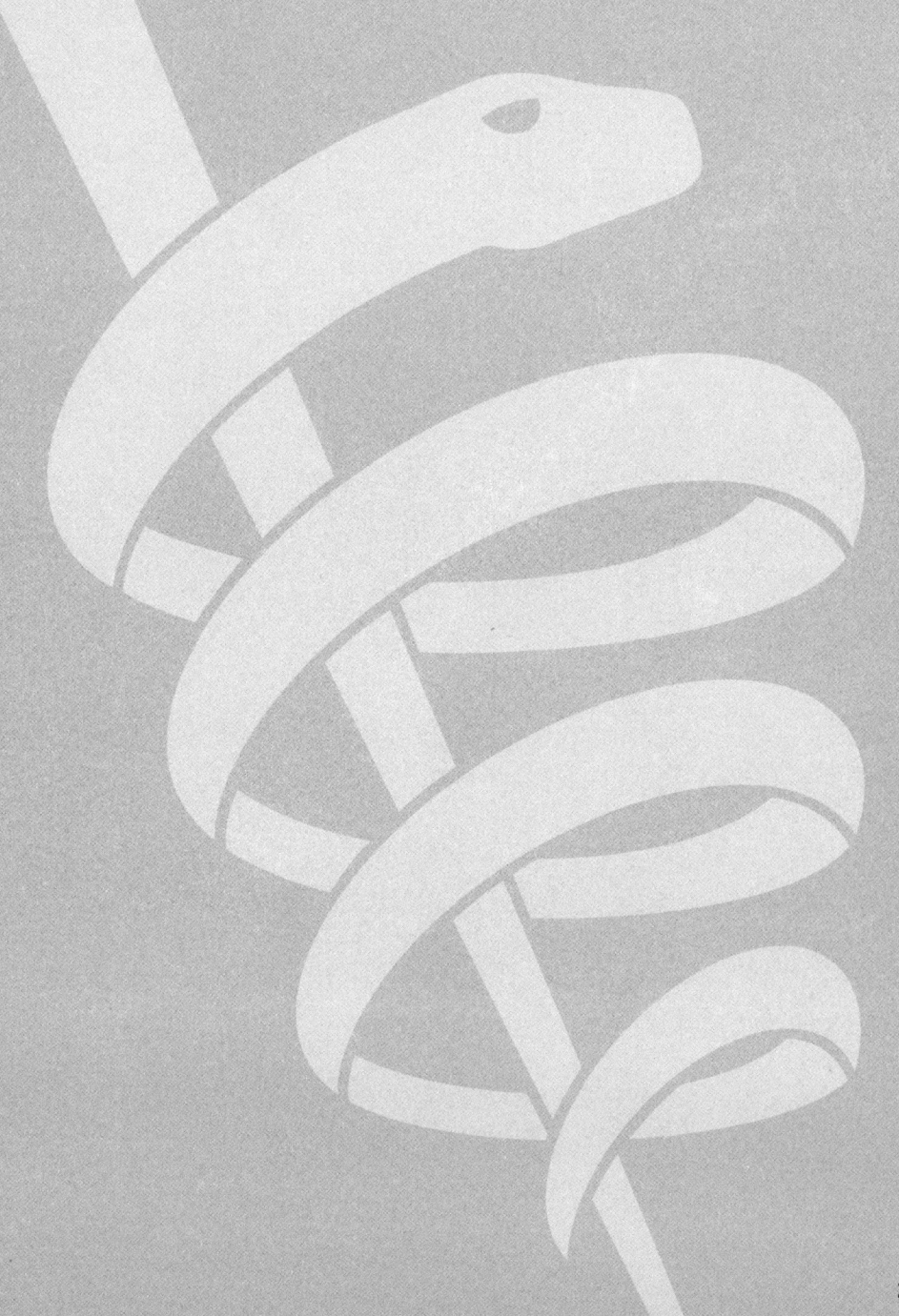

Category II Codes

Composite Codes

●0014F   Comprehensive preoperative assessment performed for cataract surgery with intraocular lens (IOL) placement (includes assessment of all of the following components) (EC)[5]:

Dilated fundus evaluation performed within 12 months prior to cataract surgery (2020F)[5]

Pre-surgical (cataract) axial length, corneal power measurement and method of intraocular lens power calculation documented (must be performed within 12 months prior to surgery) (3073F)[5]

Preoperative assessment of functional or medical indication(s) for surgery prior to the cataract surgery with intraocular lens placement (must be performed within 12 months prior to cataract surgery) (3325F)[5]

●0015F   Melanoma follow up completed (includes assessment of all of the following components) (ML)[5]:

History obtained regarding new or changing moles (1050F)[5]

Complete physical skin exam performed (2029F)[5]

Patient counseled to perform a monthly self skin examination (5005F)[5]

Rationale

Codes 0014F and 0015F represent the new Composite measures codes that were added to the Category II Codes section. Code 0014F has been added to identify specific services that are commonly performed together for the Eye Care measure set. Code 0015F identifies three services ordinarily performed together for the Melanoma measure set. As is noted in the guidelines for all codes in this section, absence of performance of any single code included as part of the set for codes 0014F and 0015F necessitates report of the individual codes instead of report of either code 0014F or 0015F.

●0513F   Elevated blood pressure plan of care documented (CKD)[1]

●0514F   Plan of care for elevated hemoglobin level documented for patient receiving Erythropoiesis-Stimulating Agent therapy (ESA) (CKD)[1]

●0516F   Anemia plan of care documented (ESRD)[1]

●0517F   Glaucoma plan of care documented (EC)[5]

●0518F   Falls plan of care documented (GER)[5]

Rationale

Codes 0513F-0518F are all Patient Management codes that are used to identify provision of a plan of care. Codes 0513F and 0514F are both used to identify measurement compliance for the Chronic Kidney Disease (CKD) measure, while codes 0516F, 0517F, and 0518F are used to identify performance measurement for the End-Stage Renal Disease (ESRD), Eye Care, and Geriatrics measures, respectively.

Each includes the phrase "documented" instead of "performed" or "provided," as documentation of the service inherently includes provision of that specific service.

Code 0513F is used as part of the Blood Pressure Management measure and is intended to help identify whether (1) the blood pressure measurement for patients aged 18 years or older is less than 130/80 mm Hg (and therefore is within the target range for risk reduction for CKD), or (2) whether the patient who has been diagnosed with advanced CKD and has a blood pressure measurement of 130/80 mm Hg or more has a documented plan of care. This code is used in conjunction with codes that specify that a blood pressure check was performed (code 2000F), and identify the specific blood pressure measurement that was obtained (codes 3074F-3080F). In addition, reporting instructions included in Appendix H in the CPT codebook notify users regarding when it is appropriate to report code 0513F (as this code identifies compliance with the measure). Additional information listed with the numerator notes that one or more of the following should be included to meet the requirements of documentation of a plan of care: (1) recheck of blood pressure at a specified future date; (2) initiation or alteration of pharmacologic therapy; and (3) documentation of the review of the patient's home blood pressure log that indicates that the patient's blood pressure is or is not well controlled. The measure specifications note the importance of performing the services included in the measure. As a result, this measure does not allow for exclusions, and use of modifiers 1P, 2P, and/or 3P when reporting service codes for this measure is restricted.

Identification of hypertension in patients with CKD is an essential part of management of the disease. Hypertension is common in patients with CKD, and if hypertension is left untreated, it will speed the progression of the disease. Recent research has shown that during office visits, approximately 20% to 30% of CKD patients do not have their blood pressure measured. Additionally, if CKD patients have an anemia/ESA visit, they are even less likely to have their blood pressure measured. In these patients, recent research has shown that 75% do not have their blood pressure measured at an anemia/ESA visit. Patients with CKD should have their blood pressure measured at each office visit so that changes can be identified and treatment initiated as soon as it is necessary. Blood pressure control is important in slowing the progression of CKD. By slowing the progression of the disease, quality of life is improved for the patient, and it results in a longer period of time before a patient requires renal replacement therapy. Patients with chronic kidney disease should have a lower target blood pressure (<130/80 mm Hg) than other patients with hypertension.

Code 0514F is used to report documentation of a plan of care for elevated hemoglobin for patients receiving erythropoiesis-stimulating agent (ESA) therapy for CKD. The measure itself (for which code 0514F is used) identifies the number of calendar months in which the targeted patient population had a documented plan of care for elevated hemoglobin level. To assist users in compliance with the intent of the measure, a definition of " . . . documented plan of care" has been included with the listing of the numerator statement in the Appendix H section for this measure. In addition, because this is a frequency measure, information has been included in the reporting instruction that identifies how often the measure should be reported. This information also notes when it is appropriate to use code 0514F. Because no exclusions are identified for this measure, the reporting instructions note that modifiers 1P, 2P, and 3P may not be used.

The clinical recommendation regarding hemoglobin (Hb) levels for CKD patients receiving ESA therapy is that Hb level should generally be in the range of 11.0 to 12.0 g/dL. Additionally, these patients should have their Hb level checked at least monthly. Given that Hb levels vary for each patient due to numerous factors, it is necessary to monitor Hb level closely to make the individualized treatment decisions required in maintaining Hb level in the target range. There is no evidence of benefit from ESA therapy when Hb levels are maintained at greater than 13.0 g/dL. Maintaining Hb at higher levels may result in potential harm to the patient, as well as incur unjustified cost. Evidence linking increased risks for patients with CKD and higher Hb levels were for target Hb levels greater than 13.0g/dL. The intention of this measure is not to suggest that the goal of ESA treatment is to reach an achieved Hb of 13.0 g/dL. Rather, as a patient safety measure, it is to realize that patients who reach Hb levels higher than 13.0 g/dL are at increased risk for adverse events, and that these elevated Hb levels need to be addressed by adjusting ESA dosage.

Code 0516F is used to identify documentation of a plan of care for anemia (for ESRD). As is true for other plan of care measures, use of this code is linked to Category II codes that identify a measurement, and the code is reported when a threshold is met that requires a specific action—namely, when the Hb measurement drops below 11 g/dL. When this happens, a plan of care should be provided for the patient, and meeting this measurement requirement sanctions use of code 0516F. Because this is a frequency measure, instructions have been included in the Appendix H document to identify how often this code should be reported. In addition, because the measure for which this code is used does not allow for exclusions, a note has been included that alerts the user that modifiers 1P, 2P, and 3P may not be used.

Anemia is a common comorbidity in patients with kidney disease, increasing in likelihood as kidney function declines. The goal of this measure is to identify anemia and develop a treatment plan that is vital to "improve patient quality of life, to improve the various physiological abnormalities associated with anemia, to decrease morbidity, to decrease hospitalization, and to improve patient survival."

Code 0517F is used to identify documentation of a plan of care for glaucoma. The measure for which this code is reported measures whether the patient aged 18 years or older with a diagnosis of primary open-angle glaucoma either has treatment that has not failed (ie, the most recent intraocular pressure [IOP] measurement was at least 15% lower than the pretreatment level) or has a plan of care documented within the last 12 months for treatments that failed. As is true for other codes used to identify documentation of a plan of care, information has been included with the listing of the numerator in the Appendix H document that identifies elements that meet the requirements for documentation of a plan of care, including (1) recheck of IOP at a specified time; (2) a change in therapy; (3) performance of additional diagnostic evaluations; (4) monitoring per patient decisions or inability to achieve due to health system reasons; and/or (5) referral to a specialist. System exclusions have been identified for this measure. Therefore, code 0517F may be reported with modifier 3P if for example, a physician is asked to report on this measure but is not the ophthalmologist or optometrist providing the primary management for primary open-angle glaucoma.

Code 0518F is used to identify documentation of a plan of care for falls in geriatric patients. The measure for which this code is used identifies whether the patient aged 65 years or older with a history of falls had a plan of care for falls documented within 12 months. A note has been included with the numerator statement listed within the Appendix H listing for this measure that notes that the plan of care must include consideration of an appropriate assistance device in addition to balance, strength, and gait training. A definition of a fall has also been included. A medical exclusion is allowed for this measure, and, therefore, reporting instructions have been included within the listing that notify the user that the modifier 1P may be appended to code 0518F to identify patients with appropriate medical exclusions. In addition, use of code 1100F determines whether code 0518F should be reported, as this code helps to differentiate whether the patient is within the target population identified by the measure.

●0519F Planned chemotherapy regimen, including at a minimum: drug(s) prescribed, dose, and duration, documented prior to initiation of a new treatment regimen (ONC)¹

●0520F Normal tissue dose constraints established within 5 treatment days from the initiation of a course of 3D conformal radiation for a minimum of 1 tissue/organ (ONC)¹

●0521F Plan of care to address pain documented (ONC)¹

Rationale

Codes 0519F, 0520F, and 0521F are all used to identify compliance with measures included as part of the Oncology measurement set. These codes are all included as part of the Patient Management series and identify utilization measures.

Code 0519F has been established to report documentation of a planned chemotherapy regimen (which includes the drug[s] prescribed, the duration, and dose of medication used) prior to initiation of a new treatment regimen. The measure in which this code is intended to be reported identifies whether the patient with a diagnosis of breast, colon, or rectal cancer who is receiving intravenous chemotherapy had a planned chemotherapy regimen documented prior to the initiation of a new treatment regimen. Because there are no exclusions sited in the measure, no exclusion modifiers may be used to identify circumstances regarding this service (ie, no use of exclusion modifiers 1P, 2P, or 3P). The importance of the need for this code is that a detailed plan for the chemotherapy regimen is a critical component of ensuring safety and high-quality care for patients with cancer of this nature.

Code 0520F is used to report establishment of normal tissue dose constraints within 5 treatment days of the initiation of 3-dimensional (3D) treatment. This is consistent with the specifications of the measure that identify whether the patient with a diagnosis of cancer receiving 3D conformal radiation therapy had documentation in the medical record that normal tissue dose constraints were established within 5 treatment days from the initiation of a course of conformal radiation for a minimum of one tissue. Reporting instructions included with this measure listing note that there are no exclusions for this measure. Therefore, modifiers 1P, 2P, and 3P may not be used with this code.

Identifying normal tissue dose constraints is an important step in the process of care for patients receiving radiation therapy treatments. Although no specific data are available, in its practice accreditation reviews, the American College of Radiation Oncology has found that normal dose constraints are included in the patient chart less frequently than reviewers expected. While dose constraint specification is an integral part of intensity-modulated radiation therapy, it is not required for 3D conformal radiation therapy. Patients treated with 3D conformal radiation therapy are often subjected to dose levels that exceed normal tissue tolerance, and precise specification of maximum doses to be received by normal tissues represents both an intellectual process for the physician during radiation treatment planning and a failsafe point for the treating therapists. In most circumstances where facilities require specification of normal tissue dose constraints prior to initiation of therapy, policies and procedures exist that prohibit exceeding those limits in the absence of written physician approval.

Code 0521F is used to report establishment of a plan of care for pain by the physician for those cancer patients receiving chemotherapy or radiation treatment who note having pain. A numerator definition has been included with the Appendix H listing to note the elements that are included as part of a documented plan of care for pain. These include (1) use of opioids, (2) a bowel regimen, (3) nonopioid analgesics, (4) psychological support, (5) patient and/or family education, and (6) reassessment of pain. Code 0521F is only used for patients who express presence of pain. As a result, a reporting instruction has been included that notes that this code is only reported when a plan of care is established and code 1125F is reported (code 1125F is used to separate the target population for inclusion in measurement). In addition, because no performance exclusions have been noted for this measure, modifiers 1P, 2P, or 3P may not be used with this code.

●**0525F**   Initial visit for episode (BkP)²

●**0526F**   Subsequent visit for episode (BkP)²

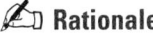 Rationale

Codes 0525F and 0526F are both used to identify performance measurement for treatment of back pain. There are multiple measures within the Back Pain clinical topic for which these codes are used, including Physical Exam After Back Pain Onset, Advice for Normal Activities for Back Pain Patients, Advice Against Bed Rest for Back Pain Patients, and Initial Visit for Back Pain. In each of these measures, codes 0525F and 0526F are used as denominator codes that separate the patient population according to whether the visit is an initial or subsequent visit for the back pain episode. As a result, the reporting instructions for these measures note that either code 0525F or 0526F is to be reported for each patient. Instructions and definitions have been included according to the specifications that are important for the measure. This includes numerator information that identifies elements necessary for the physical examination or the assessment components. A definition of "red flags" (warning signs) has also been included for measures where this term appears (eg, in the descriptor of code 1130F and in the Appropriate Imaging for Acute Back Pain[2] measure listing).

▲ **1040F** DSM-IV™ criteria for major depressive disorder documented at the initial evaluation (MDD)[1]

Rationale

Code 1040F was editorially revised, adding the words " . . . at the initial evaluation" to the descriptor to provide more information about the specific evaluation that is being measured.

▶(1080F has been deleted. To report surrogate decision maker or advance care plan documented in the medical record, report code 1123F or 1124F).◀

Rationale

Code 1080F was deleted and replaced by codes 1123F and 1124F. Use of these codes instead of code 1080F allows for more granularity in identifying specific information regarding the care plan for the elderly patient. As a result, a parenthetical note has been included for code 1080F to direct users to the appropriate codes to use to identify documentation of a surrogate decision maker or the inclusion of an advance care plan for the patient. For more information regarding the specific use for codes 1123F and 1124F, see the Rationale for these codes.

●**1116F** Auricular or periauricular pain assessed (AOE)[1]

Rationale

Code 1116F is used to report assessment of auricular or periauricular pain for acute otitis externa (AOE) patients. The measure itself targets patients 2 years and older, as is noted in the brief measure description section of the Appendix H document for the Pain Assessment measure. Because there are medical reasons for not meeting the measure specifications, a reporting instruction has been included in the Appendix H listing that allows reporting of code 1116F with modifier 1P for medical exclusions.

Pain relief is a major goal in the management of AOE. As a result, the management of diffuse AOE should include an assessment of pain, and the clinician should recommend analgesic treatment based on the severity of pain. Frequent use of analgesics is often necessary to permit patients to achieve comfort, rest, and resume normal activities. Ongoing assessment of the severity of discomfort is essential for proper management.

●1118F   GERD symptoms assessed after 12 months of therapy (GERD)[5]

Rationale
Code 1118F is used to report the assessment of gastroesophageal reflux disease (GERD) symptoms after 12 months of therapy. Although not referenced in the code descriptor, a definition of continuous therapy has been included in the Appendix H listing to provide users with information regarding service that is included as part of continuous therapy (ie, proton pump inhibitor [PPI] or histamine H2 receptor antagonist [H2RA] therapy that lasts 12 months or more to treat GERD). Similar to coding for other measures, this measure includes use of denominator codes that further delineate the patient population being measured (ie, those patients who have had continuous [12 months] therapy with PPI or H2RA [code 4185F]) from those who should not be included in the denominator for this measure (ie, those patients who have not had continuous therapy [code 4186F]). Information directing users regarding the appropriate method of reporting for GERD symptom assessment after 12 months of therapy has been included in the Reporting Instructions. In addition, information has been included in this section regarding medical exclusions for this measure. (Use of modifier 1P with code 1118F is appropriate when there is documentation of medical reasons for not assessing the GERD symptoms after 12 months of therapy.)

Because GERD is a chronic condition, continuous therapy to control symptoms and prevent complications is appropriate. Research indicates that patients on chronic therapy are able to have their dose modified or reduced based on the presence or absence of symptoms. Many patients with GERD remain on medication therapy for years, and experts suspect that not all patients are being reassessed on a regular basis to determine whether the medication is still needed. This measure attempts to capture whether a patient on chronic medication has his or her GERD symptoms assessed at least annually.

●1119F   Initial evaluation for condition (HEP C)[1]

●1121F   Subsequent evaluation for condition (HEP C)[1]

Rationale
Codes 1119F and 1121F are both denominator codes used in conjunction with code 3265F to identify Ribonucleic Acid (RNA) testing for hepatitis C viremia. The measure itself is used to determine whether the patient aged 18 years or older with a diagnosis of hepatitis C seen for an initial evaluation had hepatitis C virus (HCV) RNA testing ordered or performed during a previous encounter. Codes 1119F and 1121F are only reported when an appropriate evaluation and management (E/M) code (99201-99205, 99241-99245) is not included on the same claim form. Reporting Instructions have been included in the Appendix H document that provide direction regarding use of these codes with E/M services. Additional information has also been included regarding the appropriate use of code 3265F. (More information regarding the use of code 3265F may be found in the Rationale discussion for that code.) Because the measure allows for medical or patient

reasons for not ordering or performing HCV RNA testing, modifiers 1P and 2P may be reported in conjunction with code 3265F. These modifiers should not be appended to codes 1119F or 1121F as the modifier is ordinarily placed on the code that identifies compliance with the measure specifications; ie, the modifier is placed on the code that shows that the measure was met. Use of the modifier on this code demonstrates that (1) the patient is included as part of the target population (as demonstrated by report of denominator code 1119F), and (2) the physician has attempted to comply with the measure specifications but for a medical or patient reason (1P or 2P) the physician was unable to comply.

Testing for HCV RNA is needed to establish and confirm a diagnosis of chronic hepatitis C. Hepatitis C virus is an RNA virus of the Flaviviridae family; it replicates preferentially in hepatocytes but is not directly cytopathic, leading to persistent (chronic) infection. During chronic infection, HCV RNA reaches high levels, generally ranging from 105-107 IU/mL, but the levels can fluctuate widely. However, within the same individual, RNA levels are usually relatively stable. After initial exposure, HCV RNA can be detected in blood within 1-3 weeks and is present at the onset of symptoms. Antibodies to HCV are detected by enzyme immunoassay in only 50%-70% of patients at the onset of symptoms, increasing to more than 90% after 3 months. The clinical utility of serial HCV viral levels in a patient is predicated on continued use of the same specific quantitative assay that was used in the initial determination of the viral level. While there is little correlation between disease severity and disease progression with the absolute level of HCV RNA, quantitative determination of the HCV level provides important information on the likelihood of response to treatment in patients undergoing antiviral therapy.

●1123F Advance Care Planning discussed and documented; advance care plan or surrogate decision maker documented in the medical record (GER)[5]

●1124F Advance Care Planning discussed and documented in the medical record; patient did not wish or was not able to name a surrogate decision maker or provide an advance care plan (GER)[5]

Rationale

Codes 1123F and 1124F have both been added to the CPT codebook to more specifically identify information regarding the provision of a care plan for the patient and/or identification of a surrogate decision maker. The patient exclusion was removed from this measure. In addition, code 1080F was deleted and replaced by codes 1123F and 1124F. Use of these codes instead of code 1080F allows for more granularity in identifying specific information regarding the care plan for the elderly patient (see code 1080F for more information regarding the deletion of that code). Specifically, these codes differentiate successful provision of a care plan or identification of a surrogate decision maker from the attempted provision/ identification. Use of either code fulfills the measures requirements. As a result, no exclusion modifiers are appropriate for use with either code. To help identify this, the Reporting Instructions include information that identifies the appropriate code to use when the patient does not want to discuss an advance care plan (code 1124F). The Reporting Instructions also include information that notes that the individual reporting does not have to be the physician who documented or discussed the advance care planning with the patient. However, each physician reporting for this measure must ensure that the appropriate information is in the medical record at the time of reporting. Finally, a note has been included at the end of the Reporting Instructions that indicates that the measure applies to all health care settings including locations such as the inpatient facility or the nursing home. For each of these settings, there should be documentation in the medical record(s) that advance care planning was discussed or documented.

●**1125F** Pain severity quantified; pain present (ONC)[1]

●**1126F** Pain severity quantified; no pain present (ONC)[1]

Rationale

Codes 1125F and 1126F are both used to identify quantification of pain for oncology (ONC) patients. Each code is used within the Oncology topic in two separate measures: Pain Intensity Quantified-Medical Oncology and Radiation Oncology[1] and Plan of Care for Pain-Medical Oncology and Radiation Oncology.[1] For the second measure, these codes are used as denominator codes to further separate the population of patients included for the measure from those who should be excluded (those with no pain present), as the measure's intent is to determine whether a documented plan of care to address pain was provided for the radiation/chemotherapy visit for those cancer patients who report having pain. (If the patient has no pain, then no pain management is required.) Both measures include definitions to assist users in determining (1) quantification of pain severity (Pain Intensity Quantified measure) and (2) items or services that are included as appropriate documentation of a plan of care for pain management (Plan of Care for Pain). Because these codes are used as denominator codes in the second measure, instructions have been included to direct users in the appropriate method to report for cancer patients who have a diagnosis of pain (1125F) and how to report a documented plan of care for that patient (0521F). In addition, direction is provided to alert users to appropriate coding when no pain is present (1126F).

Neither measure allows for exclusions. As a result, modifiers 1P, 2P, and 3P may not be reported with codes 1125F, 1126F, and 0521F.

●**1127F** New episode for condition (ML)[5]

●**1128F** Subsequent episode for condition (ML)[5]

Rationale

Codes 1127F and 1128F are both used as denominator codes within the Melanoma Coordinator of Care measure. This measure is used to identify whether the patient diagnosed with a new episode of melanoma has a treatment plan documented in the chart that was communicated to the physician(s) providing continuing care within 1 month of diagnosis. Because these codes are used as denominator codes to separate the patient population into patients who have a new episode of the melanoma condition (1127F) vs patients with subsequent episodes of melanoma, instructions have been included to notify users of the appropriate codes to use to identify the population of patients who are included in the measure (1127F) and when the measure requirements have been met (5050F). In addition, because patient and system exclusions exist for this measure, modifiers 2P and 3P have been listed within the reporting instructions of the Appendix H listing for this measure to note the exclusions that may be identified.

There is no valid indication for expensive imaging studies in early-stage melanoma in the absence of signs or symptoms. There is a perception that radiologic studies are being administered for grade 0 and grade IA melanoma are clinically unnecessary and create economic burden to the patient and payer. Because diagnostic imaging is also inappropriate for patients with higher stages of melanoma, this measure is a first step in addressing the overutilization of diagnostic imaging studies in patients with melanoma.

- **1130F** Back pain and function assessed, including all of the following: Pain assessment AND functional status AND patient history, including notation of presence or absence of "red flags" (warning signs) AND assessment of prior treatment and response, *AND* employment status (BkP)[2]
- **1134F** Episode of back pain lasting 6 weeks or less (BkP)[2]
- **1135F** Episode of back pain lasting longer than 6 weeks (BkP)[2]
- **1136F** Episode of back pain lasting 12 weeks or less (BkP)[2]
- **1137F** Episode of back pain lasting longer than 12 weeks (BkP)[2]

Rationale

Codes 1130F and 1134F-1137F are all included as part of measures listed within the Back Pain clinical topic. This includes the listing of the Initial Visit for Back Pain[2] (1130F), Mental Health Assessment After Back Pain Onset[2] (1134F, 1135F), Appropriate Imaging for Acute Back Pain[2] (1134F, 1135F), and Recommendation for Exercise for Back Pain Patients[2] (1136F, 1137F) measures. Each of the codes is included as part of specific measures and serves a specific purpose according to the measure and its specifications.

Code 1130F is used to identify back pain assessment in the Initial Visit for Back Pain[2] measure to note compliance with the measure specifications (ie, that back pain and function were assessed and include a number of key elements). The elements necessary to meet the measure requirements are cited in the Appendix H measure information, while reporting instructions direct users to report code 1130F for all patients for whom the assessment (with all necessary elements) was performed.

Codes 1134F and 1135F are both used as denominator codes to separate the patient population within the Mental Health Assessment After Back Pain Onset[2] measure according to those patients who should be included for measurement (ie, those who have had back pain for longer than 6 weeks) vs those who should not be included for measurement (ie, patients who have episodes of back pain lasting 6 weeks or less). The measure itself is used to determine whether the patient with a diagnosis of back pain received a mental health assessment and requires that documentation of a mental health assessment be present in the medical record prior to the back surgery or steroidal injection procedure. This information is listed in the measure statement found in the Appendix H measure listing. In addition, the denominator information included in the appendix notes that patients undergoing back surgery or epidural steroid injection are also included as part of the measure population. To provide clarification regarding appropriate use of codes 1134F, 1135F, and 2044F (used to identify compliance with the measure), specific reporting instructions have been included to note when each code should or should not be reported. The reporting instructions for this measure note that it is not necessary to report one of the denominator codes if the provider is reporting at the time of the surgical procedure/intervention. If reporting at the time of the evaluation and management visit, then the denominator codes should be used to indicate the duration of the pain. This measure also notes that exclusions are not included as part of the measure, and therefore modifiers 1P, 2P, and 3P may not be used with this code.

Codes 1134F and 1135F are also used as denominator codes to separate the patient populations for the Appropriate Imaging for Acute Back Pain[2] measure. This is an overuse measure, included to designate elements or procedures that are inappropriate to report according to the measure specifications. For this measure, codes 1134F and 1135F serve to separate the patient population into those patients who are the target of the measure (ie, those patients who have had pain that lasted longer than 6 weeks) vs those patients who are not part of the target population (ie, patients with an episode of back pain lasting 6 weeks or less). Codes 3330F and 3331F are used to identify compliance with the measure (3331F) or the lack thereof (3330F). (For more information regarding use of codes 3330F and 3331F, see the Rationale listing for these codes.)

Codes 1136F and 1137F are both used as denominator codes within the Recommendation for Exercise for Back Pain Patients[2] measure. The measure determines whether a patient received instructions for therapeutic exercise with follow-up by the physician or was counseled to perform supervised exercise during an episode of back pain lasting longer than 12 weeks. Codes 1136F and 1137F are used to separate patients who had back pain that lasted 12 weeks or less (1136F, not part of the measure population) from those who had back pain that lasted longer than 12 weeks (1137F, part of the target population). As a result, one of these codes should be reported for each patient, as is noted in the Appendix H reporting instructions for this measure. In addition, both codes 4240F and 4242F are used to identify alternative methods of complying with the measure specifications, using code 4240F to identify instructions in therapeutic exercise with follow-up by the physician or code 4242F to identify provision of counseling for a supervised exercise program for the patient (also noted in the reporting instructions for the measure). Because no exclusions are cited for this measure, modifiers 1P, 2P, and 3P may not be reported with any of the codes listed in this measure.

2000F Blood pressure measured (CAD, CKD, HF, HTN)[1], (DM)[2,4]

2001F Weight recorded (HF, PAG)[1]

2020F Dilated fundus evaluation performed within six 12 months prior to cataract surgery (EC)[5]

2024F Seven standard field stereoscopic photos with interpretation by an ophthalmologist or optometrist documented and reviewed (DM)[2,4]

2026F Eye imaging validated to match diagnosis from seven standard field stereoscopic photos results documented and reviewed (DM)[2,4]

Rationale

Codes 2000F, 2001F, 2020F, 2024F, and 2026F are all included in *CPT Changes 2009* to reflect changes to the listed information for each code that do not reflect a change in the intent of the code. This is due to the fact that the descriptor language for each of the codes remains intact and unchanged; therefore, the intent of the code remains the same. Instead, the change made to the code listing reflects either (1) a change to the suffix(es) listed with the code that identifies additional measures for which this code may be listed/used or (2) the addition of a superscript that identifies the measure developer/endorser for the measure for which the code was developed. In both cases, the addition of the information simply expands the usage of the code by allowing the code to be reported for additional measures. As a result, the delta symbol (▲) is not included with the code listing when only the superscript or a suffix acronym is added/deleted from the code language.

●**2035F** Tympanic membrane mobility assessed with pneumatic otoscopy or tympanometry (OME)[1]

Rationale

Code 2035F has been added to identify a tympanic membrane mobility assessment with pneumatic otoscopy or with tympanometry. This code is currently used to identify compliance with a single measure included as part of the Acute Otitis Externa/Otitis Media with Effusion (OME) clinical topic. Because there are medical and patient reasons included in the measure specifications for not performing the assessment, reporting instructions have been included that direct users regarding the appropriate use of modifiers 1P and 2P with this code.

Correctly diagnosing middle ear effusion is essential for proper management. Otitis media with effusion is often characterized by a cloudy tympanic membrane with distinctly impaired mobility that can best be determined with pneumatic otoscopy or tympanometry. Clinicians should use pneumatic otoscopy as the primary diagnostic method for OME.

●**2040F** Physical examination on the date of the initial visit for low back pain performed, in accordance with specifications (BkP)[2]

●**2044F** Documentation of mental health assessment prior to intervention (back surgery or epidural steroid injection) or for back pain episode lasting longer than 6 weeks (BkP)[2]

Code 2040F is used to report a physical examination on the date of the initial visit for low back pain. It is included as part of reporting for the Physical Exam after Back Pain Onset[2] measure, which determines whether a patient with a diagnosis of back pain received a physical examination during the initial visit for the episode of back pain. Since there are varied indications within the specifications for this measure, additional information from the measure has been included within the Appendix H listing to assist users in identifying the intent of the measure, which will aid them in appropriate use of code 2040F. To notify users that special information exists for this measure (and use of this code), the descriptor for code 2040F includes a special reference to specification information. A reference is also made in the reporting instructions to view the actual specifications.

Code 2044F is listed to identify compliance with the Mental Health Assessment After Back Pain Onset measure, which identifies whether a patient with a diagnosis of back pain received a mental health assessment. For more information regarding use of this code, please see the Rationale for codes 1134F and 1135F.

3014F Screening mammography results documented and reviewed (PV)[1,2]

3017F Colorectal cancer screening results documented and reviewed (PV)[1,2]

3060F Positive microalbuminuria test result documented and reviewed (DM)[2,4]

3061F Negative microalbuminuria test result documented and reviewed (DM)[2,4]

3062F Positive macroalbuminuria test result documented and reviewed (DM)[2,4]

3066F Documentation of treatment for nephropathy (eg, patient receiving dialysis, patient being treated for ESRD, CRF, ARF, or renal insufficiency, any visit to a nephrologist) (DM)[2,4]

3072F Low risk for retinopathy (no evidence of retinopathy in the prior year) (DM)[2,4]

▲ **3073F** Pre-surgical (cataract) axial length, corneal power measurement and method of intraocular lens power calculation documented (must be performed within twelve months prior to surgery) (EC)[5]

3074F Most recent systolic blood pressure < 130 mm Hg (DM)[2,4] (HTN, CKD)[1]

3075F Most recent systolic blood pressure 130 to 139 mm Hg (DM)[2,4] (HTN, CKD)[1]

3077F Most recent systolic blood pressure ≥ 140 mm Hg (DM)[2,4] (HTN, CKD)[1]

3078F Most recent diastolic blood pressure < 80 mm Hg (DM)[2,4] (HTN, CKD)[1]

3079F Most recent diastolic blood pressure 80 - 89 mm Hg (DM)[2,4] (HTN, CKD)[1]

3080F Most recent diastolic blood pressure ≥ 90 mm Hg (DM)[2,4] (HTN, CKD)

3100F Carotid image study report includes direct or indirect reference to measurements of distal internal carotid diameter as the denominator for stenosis measurement (STR, RAD)[5]

Rationale

Codes 3014F, 3017F, 3060F, 3061F, 3062F, 3066F, 3074-3080F, and 3100F are all included in *CPT Changes 2009* to reflect changes to the listed information for that code that do not reflect a change in the intent of the code. This is due to the fact that the descriptor language for each of the codes remains intact and unchanged; therefore, the intent of the code remains the same. Instead, the change made to the code listing reflects either (1) a change to the suffix listed with the code, that identifies additional measures for which this code may be listed, or (2) the measure developer/endorser for the measure for which the code was developed. In both cases, the addition of the information simply expands the usage of the code by allowing the code to be reported for additional measures. As a result, the delta symbol (▲) is not included with the code listing when only the superscript or a suffix acronym is added/deleted from the code language.

Code 3073F has been revised, exchanging the word "six" for "12" to note that the calculations have to be performed 12 months prior to cataract surgery. This information reflects a change to the measure specifications for both the Documentation of Presurgical Axial Length, Corneal Power Measurement and Method of Intraocular Lens Power Calculation measure and the Comprehensive Preoperative Assessment for Cataract Surgery with Intraocular Lens (IOL) Placement measure.

●3215F   Patient has documented immunity to Hepatitis A (HEP-C)[1]

●3216F   Patient has documented immunity to Hepatitis B (HEP-C)[1]

▶Code 3217F has been deleted.◀

●3218F   RNA testing for Hepatitis C documented as performed within six months prior to initiation of antiviral treatment for Hepatitis C (HEP-C)[1]

▶Code 3219F has been deleted.◀

●3220F   Hepatitis C quantitative RNA testing documented as performed at 12 weeks from initiation of antiviral treatment (HEP-C)[1]

Rationale

Codes 3215F-3220F each relate information for reporting on the Hepatitis C measures. Codes 3215F and 3216F are included in separate measures within the Hepatitis C clinical topic and are both used identify patient immunity for either hepatitis A (3215F) or hepatitis B (3216F). Both are also chosen from a set of codes used for the measure specified to identify whether (1) the indicated vaccine was recommended; (2) it was received; or (3) the patient has an immunity to the virus, and to note compliance with the measure.

Two of the notations in the CPT codebook represent a deletion of codes: 3217F and 3219F. These codes were deleted shortly after they were posted to the CPT Web site in favor of a single code that includes language that more appropriately represents the measure that was developed (3218F). The measure identifies whether the patient aged 18 years and older with a diagnosis of chronic hepatitis C who is receiving antiviral treatment had quantitative hepatitis C virus Ribonucleic Acid (RNA) testing performed within 6 months prior to initiation of treatment. This measure includes use of denominator codes 4150F, Patient receiving antiviral treatment for Hepatitis C, and 4151F, Patient not receiving antiviral treatment for hepatitis C, which differentiate the target patient population (as identified by code 4150F) from those patients who should not be included as part of the denominator/target population (4151F). As a result, reporting instructions have been included that identify when code 3218F (which identifies compliance with the measures specifications through documentation of RNA testing for hepatitis C) should be additionally reported. Only medical exclusions exist for this measure. As a result, reporting instructions have been included to identify that code 3218F may be reported with modifier 1P only when appropriate medical exclusions apply, such as when the patient is first seen by the physician after initiation of treatment.

●3230F Documentation that hearing test was performed within 6 months prior to tympanostomy tube insertion (OME)[1]

Rationale

Code 3230F is used to report compliance for information included as part of the Otitis Media Externa (OME) measure. This code specifically is used to note whether the patient aged 2 months through 12 years with a diagnosis of OME who underwent tympanostomy tube insertion had a hearing test performed within 6 months prior to tympanostomy tube insertion. Medical and system exclusions exist for this measure. As a result, modifiers 1P and 3P may be appended to code 3230F to identify allowances for exclusions from this measure's specifications. This information has been included in the reporting instructions. Other information included in the reporting instructions includes (1) instructions regarding timing for when this code should be reported, (2) chart documentation necessary, and (3) information regarding report for multiple providers.

Otitis media externa is often accompanied by hearing loss, which can impair early language acquisition especially in severe cases, which often require tympanostomy tube insertion. Therefore, it is imperative that any patient for whom tympanostomy tube insertion is indicated have his or her hearing tested.

●3260F pT category (primary tumor), pN category (regional lymph nodes), and histologic grade documented in pathology report (PATH)[1]

Rationale

Code 3260F is used to report histological grade for resections provided for cancer reporting for both breast and colorectal cancer. The measure for each anatomic area specifies whether the breast or colorectal cancer pathology report included the pT category, the pN category, and the histologic grade. This is important, because this information is used to assist in therapeutic decision making for the patient. As a result, reporting instructions note that information regarding this measure should be reported each time a resection pathology report is prepared for either clinical condition. In addition, only medical exclusions exist for this measure, and modifier 1P may be reported only to identify medical reasons for not meeting the measure specifications (such as noncarcinoma resections and reexcisions that are tumor free).

Therapeutic decisions for breast and/or colon cancer management are stage driven and cannot be made without a complete set of pathology descriptors.

Incomplete cancer resection pathology reports may result in misclassification of patients, rework and delays, and suboptimal management. The College of American Pathologists (CAP) has produced evidence-based checklists of essential pathologic parameters that are recommended to be included in cancer resection pathology reports. These checklists have been endorsed as a voluntary standard by the National Quality Forum and are considered the reporting standard by the Commission on Cancer of the American College of Surgeons. The CAP recently conducted a structured audit of adequacy of breast cancer pathology reports at 86 institutions. Overall, 35% of eligible reports were missing at least one of the 10 CAP-recommended breast cancer elements. Cancer Care Ontario conducted a similar study in 2005 and found that 25% of breast cancer pathology reports did not include all of the information required by the CAP standards. While the exact percentage of pathology reports for breast cancer resection that are missing the pT category, the pN category, and the histologic grade is unknown, these are essential elements in breast and colon cancer treatment decisions and should be included in every pathology report when possible.

● **3265F**   Ribonucleic acid (RNA) testing for Hepatitis C viremia ordered or results documented (HEP C)[1]

● **3266F**   Hepatitis C genotype testing documented as performed prior to initiation of antiviral treatment for Hepatitis C (HEP C)[1]

Rationale

Codes 3265F and 3266F are both testing procedure codes used for measures included in the Hepatitis C clinical condition set. Code 3265F is used to identify whether Hepatitis C patients had hepatitis C virus (HCV) RNA testing ordered or whether a hepatitis C test was previously performed for the patient. Since the measure is used to determine RNA testing for hepatitis C during the initial evaluation, denominator codes have also been included within the measure to differentiate the targeted patient population (ie, those patients with hepatitis C who were seen for an initial evaluation—1119F) from those who should not be included within the measure (subsequent patient evaluation visits for hepatitis C patients—1121F). The reporting instructions include directions educate the user regarding the appropriate use of code 3265F and modifiers 1P and 2P.

Code 3266F is used to report whether patients with chronic hepatitis C receiving antiviral treatment had HCV genotype testing performed prior to initiation of treatment. Denominator codes are used with the measure associated with this code, separating patients who are receiving antiviral treatment (4150F) from those who are not receiving antiviral treatment for hepatitis C (4151F). Separation of these patients then allows measurement of the appropriate patients and use of code 3266F for those patients receiving antiviral treatment who have had HCV genotype testing performed prior to treatment. The reporting instructions include information that restricts use of exclusion modifiers with this code.

The HCV RNA testing is needed to establish and confirm the diagnosis of chronic hepatitis C. Hepatitic C virus is an RNA virus of the Flaviviridae family; it replicates preferentially in hepatocytes but is not directly cytopathic, leading to persistent infection. During chronic infection, HCV RNA reaches high levels, generally ranging from 105-107 IU/mL, but the levels can fluctuate widely. However, within the same individual, RNA levels are usually relatively stable. After initial exposure, HCV RNA can be detected in blood within 1-3 weeks and is present at the onset of symptoms. Antibodies to HCV are detected by enzyme immunoassay in only 50%-70% of patients at the onset of symptoms, increasing to more than 90% after 3 months. The clinical utility of serial HCV viral levels in a patient is predicated on continued use of the same specific quantitative assay that was used in the initial determination of the viral level. While there is little correlation between disease severity or disease progression and the absolute level of HCV RNA, quantitative determination of the HCV level provides important information on the likelihood of response to treatment in patients undergoing antiviral therapy. Data elements required for the measure can be captured and the measure is actionable by the physician.

Genotype testing prior to initiation of therapy is used to guide treatment decisions regarding duration of therapy and likelihood of response. There are six HCV genotypes and more than 50 subtypes. These genotypes differ by as much as 31-34% in their nucleotide sequences, whereas subtypes differ by 20%-23% based on full-length genomic sequence comparisons. Genotype determinations influence treatment decisions. Patients with genotypes 2 or 3 have better response rates to retreatment than those with genotype 1.

●3268F Prostate-specific antigen (PSA), AND primary tumor (T) stage, AND Gleason score documented prior to initiation of treatment (PRCA)[1]

●3269F Bone scan performed prior to initiation of treatment or at any time since diagnosis of prostate cancer (PRCA)[1]

●3270F Bone scan not performed prior to initiation of treatment nor at any time since diagnosis of prostate cancer (PRCA)[1]

●3271F Low risk of recurrence, prostate cancer (PRCA)[1]

●3272F Intermediate risk of recurrence, prostate cancer (PRCA)[1]

●3273F High risk of recurrence, prostate cancer (PRCA)[1]

●3274F Prostate cancer risk of recurrence not determined or neither low, intermediate nor high (PRCA)[1]

Rationale

Codes 3268F-3274F are all used to identify varied measure information for the Prostate Cancer clinical topic, including information regarding the initial evaluation, overuse of bone scans for low-risk patients, and prescription of adjuvant hormonal therapy for high-risk patients. Generally, the measures for which these codes are used denote compliance in providing certain services for the patients who fit the category. However, one of the measures (bone scan overuse) is included to ensure measurement of services that should not be provided for certain patients—that is, to provide measurement of certain services that are overused or are inappropriate given the population of patients for whom the service is provided.

Code 3268F is used to report documentation of the (1) prostate-specific antigen (PSA), (2) primary tumor (T) stage, and (3) Gleason score prior to the initiation of treatment for prostate cancer patients. The measure for which this code is reported (Initial Evaluation) is used to determine whether a patient with prostate cancer receiving interstitial prostate brachytherapy, external beam radiotherapy to the prostate, radical prostatectomy, or cryotherapy had documented evaluation of PSA, primary tumor stage, and Gleason score. Upon review of the information included in the Appendix H listing for this measure, users will note that certain words are emphasized within the text of the measure "snapshot" listed. These words are emphasized to alert users to the importance of including all of the testing procedures listed (using the capitalized "AND") and the importance of including all of the testing procedures if any of the treatments listed are provided for the prostate cancer patient (ie, use of the capitalized "OR"). To further accentuate this, the descriptor language information also includes emphasized text to alert users to the importance of including all of the listed elements to use the code and meet the measure requirements. This information is also further demonstrated with the reporting instructions included for this measure. The measure does allow for medical exclusions and therefore directs users to report modifier 1P with code 3268F when such exclusions apply.

Codes 3269F-3274F are all used within two separate measures provided for prostate cancer patients. Codes 3269F and 3270F are both used as part of an overuse measure, namely, use of bone scans for staging of low-risk patients. Code 3269F denotes that a bone scan was performed for the prostate cancer patient either prior to initiation of treatment or any time after the prostate cancer diagnosis. Code 3270F notes the converse application, indicating absence of a bone scan procedure. Use of these codes requires stratification of the population of patients according to risk. Therefore, codes 3271F-3274F are used as denominator codes that identify the risk level of recurrence for prostate cancer. Codes 3271F-3273F portray increasing levels of risk, while code 3274F notes an undetermined level of risk of recurrence or that the risk of recurrence is neither low, intermediate, nor high. Unlike other measures, overuse measures provide a different set of instructions for use and exclusions. Exclusions for this measure consist of documentation of medical reasons for having a bone scan performed, including documentation of pain, provision of salvage therapy, or other medical reasons. The exclusions notation also lists system reasons for having a bone scan done, such as a bone scan that was ordered by someone other than the reporting physician. In addition, a definition for salvage therapy is included as well as a special reference to the technical specifications to afford users knowledge regarding what salvage therapy is and why it is included as an exclusion that permits bone scanning for this population of patients. The technical specification reference directs users to the developers' Web site for additional information to identify definitions of low risk, intermediate risk, and high risk for recurrence of prostate cancer.

Finally, in the reporting instructions listing, users are directed regarding the appropriate method to report nonprovision of a bone scan for low-risk patients. Users are also directed in the appropriate method and codes to use to identify exclusions (ie, by appending modifier 1P or 3P to code 3269F and not to code 3270F).

Codes 3271F-3274F are also used as denominator codes to differentiate the patient population for the Adjuvant Hormonal Therapy for High-Risk Patients measure. This measure notes whether a patient with a diagnosis of prostate cancer at high risk of recurrence and receiving external beam radiotherapy to the prostate was prescribed adjuvant hormonal therapy (gonadotropin-releasing hormone agonist or antagonist). Code 4164F is used in this measure to indicate compliance with the measure specifications, as is noted in the reporting instructions provided with the measure "snapshot" included in the Appendix H document. Exclusions for medical (1P) and patient (2P) reasons are also included in these instructions.

The initial assessment of all prostate cancer patients should include the three evaluations required in the Initial Evaluation measure. If receiving external beam radiotherapy, prostate cancer patients with a high risk of recurrence should also be prescribed hormonal therapy. This has been shown to increase the effectiveness of the radiotherapy, as is noted in the specifications for the Adjuvant Hormonal Therapy for High-Risk Patients measure.

A bone scan is generally not required for staging prostate cancer in men with a low risk of recurrence. The overuse measure Bone Scan for Staging Low-Risk Patients[1] is written as a negative measure so that the performance goal is 100%, consistent with the other measures for this condition.

●**3278F**   Serum levels of calcium, phosphorus, intact Parathyroid Hormone (PTH) and lipid profile ordered (CKD)[1]

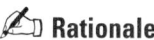 **Rationale**

Code 3278F is the only code included in the Laboratory Testing (Calcium, Phosphorus, and Intact Parathyroid Hormone [PTH], and Lipid Profile) measure for the Chronic Kidney Disease (CKD) clinical topic. The measure notes whether the patient aged 18 years or older with the diagnosis of advanced CKD (ie, stage 4 or 5 CKD and not receiving renal replacement therapy) had serum levels of calcium, phosphorus, and intact PTH measured and lipid profile laboratory testing ordered at least once during the 12-month reporting period. Use of this code indicates compliance with the measure specifications, which allow for medical and patient exclusions via use of modifiers 1P and 2P with code 3278F.

Bone disease is a common complication of CKD. Patients with CKD should be monitored for calcium and phosphate imbalances and secondary hyperparathyroidism, as these are associated with increased cardiovascular mortality.

●**3279F**   Hemoglobin level greater than or equal to 13 g/dL (CKD, ESRD)[1]

●**3280F**   Hemoglobin level 11 g/dL to 12.9 g/dL (CKD, ESRD)[1]

●**3281F**   Hemoglobin level less than 11 g/dL (CKD, ESRD)[1]

✍ Rationale

Codes 3279F, 3280F, and 3281F are all used to differentiate the patient populations for two measures included in two different clinical topics: The Plan of Care—Elevated Hemoglobin for Patients Receiving Erythropoiesis-Stimulating Agents (ESA)[1] included within the Chronic Kidney Disease (CKD) clinical topic and the Plan of Care for Anemia[1] measure included in the End Stage Renal Disease (ESRD) clinical topic. For the Plan of Care measure for CKD, these codes are used to identify different thresholds of hemoglobin (Hb) levels that are achieved for patients receiving ESA therapy (the ESA therapy being identified by use of code 4171F; for more regarding use of codes 4171F and 4172F, see the Rationale for these codes). In addition, code 0514F is reported for those patients with an elevated Hb for whom a plan of care is provided. (See the Rationale for more information regarding use of code 0514F.) These codes provide the same action for the Plan of Care for Anemia[1] patients for the ESRD clinical topic, utilizing code 0516F to identify the provision of a plan of care when that service is provided for patients whose Hb levels fall below the 11 g/dL threshold. In addition, the reporting instructions note that there are no exclusions for this measure, and modifiers 1P, 2P, and 3P, may not be used to identify exclusions for it.

The clinical recommendation regarding Hb levels for CKD patients receiving ESA therapy is that Hb level should generally be in the range of 11.0-12.0 g/dL. Additionally, these patients should also have their Hb level checked at least monthly. Given that Hb levels vary for each patient due to numerous factors, it is necessary to monitor Hb level closely to make the individualized treatment decisions required in maintaining Hb level in the target range. There is no evidence of benefit from ESA therapy when Hb levels are maintained at greater than 13.0 g/dL. Maintaining Hb at higher levels may result in potential harm to the patient, as well as incur unjustified cost. Evidence linking increased risks for patients with CKD and higher Hb levels were for target Hb levels greater than 13.0g/dL. The intention of this measure is not to suggest that the goal of ESA treatment is to reach an achieved Hb of 13.0 g/dL. Rather, as a patient safety measures, it is to realize that patients who reach Hb levels higher than 13.0 g/dL are at increased risk for adverse events, and that these elevated Hb levels need to be addressed by adjusting ESA dosage.

Anemia is a common comorbidity in patients with kidney disease, increasing in likelihood as kidney function declines. The goal of this measure is to identify anemia and develop a treatment plan that is vital to decrease morbidity and hospitalization and to improve quality of life, the various physiologic abnormalities associated with having anemia, and patient survival.

●**3284F** Intraocular pressure (IOP) reduced by a value of greater than or equal to 15% from the pre-intervention level (EC)[5]

●**3285F** Intraocular pressure (IOP) reduced by a value less than 15% from the pre-intervention level (EC)[5]

Rationale

Codes 3284F and 3285F are used to report intraocular pressure reduction for glaucoma patients. The measure for which these codes are reported determines whether patients treated for glaucoma either (1) have a treatment that has not failed (and therefore have an intraocular pressure [IOP] value that is at least 15% greater than the preintervention level) or (2) have a plan of care documented within 12 months of the treatment that *has* failed. For patients who do not meet the threshold for a successful intervention, code 0517F is reported only if a plan of care is documented in the record. To assist users, special instructions have been placed in the Appendix H measure listing that note items that are included as part of a plan of care, which include: (1) recheck of IOP at specified time; (2) change in therapy; (3) performance of additional diagnostic evaluations; (4) monitoring per patient decisions or not being able to achieve the desired level due to health system reasons, and/or (5) referral to a specialist. Reporting instructions for this measure note that system exclusions may be used if a physician is asked to report on this measure but is not the ophthalmologist or optometrist providing the primary management for primary open-angle glaucoma.

Results of several randomized clinical trials (Early Manifest Glaucoma Trial [EMGT], Collaborative Initial Glaucoma Treatment Study [CIGTS], Advanced Glaucoma Intervention Study, and Collaborative Normal Tension Glaucoma Study) all demonstrate that reduction of IOP of at least 18% reduces the rate of worsening of visual fields by at least 40%. The various studies, however, achieved different levels of mean IOP lowering in realizing their benefit in patient outcomes, ranging from 18% in the "normal pressure" subpopulation of the EMGT to 42% in the CIGTS study (level I studies). As such, an appropriate "failure" indicator is to not achieve at least a 15% IOP reduction. The rationales for a failure indicator are that (1) the results of different studies can lead experienced clinicians to believe that different levels of IOP reduction are appropriate; (2) it is necessary to minimize the impact of adverse selection for those patients whose IOPs are more difficult to control; and (3) each patient's clinical course may require IOP reduction that may vary from 18-40% or more.

●**3288F**   Falls risk assessment documented (GER)[5]

Rationale

Code 3288F is used to identify documentation of a falls risk assessment. The measure in which this code is used identifies whether the patient aged 65 years or older with a history of falls had a risk assessment for falls completed within 12 months. The Appendix H numerator information defines the elements for risk assessment and includes a definition of "fall." In addition, the reporting instructions direct users to report code 3288F with code 1100F for patients in whom a falls risk assessment is performed.

Screening for specific medical conditions may direct the therapy. Although the clinical guidelines and supporting evidence call for an evaluation of many factors, it was felt that for the purposes of measuring performance and facilitating implementation, this initial measure must be limited in scope. For this reason, the work group defined an evaluation of balance and gait as a core component that must be completed in all patients with a history of falls as well as four additional evaluations, at least one of which must be completed within the 12-month period. Data elements required for the measure can be captured and the measure is actionable by the physician.

- **3290F** Patient is D (Rh) negative and unsensitized (PRENATAL)[1]
- **3291F** Patient is D (Rh) positive or sensitized (PRENATAL)[1]
- **3292F** HIV testing ordered or documented and reviewed during the first or second prenatal visit (PRENATAL)[1]

Rationale

Codes 3290F, 3291F, and 3292F are used to identify services included as part of the Prenatal Care clinical topic and to note patient sensitivity to certain Rh factors (codes 3290F and 3291F) or the order of or documentation and review of human immunodeficiency virus (HIV) testing during the first two visits of the prenatal care.

Codes 3290F and 3291F are included as part of the Anti-Immune D Globulin measure for the Prenatal Care clinical topic, and they note whether the patient is D (Rh) negative and unsensitized (code 3290F) or positive or sensitized to the D (Rh) factor (code 3291F). The testing and results provide information to the physician regarding whether treatment is necessary to guard against an adverse immune response by the mother toward the forming fetus, and code 4178F is reported to identify anti-D immune globulin administration between the 26th and 30th weeks of gestation. Only medical and patient reasons exist for not providing the Rh factor testing according to the timing noted in the measure specifications. Therefore, modifiers 1P and 2P may be used to identify medical reasons (such as absence of the testing due to the known presence of HIV) or patient reasons for not providing the testing within the first two visits for prenatal care as is noted in the reporting instructions.

Code 3292F is used to identify HIV testing that was ordered or documented and reviewed by the provider. It is used as part of the Screening for Human Immunodeficiency Virus (HIV)[1] measure and is intended to note whether a patient who gave birth during the 12-month period, who was seen for continuing prenatal care, was screened for HIV infection during the first or second prenatal care visit. Only medical and patient reasons exist for not performing this test during the noted timeframe. Therefore, this exclusion information has been captured in the Appendix H measure listing in the exclusion statement as well as in the reporting instructions.

Rh sensitization is a serious complication of pregnancy that places the lives of both mother and child at risk. This complication can be avoided through the prophylactic administration of anti-D immune globulin. In regard to HIV testing, while the number of perinatally transmitted cases of HIV has decreased, perinatal transmission still accounts for the majority of new cases of HIV in children.

Benefits of knowing a woman's HIV status early in pregnancy have been well documented and allow the health care provider to initiate treatment early in the pregnancy, thereby decreasing the risk of transmission of HIV to the child. As a result, the measure specifications and codes developed from these measures assist in compliance with these measures.

●3300F   American Joint Committee on Cancer (AJCC) stage documented and reviewed (ONC)[1]

●3301F   Cancer stage documented in medical record as metastatic and reviewed (ONC)[1]

●3302F   AJCC Cancer Stage 0, documented (ONC)[1], (ML)[5]

●3303F   AJCC Cancer Stage IA, documented (ONC)[1], (ML)[5]

●3304F   AJCC Cancer Stage IB, documented (ONC)[1], (ML)[5]

●3305F   AJCC Cancer Stage IC, documented (ONC)[1], (ML)[5]

●3306F   AJCC Cancer Stage IIA, documented (ONC)[1], (ML)[5]

●3307F   AJCC Cancer Stage IIB, documented (ONC)[1], (ML)[5]

●3308F   AJCC Cancer Stage IIC, documented (ONC)[1], (ML)[5]

●3309F   AJCC Cancer Stage IIIA, documented (ONC)[1], (ML)[5]

●3310F   AJCC Cancer Stage IIIB, documented (ONC)[1], (ML)[5]

●3311F   AJCC Cancer Stage IIIC, documented (ONC)[1], (ML)[5]

▲3312F   AJCC Cancer Stage IVA, documented (ONC)[1], (ML)[5]

(Codes 3313F and 3314F have been deleted)

Rationale

Codes 3300F-3312F are all codes that relate to cancer staging and are listed within four measures: the overuse measure Overutilization of Imaging Studies in Stage 0-IA Melanoma,[5] included within the Melanoma clinical topic, and the Cancer Stage Documented,[1] Hormonal Therapy for Stage IC-IIIC, ER/PR Positive Breast Cancer,[1] and Adjuvant Chemotherapy for Stage IIIA through Stage IIIC Colon Cancer Patients[1] measures included in the Oncology clinical topic. These codes all utilized American Joint Committee on Cancer (AJCC) staging levels to identify the stage (severity) of the cancer involvement.

Codes 3300F and 3301F are both cancer staging codes that identify the documentation and review of the cancer stage. They are used for measurement within the Cancer Stage Documented measure. It is used to determine whether the patient with a diagnosis of breast, colon, or rectal cancer who is receiving chemotherapy or radiation therapy had either a baseline AJCC cancer stage or documentation that the cancer is metastatic in the medical record. As is noted in the descriptor for each of these codes, code 3300F is reported to identify documentation and review of the cancer stage and code 3301F is used to identify documentation of the cancer stage as metastatic. The reporting instructions note that documentation of the cancer stage has no exclusions. As a result, modifiers 1P, 2P, and 3P may not be reported with these codes.

For the most up-to-date version of codes 3302F-3312F, please visit the CPT website.

Codes 3302F-3312F all identify documentation of different cancer stages, beginning with code 3302F for AJCC cancer stage 0 and continuing through code 3312F for AJCC cancer stage IV. Code 3312F was slightly revised after its initial posting on the American Medical Association Web site, removing an additional stage identifier included in the descriptor (deleting the "A" from "IVA"), as this was additional information that was not required for appropriate code identification of the cancer stage. These codes are included as part of three different measures: the Overutilization of Imaging Studies in Stage 0-IA Melanoma[5] measure, the Hormonal Therapy for Stage IC-IIIC, ER/PR Positive Breast Cancer[1] measure, and the Adjuvant Chemotherapy for Stage IIIA through Stage IIIC Colon Cancer patients[1] measure. All three measures use these codes to establish thresholds for identifying when services should or should not be provided.

Two of the measures (the Hormonal Therapy for Stage IC-IIIC, ER/PR Positive Breast Cancer[1] and the Adjuvant Chemotherapy for Stage IIIA through Stage IIIC Colon Cancer Patients[1] measure) use these codes to designate when certain services should be provided. Reporting instructions for these measures direct users to report additional codes if the thresholds are met. For the Hormonal Therapy for Stage IC-IIIC measure, users are directed to report one of the cancer-staging codes for each patient and to additionally report codes 3315F or 3316F if the patient is within the stage IC to IIIC range (ie, codes 3305F-3311F). If the patient is positive for estrogen receptor (ER) or progesterone receptor (PR) for breast cancer (code 3315F) and tamoxifen or an aromatase inhibitor is prescribed, then the measure reporting instructions note that code 4179F should also be reported to identify that the physician has provided the service that meets the requirements of the measure. Coding for the Adjuvant Chemotherapy for Stage IIIA through Stage IIIC Colon Cancer Patients[1] measure is done in a similar manner, using codes 3302F-3311F to identify the cancer stage (codes 3309F-3311F identifying the possible target population) and code 4180F for stage IIIA through stage IIIC colon cancer patients for whom adjuvant chemotherapy was prescribed or previously received. There are also other instructions included with both of these measures that instruct users regarding use of modifiers 1P, 2P, and 3P for appropriate exclusion circumstances for each measure. The Over-utilization of Imaging Studies in Stage 0-IA Melanoma measure is used to designate overuse of imaging studies for certain melanoma patients (stage 0 or IA melanoma). For this measure, the established threshold noted in the measure and identified by use of the codes included is used to identify when the imaging study should not be used (the measure statement cites that the measure determines whether the patient with AJCC stage 0 or IA melanoma, without signs or symptoms, did not have imaging studies ordered). The information included in Appendix H with this measure cites exclusions that would validate provision of the imaging procedures including medical (such as the presentation of patient signs or symptoms that justify imaging) and system (such as the ordering of imaging for clinical trial enrollment of the order of the imaging procedure by another physician) reasons for performing the imaging procedure. In these cases, the reporting instructions included with the measure listing specify the codes for which modifier use is appropriate, noting use of modifiers with code 3319F. It also warns users against incorrect use of modifiers with code 3320F.

There is no valid indication for expensive imaging studies in early-stage melanoma in the absence of signs or symptoms. There is a perception that radiologic studies are being administered for grade 0 and grade I melanoma that are clinically unnecessary and create economic burden to the patient and payer. While diagnostic imaging is inappropriate for patients with higher stages of melanoma as well, this measure is a first step in addressing the overutilization of diagnostic imaging studies in patients with melanoma.

Despite evidence suggesting the role of adjuvant endocrine therapy in lowering the risk of tumor recurrence, many female patients who should be receiving this therapy are not. The Hormonal Therapy for Stage IC-IIIC, ER/PR Positive Breast Cancer[1] measure assesses whether patients with a certain stage of breast cancer (IC-III) and ER/PR positivity are currently receiving the therapy.

Note: The reporting/managing physician does not need to have actually written the prescription; however the reporting/managing physician must verify that the patient already has been prescribed the hormonal therapy by another physician.

Patients with stage IIIA through stage IIIC colon cancer do not always receive the recommended treatment of adjuvant chemotherapy. The Adjuvant Chemotherapy for Stage IIIA Through Stage IIIC Colon Cancer Patients[1] measure is intended to determine whether and how often chemotherapy is administered. The specific chemotherapy drugs specified in this measure reflect the most current guidelines of the National Comprehensive Cancer Network.

●**3315F**   Estrogen receptor (ER) or progesterone receptor (PR) positive breast cancer (ONC)[1]

●**3316F**   Estrogen receptor (ER) and progesterone receptor (PR) negative breast cancer (ONC)[1]

●**3317F**   Pathology report confirming malignancy documented in the medical record and reviewed prior to the initiation of chemotherapy (ONC)[1]

●**3318F**   Pathology report confirming malignancy documented in the medical record and reviewed prior to the initiation of radiation therapy (ONC)[1]

Rationale

Codes 3315F-3318F are all used to identify compliance for two different measures within the Oncology clinical condition set. Each pair of codes also serves different purposes within their respective measures to identify important factors regarding the measure.

Codes 3315F and 3316F are codes that are reported for the Hormonal Therapy for Stage IC-IIIC, ER/PR Positive Breast Cancer[1] measure. The purpose of this measure is to identify whether female patients aged 18 years and older with stage IC through stage IIIC, estrogen receptor (ER)– or progesterone receptor (PR)–positive breast cancer were prescribed tamoxifen or an aromatase inhibitor within the

12-month reporting period. Within this measure, these codes are used as denominator codes to separate the patients who are estrogen or progesterone receptor positive (identified by code 3315F) from those who are are estrogen or progesterone receptor negative (identified by code 3316F) and therefore not part of the target population. The reporting instructions direct users regarding the appropriate use of all of the codes included in this measure including the staging codes 3302F-3312F (see Rationale for codes 3302F-3312F for more information regarding use of these codes), noting use of code 3315F or 3316F if the threshold stages (stage IC through stage IIIC [identified by use of codes 3305F-3311F]) are reached. In these cases, the instructions indicate that if a patient with stage IC through stage IIIC is ER or PR positive (code 3315F), and tamoxifen or an aromatase inhibitor is prescribed, then code 4179F should be additionally reported to identify this circumstance, which denotes compliance with the measure for the target population (as noted in the measure statement). The reporting instruction also states that exclusions exist for use of code 4179F, indicating that modifiers 1P, 2P, or 3P should be reported in addition to code 4179F for these exclusion types. In addition, if reporting exclusion and initial stage or the ER/PR status is unknown, then there is no requirement to report staging codes for the AJCC cancer stage.

Codes 3317F and 3318F are both reported as part of the Pathology Report—Medical Oncology and Radiation Oncology[1] measure. This measure identifies whether the patient with a diagnosis of cancer receiving chemotherapy has a pathology report in the medical record that confirms malignancy prior to the initiation of therapy. As a result, these codes serve a purpose that is somewhat similar to overuse measure codes, since the measure itself notes that a pathology report should be in the medical record prior to the initiation of therapy. In this way, it is not discouraging provision of treatment but instead is ensuring that the appropriate steps are taken prior to the initiation of radiation or chemotherapy treatment. The reporting instructions included with this measure also cite special information regarding the use of these codes, noting that if the patient is seen for the first time by the reporting physician after treatment has been initiated, the pathology report should be documented before the reporting physician *continues* treatment. It further clarifies this by noting that the physician continuing the treatment(s) should report as if treatment is being initiated. Exclusions are also allowed for report of this measure, identifying use of codes 3317F or 3381F with modifier 1P (eg, for palliative treatment of metastatic illness).

Despite evidence suggesting the role of adjuvant endocrine therapy in lowering the risk of tumor recurrence, many female patients who should be receiving hormonal therapy for stage IC through IIIC, ER/PR-positive breast cancer are not.

●3319F   One of the following diagnostic imaging studies ordered: (chest X-ray, CT, Ultrasound, MRI, PET, or nuclear medicine scans) (ML)[5]

●3320F   None of the following diagnostic imaging studies ordered: (chest X-ray, CT, Ultrasound, MRI, PET, or nuclear medicine scans) (ML)[5]

✍ Rationale

Codes 3319F and 3320F are both used to report whether the patient with American Joint Committee on Cancer (AJCC) stage 0 or IA melanoma, without signs or symptoms, did not have imaging studies ordered. They are both included within the Overutilization of Imaging Studies in Stage 0-IA Melanoma[5] measure, which is an overuse measure for imaging. The codes themselves note whether one of a number of diagnostic imaging studies was performed (3319F) or not (3320F). These codes require use of one of the cancer staging codes in the 3302F-3312F series to sort the patient population that is being measured according to those cancer stage patients who should not have the imaging procedures done. For more information regarding the appropriate use of codes 3302F through 3312F for cancer stage reporting and this measure, see the Rationale for these codes.

●3325F Preoperative assessment of functional or medical indication(s) for surgery prior to the cataract surgery with intraocular lens placement (must be performed within twelve months prior to cataract surgery) (EC)[5]

✍ Rationale

Code 3325F is used to report the preoperative assessment for cataract surgery within a 12-month period prior to the surgery. The assessment should identify functional or medical indications. This code is used within the Cataracts: Comprehensive Pre-operative Assessment for Cataract Surgery With Intraocular Lens (IOL) Placement[5] measure, which identifies whether the patient aged 18 years or older who had cataract surgery with intraocular lens (IOL) placement received a comprehensive preoperative assessment prior to the cataract surgery with IOL placement within 12 months prior to surgery. This measure includes use of a composite code that identifies the completion of multiple services when it is reported, but requires that all services listed within the code descriptor be performed. Because no exclusions are cited for this measure, modifiers 1P, 2P, and 3P may not be used with any of the codes included within this measure listing.

To ensure that cataract surgery is appropriate and safe to perform, the operating surgeon is obligated to ensure (1) that there is a patient-centered problem that cataract surgery will address and improve (ie, that there is likely to be an appropriate outcome of surgery); (2) that the safety of the procedure is maximized through appropriate IOL choice to reduce "wrong power IOL" surgery; and (3) that there are no other conditions that would impact either the appropriateness or the safety of surgery through a comprehensive eye examination, including dilation.

The purpose of the comprehensive evaluation of a patient whose chief complaint might be related to a cataract is to determine the presence of a cataract, confirm that a cataract is a significant factor related to the visual impairment and symptoms described by the patient, and exclude or identify other ocular or systemic conditions that might contribute to visual impairment or affect the cataract surgical plan or ultimate outcome. During the preoperative evaluation, other ocular conditions could be found in the course of fundus evaluation that would lead to identification of possible contraindications for surgery.

● **3330F** Imaging study ordered (BkP)[2]

● **3331F** Imaging study not ordered (BkP)[2]

Rationale

Codes 3330F and 3331F are both used to report regarding imaging studies for back pain. These codes are included as part of the Appropriate Imaging for Acute Back Pain[2] measure, which is an overuse measure that identifies when imaging services are inappropriate and should not be reported for back pain. The measure description included in the Appendix H document includes a term that is defined later within the measure listing. "Red flags" are defined as "warning signs" or "signs or symptoms that would warrant [use of] imaging" and include a number of different elements that warn the provider that use of imaging is warranted, including (1) a history of cancer or unexplained weight loss, (2) current infection or immunosuppression, (3) fracture or suspected fracture, and (4) cauda equina syndrome or progressive neurologic deficit. Because this is an overuse measure, codes are used to separate the patient population according to those who are subject to the measure and require absence of imaging to meet the measure (code 1134F) and those who are not to be included as part of the measure and therefore are exempt from further identification (code 1135F, or those patients who would require imaging due to the implicated illness that may be present). Instructions included in the measure statement listing also note that use of code 1134F requires additional reporting of either code 3330F (to note that the imaging study was inappropriately ordered) or code 3331F (to note that the imaging study was not ordered as is appropriate). In addition, the reporting instructions note that code 3330F may be reported with modifier 1P to indicate specific medical exclusions that would warrant the provision of the imaging when done (as is noted in the measure listing provided in Appendix H of the CPT codebook).

▲ **3340F** Mammogram assessment category of "incomplete: need additional imaging evaluation", documented (RAD)[5]

▲ **3341F** Mammogram assessment category of "negative", documented (RAD)[5]

▲ **3342F** Mammogram assessment category of "benign", documented (RAD)[5]

▲ **3343F** Mammogram assessment category of "probably benign", documented (RAD)[5]

▲ **3344F** Mammogram assessment category of "suspicious", documented (RAD)[5]

▲ **3345F** Mammogram assessment category of "highly suggestive of malignancy", documented (RAD)[5]

● **3350F** Mammogram assessment category of "known biopsy proven malignancy", documented (RAD)[5]

Rationale

Codes 3340F-3350F have all been added for the first time to the CPT codebook but have been revised since their initial posting on the American Medical Association Web site. Originally, codes 3340F-3345F each included language in their descriptors that referenced the Breast Imaging Reporting and Data System (BI-RADS), which is a proprietary categorization for mammogram readings. Each of the descriptors for these specific codes has been revised to remove this proprietary language, substituting the more generic term "Mammogram assessment category" with the appropriate level of assessment for each category. The intent of use for these codes is to identify different assessment categories for mammogram readings. The removal of proprietary names from the codes allows other mammogram assessment types to be identified by use of these codes.

The codes are included as part of three separate measures listed in Appendix H for the Radiology clinical topic: Inappropriate Use of "Probably Benign" Assessment Category in Mammography Screening,[5] Communication of Suspicious Findings From the Diagnostic Mammogram to the Practice Managing Ongoing Care,[5] and Communication of Suspicious Findings From the Diagnostic Mammogram to the Patient.[5] The first measure is used to determine whether the patient had a final report for a screening mammogram that was classified as "probably benign." As is noted in the code descriptors for this measure, these codes are used to identify a range of categorization for mammogram assessment that includes "incomplete," "negative," "benign," "probably benign," "suspicious," "highly suggestive of malignancy," and "known biopsy proven malignancy." A definition for the category "probably benign" has also been included, noting that this includes the Mammography Quality Standards Act assessment category of "probably benign"; BI-RADS category 3; or a Food and Drug Administration–approved equivalent assessment category. The technical specifications for this measure are also cited to allow additional identification of the appropriate information for this level of category. The second and third measures determine whether the patient undergoing a diagnostic mammogram classified as "suspicious" or "highly suggestive of malignancy" has documentation of direct communication of findings from the diagnostic mammogram to the practice within 3 business days of examination interpretation or to the patient within 5 business days. Codes 3340F-3350F are used in these measures as denominator codes to separate the patient populations according to thresholds designated in each measure. Since these descriptions also included the proprietary language, they were changed to reflect nonproprietary, generic language. Other information regarding the first measure was also revised to reflect changes to the measure itself to remove reference of communication to the patient and replace it with communication to the practice that manages ongoing care or to the treating or referring physician or representative. Information has also been included with the numerator and denominator statements for this measure to define direct communication and "suspicious" and "highly suggestive of malignancy" as referenced in these statements. Reporting instructions provided within the Appendix H listing of both measures direct users regarding appropriate use of codes that identify compliance with the measure, using code 5060F in the first measure to allow report of communication within 3 days of suspicious findings to the practice managing care and code 5062F in the second measure to allow report of communication within 5 days of suspicious findings to the patient.

Note: Codes 5060F and 5062F both included proprietary language that was removed from each descriptor. The language now reflects generic nonproprietary wording that allows other mammogram assessment types to be identified by use of these codes.

- ●**3351F**   Negative screen for depressive symptoms as categorized by using a standardized depression screening/assessment tool (MDD)[2]
- ●**3352F**   No significant depressive symptoms as categorized by using a standardized depression assessment tool (MDD)[2]
- ●**3353F**   Mild to moderate depressive symptoms as categorized by using a standardized depression screening/assessment tool (MDD)[2]
- ●**3354F**   Clinically significant depressive symptoms as categorized by using a standardized depression screening/assessment tool (MDD)[2]

Rationale

Codes 3351F-3354F are all included as part of a single measure listed within the Major Depressive Disorder clinical condition. These codes are used to identify progressively higher symptoms for categorizing major depressive disorder. As a result, these codes designate a threshold identified within the measure (patients who are in a high-risk category) that specifies the target population for measurement purposes. The denominator information listed in Appendix H indicates that patients who have positive screens for depressive symptoms but who do not receive further assessment of depressive symptoms with a standardized tool do not count toward the numerator. This is noted to alert users that additional services should be provided for these patients; provision of screening for these patients that produces positive results is not enough to meet the measure requirements, as further testing of this patient with a standardized tool for screening is expected. The measure further alerts users that documentation of any of the levels of progression for screening counts toward meeting the measure requirements. This information is noted within the four codes used for this measure. Additional information is also included to identify high-risk categories that would inherently be included as part of this measure and should therefore be categorized and measured for compliance, including certain specific conditions that place a patient at risk, such as diabetes, persistent asthma, chronic obstructive pulmonary disease, and low back pain. Because no exclusions are cited for this measure, modifiers 1P, 2P, and 3P may not be used with any codes included in this measure.

4000F   Tobacco use cessation intervention, counseling (COPD, CAP, CAD)[1] (DM)[4] (PV)[2]

4001F   Tobacco use cessation intervention, pharmacologic therapy (COPD, CAP, CAD)[1] (DM)[4] (PV)[2]

Code 4007F has been deleted. To report age related eye disease study (AREDS) formulation prescribed or recommended, use code 4177F

4009F   Angiotensin converting enzyme (ACE) inhibitor or Angiotensin Receptor Blocker (ARB) therapy prescribed (HF, CAD CKD)[1], (DM)[2]

4037F   Influenza immunization ordered or administered (COPD, PV, CKD, ESRD)[1]

▲ **4040F** Pneumococcal vaccine administered or previously received (COPD)[1], (PV)[2]

4051F Referred for an arteriovenous (AV) fistula (ESRD, CKD)[1]

4120F Antibiotic prescribed or dispensed (URI, PHAR, A-BRONCH)[2]

4124F Antibiotic neither prescribed nor dispensed (URI, PHAR, A-BRONCH)[2]

🖉 Rationale

Codes 4000F, 4001F, 4009F, 4037F, 4051F, 4120F, and 4124F are all included in *CPT Changes 2009* to reflect changes to the listed information for these codes that do not reflect an alteration in the intent of use for the codes. This is because the descriptor language for each of the codes remains intact and unchanged; therefore, the intent of the code remains the same. Instead, the change made to the code listing reflects either (1) a change to the suffix(es) listed with the code that identifies additional measures for which this code may be listed/used or (2) the addition of a superscript that identifies the measure developer/endorser for the measure for which the code was developed. In both cases, the addition of the information simply expands the usage of the code by allowing the code to be reported for additional measures. As a result, the delta symbol (▲) is not included with the code listing when only the superscript or a suffix acronym is added/deleted from the code language.

Code 4040F was revised to reflect an editorial correction to the measure language deleting the word "ordered" and inserting the word "administered" to instead reflect that the vaccine was administered or previously received. The code is still included as part of the Chronic Obstructive Pulmonary Disease (COPD) and Preventive Care (PV) clinical topics.

● **4130F** Topical preparations (including OTC) prescribed for acute otitis externa (AOE)[1]

● **4131F** Systemic antimicrobial therapy prescribed (AOE)[1]

● **4132F** Systemic antimicrobial therapy not prescribed (AOE)[1]

🖉 Rationale

Codes 4130F-4132F are used to report measure compliance in the Acute Otitis Externa (AOE) clinical topic. Code 4130F is used as part of a separate measure from codes 4131F and 4132F within this measure topic, as is reflected in the Appendix H document.

Code 4130F is used in the Acute Otitis Externa—Topical Therapy[1] measure to identify prescription of topical preparations for AOE. The measure determines whether the patient aged 2 years or older with a diagnosis of AOE was prescribed topical preparations. This is important, as topical preparations used to treat AOE are active against the most common bacterial pathogens in AOE, *Pseudomonas aeruginosa* and *Staphylococcus aureus* (topical preparations have demonstrated efficacy in the treatment of AOE with resolution in about 65-90% of patients). Both medical and patient exclusions exist for this measure. As a result, the reporting instructions included in the Appendix H document note that modifiers 1P and 2P may be used in addition to code 4130F.

Codes 4131F and 4132F are both used as part of measures that have similar purposes for two different patient populations. Code 4131F and 4132F are used in the Systemic Antimicrobials—Avoidance of Inappropriate Use[1] measure to identify whether the patient aged 2 months through 12 years with a diagnosis of otitis media with effusion was *not* prescribed systemic antimicrobials. These codes are used for a similar purpose in the Systemic Antimicrobial Therapy—Avoidance of Inappropriate Use[1] measure, as the actual measure is for AOE and also differs according to the ages identified within these measures. Both measures are overuse measures and are intended to measure restriction of use of antimicrobials. These measures, however, do allow use of antimicrobials under certain medical circumstances. As a result, the reporting instructions for these measures note that the 1P modifier may be appended to code 4131F for valid medical reasons. The instructions for both measures specifically identify use of the modifier in addition to code 4131F, as this demonstrates that systemic antimicrobial therapy *was* prescribed (as identified by code 4131F), and that a medical reason exists for why this code was used (as identified by modifier 1P). If the antimicrobial agent was *not* prescribed, then code 4132F is used to identify this circumstance.

Many patients with AOE receive systemic antimicrobial therapy despite its limited utility, often in addition to topical therapy. There are no data on the efficacy of systemic therapy with the use of appropriate antibacterials and stratified by severity of the infection. Moreover, orally administered antibiotics have significant adverse effects that include rashes, vomiting, diarrhea, allergic reactions, altered nasopharyngeal flora, and development of bacterial resistance. The use of systemic antimicrobial therapy to treat AOE should be limited to those clinical situations in which it is indicated.

●**4133F**   Antihistamines or decongestants prescribed or recommended (OME)[1]

●**4134F**   Antihistamines or decongestants neither prescribed nor recommended (OME)[1]

●**4135F**   Systemic corticosteroids prescribed (OME)[1]

●**4136F**   Systemic corticosteroids not prescribed (OME)[1]

Rationale

Codes 4133F-4136F are used as part of overuse measures. These include the Otitis Media With Effusion Antihistamines or Decongestants—Avoidance of Inappropriate Use[1] measure and the measure for Otitis Media With Effusion Systemic Steroids—Avoidance of Inappropriate Use.[1] The difference between these measures is the material that is intended for restriction within the measure (antihistamines/decongestants or systemic steroids). For these measures, codes 4133F-4136F are all used to identify whether the antihistamines or decongestants or systemic corticosteroids were not prescribed according to the intent of the measures. These measures also allow for medical exclusion by noting use of modifier 1P with codes 4133F and/or 4135F in the reporting instructions for each measure.

Otitis media with effusion usually resolves spontaneously, with indications for therapy only if the condition is persistent and clinically significant benefits can be achieved. Antimicrobials have no proven long-term effectiveness and have potential adverse effects for this condition.

●**4150F**   Patient receiving antiviral treatment for Hepatitis C (HEP C)[1]

●**4151F**   Patient not receiving antiviral treatment for Hepatitis C (HEP C)[1]

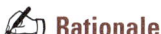 **Rationale**

Codes 4150F and 4151F both identify information related to compliance with a number of measures, including Hepatitis C Ribonucleic Acid (RNA) Testing Before Initiating Therapy,[1] HCV Genotype Testing Prior to Therapy,[1] Combination Antiviral Therapy,[1] HCV Quantitative RNA Testing at Week 12 of Therapy,[1] and Counseling Regarding Use of Contraception Prior to Antiviral Therapy,[1] all of which are measures included as part of the hepatitis C clinical condition. In each measure, they are used as denominator codes, which are codes that differentiate the patient population for these measures, ie, they differentiate the patients who have received antiviral treatment for hepatitis C (code 4150F) and are therefore eligible for measurement from those who have not received the treatment (code 4151F) and should not be included for measurement. This separation allows users the ability to determine and report whether the measured action has been taken for the desired patient population. Because some of these measures allow for exclusion, the reporting instructions note the appropriate modifier(s) to use for the appropriate code (outside of codes 4150F and 4151F) and, in some cases, give examples of the types of circumstances that would qualify for use of the modifier. Other reporting instructions within some measures specify exclusion of use of the modifier for any codes included within that measure.

For each measure, codes listed to note compliance with the measure's specifications have also been included in the listing. These include codes 3218F, 3220F, 3266F, 4153F, and 4159F.

●**4152F**   Documentation that combination peginterferon and ribavirin therapy considered (HEP-C)[1]

●**4153F**   Combination peginterferon and ribavirin therapy prescribed (HEP-C)[1]

●**4154F**   Hepatitis A vaccine series recommended (HEP-C)[1]

●**4155F**   Hepatitis A vaccine series previously received (HEP-C)[1]

●**4156F**   Hepatitis B vaccine series recommended (HEP-C)[1]

●**4157F**   Hepatitis B vaccine series previously received (HEP-C)[1]

●**4158F**   Patient education regarding risk of alcohol consumption performed (HEP-C)[1]

●**4159F**   Counseling regarding contraception received prior to initiation of antiviral treatment (HEP-C)[1]

🖉 Rationale

Codes 4154F, 4155F, 4156F, 4157F, and 4158F are all included as part of the Hepatitis C clinical topic. Codes 4154F and 4155F are used as part of the Hepatitis A Vaccination[1] measure, which determines whether the patient aged 18 years or older with a diagnosis of hepatitis C was offered or received hepatitis A vaccination, or has documented immunity. Each of the codes within this measure (4154F, 4155F, and 3215F) identify compliance with some part of the measure. Codes 4156F and 4157F note compliance within the measure for Hepatitis B Vaccination, which determines whether the patient aged 18 years or older with a diagnosis of hepatitis C was offered or received hepatitis B vaccination, or has documented immunity. Code 4158F is used within the Education Regarding Risk of Alcohol Consumption[1] measure, which notes whether the patient aged 18 years or older with a diagnosis of hepatitis C received education regarding the risk of alcohol consumption at least once within the 12-month reporting period. Although some of the measures relate to other types of hepatitis (ie, A and B), each of the measures in this clinical topic relates back to factors that denote compliance for hepatitis C. As a result, the codes included in these measures and within this clinical topic identify compliance with the Hepatitis clinical topic.

Codes 4152F, 4153F, and 4159F are used to identify compliance for the Consideration for Antiviral Therapy[1] (codes 4152F and 4153F), Combination Antiviral Therapy[1] (code 4153F), and Counseling Regarding Use of Contraception Prior to Antiviral Therapy[1] (code 4159F) measures. For the Consideration for Antiviral Therapy[1] measure, use of either code 4152F or 4153F identifies compliance with the measure, while separate use of code 4153F or 4159F identifies compliance with the Consideration for Antiviral Therapy[1] and Counseling Regarding Use of Contraception Prior to Antiviral Therapy[1] (code 4159F) measures. Codes 4150F and 4151F are used as denominator codes for each of these measures. For more information regarding use of code 4159F, see the Rationale for codes 4150F and 4151F.

●**4163F** Patient counseling at a minimum on all of the following treatment options for clinically localized prostate cancer: active surveillance, AND interstitial prostate brachytherapy, AND external beam radiotherapy, AND radical prostatectomy, provided prior to initiation of treatment (PRCA)[1]

●**4164F** Adjuvant (ie, in combination with external beam radiotherapy to the prostate for prostate cancer) hormonal therapy (gonadotropin-releasing hormone [GnRH] agonist or antagonist) prescribed/administered (PRCA)[1]

Code 4163F is used to report whether prostate cancer patients with clinically localized disease received counseling regarding certain specific treatment options for their disease. It is included as part of the Prostate Cancer clinical topic within the Treatment Options for Patients With Clinically Localized Disease[1] measure. This measure allows for medical exclusions and includes a definition of salvage therapy.

Code 4164F is used to identify compliance with the Adjuvant Hormonal Therapy for High-Risk Patients.[1] For more information regarding use of this code and other codes included as part of this measure, see the Rationale listing for codes 3271F through 3274F.

●4165F 3-dimensional conformal radiotherapy (3D-CRT) or intensity modulated radiation therapy (IMRT) received (PRCA)[1]

Rationale

Code 4165F is used to report performance measurement for the 3-Dimensional Radiotherapy[1] measure within the Prostate Cancer clinical topic. It is used to determine whether a patient with prostate cancer who is receiving external beam radiotherapy to the prostate *only* (no metastases) received 3-dimensional conformal radiotherapy or intensity-modulated radiation therapy. Use of this code requires use of denominator code 4200F or 4201F to sort the patient population into those patients who received external beam therapy for regions other than the prostate (code 4201F) and those within the target population, ie, patients who received external beam radiotherapy to the prostate only (code 4200F). Reporting instructions direct users to report code 4165F to identify compliance with the measure when patients within the target population received 3-dimensional conformal radiotherapy or intensity-modulated radiation therapy. The reporting instructions also notify users of the absence of exclusions for this measure. As a result, no exclusions are reportable for this measure and modifiers 1P, 2P, and 3P may not be used with any of the codes included with this measure.

Current computer-aided radiotherapy techniques improve the precision of the irradiation of cancerous tissue and should be employed for all patients receiving external beam radiotherapy to the prostate.

●4167F Head of bed elevation (30-45 degrees) on first ventilator day ordered (CRIT)[1]

●4168F Patient receiving care in the intensive care unit (ICU) and receiving mechanical ventilation, 24 hours or less (CRIT)[1]

●4169F Patient either not receiving care in the intensive care unit (ICU) OR not receiving mechanical ventilation OR receiving mechanical ventilation greater than 24 hours (CRIT)[1]

Rationale

Codes 4167F-4169F are all used as part of a single measure included in the Anesthesiology/Critical Care clinical topic. This measure (Prevention of Ventilator-Associated Pneumonia—Head Elevation[1]) determines whether the patient aged 18 years or older receiving care in the intensive care unit (ICU) who received mechanical ventilation had an order on the first ventilator day for head of bed elevation (30-45 degrees). Codes 4168F and 4169F are used as denominator codes that differentiate the patients being targeted by the measure (those patients receiving care in the ICU and receiving mechanical ventilation—code 4168F) from those who are to be excluded from measurement (patients not receiving care in the ICU, not receiving mechanical ventilation, or receiving mechanical ventilation for more than 24 hours—code 4169F). For those patients who are within the correct population, code 4167F may be used to identify that the head of the patient's bed was elevated 30-45 degrees on the first ventilator day that the procedure was ordered. Medical exclusions are allowed for this measure, and modifier 1P may be used with code 4167F for patients who meet these exclusion criteria.

- **●4171F** Patient receiving erythropoiesis-stimulating agents (ESA) therapy (CKD)[1]

- **●4172F** Patient not receiving erythropoiesis-stimulating agents (ESA) therapy (CKD)[1]

Rationale

Codes 4171F and 4172F are both used as part of the Plan of Care—Elevated Hemoglobin for Patients Receiving Erythropoiesis-Stimulating Agents (ESA)[1] measure within the Chronic Kidney Disease clinical topic. Although other codes more specifically separate the targeted patient population according to specific thresholds designated within the measure (via use of codes 3279F, 3280F, and 3281F; see Rationale for these codes for more regarding their use), codes 4171F and 4172F are used as denominator codes to designate the target patient population, directing users to report code 4171F for patients who receive therapy with erythropoiesis-stimulating agents. Because exclusions are not included as part of the measure, modifiers 1P, 2P, and 3P may not be reported with these codes for this measure, as is noted in the reporting instructions.

- **●4174F** Counseling about the potential impact of glaucoma on visual functioning and quality of life, and importance of treatment adherence provided to patient and/or caregiver(s) (EC)[5]

- **●4175F** Best-corrected visual acuity of 20/40 or better (distance or near) achieved within the 90 days following cataract surgery (EC)[5]

- **●4176F** Counseling about value of protection from UV light and lack of proven efficacy of nutritional supplements in prevention or progression of cataract development provided to patient and/or caregiver(s) (NMA—No Measure Associated)

- **●4177F** Counseling about the benefits and/or risks of the Age-Related Eye Disease Study (AREDS) formulation for preventing progression of age-related macular degeneration (AMD) provided to patient and/or caregiver(s) (EC)[5]

Rationale

Codes 4174F, 4175F, and 4177F are all included as part of the Eye Care clinical topic. Each code, however, is included as part of separate measures within this clinical topic and identifies either provision of counseling (codes 4174F and 4177F) or the achievement of a particular level of visual acuity after cataract surgery (code 4175F).

Codes 4174 and 4177F are both used to identify counseling provided to the patient regarding primary open-angle glaucoma (code 4174F) or antioxidant supplement for age-related macular degeneration (code 4177F). For both codes, system exclusions exist, and modifier 3P may be appended to these codes to identify system exclusions such as when the physician reporting the code is not the physician performing the service specified in the measure. In addition, report of code 4174F for counseling for primary open-angle glaucoma allows for medical exclusions as well, as is indicated in the reporting instructions for this measure. Code 4177F is a replacement code for code 4007F, which was deleted. Code 4177F was developed to more accurately reflect the intent of the measure. (For more information regarding the deletion of code 4007F, see the Rationale for that code.)

Code 4175F is used to report a visual acuity correction of at least 20/40 within 90 days of the cataract surgery. It is included as part of the Cataracts: 20/40 or Better Visual Acuity Within 90 Days Following Cataract Surgery[5] measure, which determines whether the patient aged 18 years or older who had cataract surgery and had no significant ocular conditions impacting the visual outcome of surgery had best-corrected visual acuity of 20/40 or better (distance or near) achieved within 90 days following the cataract surgery. This measure is different from most other measures as it requires use of *International Classification of Diseases, Ninth Revision*, codes to identify exclusions. The reporting instructions identify this and note that modifiers 1P, 2P, and 3P should not be used with this code. In addition, a special note has been included in the reporting instructions to reference the complete listing of the measure and its specifications for a detailed list of qualifying conditions.

Code 4176F was previously included as part of the Eye Care Clinical Topic. However, the single measure in which this code was included has been removed. The code itself has been retained in the CPT codebook in the Category II code section, but as a result of the deletion of the measure, it does not appear as part of any other clinical topic or measure. As a result, since this code is not included as part of any other measure in Appendix H, this code has been identified as "NMA—No Measure Associated" and will be maintained in the codebook until it is included within a measure listing or is deleted due to lack of a need for use.

●4178F   Anti-D immune globulin received between 26 and 30 weeks gestation (PRENATAL)[1]

Rationale

Code 4178F is used as part of the Prenatal clinical topic. It identifies compliance with the Anti-D Immune Globulin[1] measure, which determines whether the D (Rh)–negative and unsensitized patient who gave birth during the 12-month period, who was seen for continuing prenatal care, received anti-D immune globulin at 26-30 weeks' gestation. Medical, patient, and system exclusions exist for this measure, and the reporting instructions therefore note allowance of use of modifiers 1P, 2P, and 3P with this code. The reporting instructions also note use of code 4178F to identify Rh-negative patients who are unsensitized and who are administered the anti-D immune globulin within the 26th to 30th weeks of gestation.

●4179F   Tamoxifen or aromatase inhibitor (AI) prescribed (ONC)[1]

Rationale

Code 4179F is used to report prescription of tamoxifen or an aromatase inhibitor and is used as part of the Hormonal Therapy for Stage IC-IIIC, ER/PR Positive Breast Cancer[1] measure in the Oncology series. Use of this code identifies compliance with this measure for the target population. For more information regarding use of code 4179F, see the Rationale for codes 3315F-3316F.

- **4180F** Adjuvant chemotherapy prescribed or previously received for Stage IIIA through Stage IIIC colon cancer (ONC)[1]
- **4181F** Conformal radiation therapy received (NMA—No Measure Assoc.)
- **4182F** Conformal radiation therapy not received (NMA—No Measure Assoc.)

✎ Rationale

Code 4180F is used to report measurement for the Adjuvant Chemotherapy for Stage IIIA Through Stage IIIC Colon Cancer Patients[1] measure, which is part of the Oncology clinical topic. Use of this code notes compliance for this measure, as the measure determines whether the patient aged 18 years or older with stage IIIA through stage IIIC colon cancer was prescribed or previously received adjuvant chemotherapy within the 12-month reporting period. The numerator information listed in Appendix H notes that special guidelines referenced within the actual measure denote special recommended therapies for these circumstances. In addition, medical, patient, and system exclusions exist, and as a result, modifiers 1P, 2P, and 3P may be used to identify exclusionary circumstances when reporting for this measure.

Codes 4181F and 4182F are both codes that were previously included in the Appendix H listing. However, the measure in which these codes were included was removed. As a result, the codes no longer appear in the Appendix H listing. The codes themselves, however, have been retained in the Category II code section of the CPT codebook. As a result of the deletion, because these codes are not included as part of any other measure in Appendix H, the codes have been identified as "NMA—No Measure Associated" and will be maintained in the codebook until they are included within a measure listing or are deleted due to lack of a need for use.

- **4185F** Continuous (12-months) therapy with proton pump inhibitor (PPI) or histamine H2 receptor antagonist (H2RA) received (GERD)[5]
- **4186F** No continuous (12-months) therapy with either proton pump inhibitor (PPI) or histamine H2 receptor antagonist (H2RA) received (GERD)[5]

✎ Rationale

Codes 4185F and 4186F are included as part of the Gastroesophageal Reflux Disease clinical topic. For information regarding use of these codes, see the discussion included for code 1118F.

- **4187F** Disease modifying anti-rheumatic drug therapy prescribed or dispensed (RA)[2]

🖉 Rationale

Code 4187F is used to report the prescription, dispensing, or administration of disease-modifying antirheumatic drugs for patients with rheumatoid arthritis. It is included as part of the Disease-Modifying Antirheumatic Drug Therapy in Rheumatoid Arthritis[2] measure in the Rheumatoid Arthritis clinical condition. Medical exclusions exist for this measure, and therefore, reporting instructions note that modifier 1P may be used to identify medical exclusions when appropriate exclusions exist. In addition, an additional definition has been included to note that *dispensed* encompasses administered disease-modifying antirheumatic drug therapy.

●4188F Appropriate angiotensin converting enzyme (ACE)/angiotensin receptor blockers (ARB) therapeutic monitoring test ordered or performed (AM)[2]

●4189F Appropriate digoxin therapeutic monitoring test ordered or performed (AM)[2]

●4190F Appropriate diuretic therapeutic monitoring test ordered or performed (AM)[2]

●4191F Appropriate anticonvulsant therapeutic monitoring test ordered or performed (AM)[2]

🖉 Rationale

Codes 4188F-4191F are all used to report measurement for the annual monitoring measure set. This is a new clinical topic and includes a single measure that identifies Annual Monitoring for Patients on Angiotensin Converting Enzyme (ACE) Inhibitors or Angiotensin Receptor Blockers (ARB).[2] These codes are used to note compliance with the measure for the order or performance of an appropriate (1) angiotensin converting enzyme or angiotensin receptor blocker, (2) digoxin, (3) diuretic, or (4) anticonvulsant therapy monitoring test (codes 4188F-4191F, respectively). Denominator codes have been included with this measure, which include codes 4210F, 4220F, 4221F, and 4230F. Each of these codes corresponds to use of one of the compliance codes listed above, directly indicating whether the patient should be included as part of the target population. Codes 4210F, 4220F, 4221F, and 4230F do this through use of descriptor language that denotes a single code for each therapeutic agent listed. The denominator codes also cite time as a factor for use of these codes, noting that the target population includes medication therapy assigned for 6 months or more. To assist users with reporting allowed medical exclusions, reporting instructions have been included that identify use of modifier 1P with codes 4188F-4191F only, as these codes are used to identify the targeted action desired for this measure.

●4200F External beam radiotherapy to prostate only (PRCA)[1]

●4201F External beam radiotherapy for prostate cancer to region(s) other than prostate only (PRCA)[1]

●4210F Angiotensin converting enzyme (ACE) or angiotensin receptor blockers (ARB) medication therapy for 6 months or more (AM)[2]

●4220F Digoxin medication therapy for 6 months or more (AM)[2]

- **4221F** Diuretic medication therapy for 6 months or more (AM)[2]
- **4230F** Anticonvulsant medication therapy for 6 months or more (AM)[2]

✍ Rationale

Codes 4200F and 4201F are used as denominator codes for the Prostate Cancer clinical topic, while codes 4210F, 4220F, 4221F, and 4230F are used as denominator codes within the Annual Monitoring clinical topic. For more information regarding use of these codes, see the Rationale for codes 4200F, 4201F, and 4188F through 4191F.

- **4240F** Instruction in therapeutic exercise with follow-up by the physician provided to patients during episode of back pain lasting longer than 12 weeks (BkP)[2]
- **4242F** Counseling for supervised exercise program provided to patients during episode of back pain lasting longer than 12 weeks (BkP)[2]
- **4245F** Patient counseled during the initial visit to maintain or resume normal activities (BkP)[2]
- **4248F** Patient counseled during the initial visit for an episode of back pain against bed rest lasting 4 days or longer (BkP)[2]

✍ Rationale

Codes 4240F, 4242F, 4245F, and 4248F are all used to report performance measurement for the Back Pain clinical topic. They are included as part of 3 separate measures within this topic, including Recommendation for Exercise for Back Pain Patients,[2] Advice for Normal Activities for Back Pain Patients,[2] and Advice Against Bed Rest for Back Pain Patients. In each of these measures, denominator codes are used to specify the target population for the measure. The measures, however, use different codes to define the denominator (target population).

Codes 4240F and 4242F are used to identify compliance as part of the Recommendation for Exercise for Back Pain Patients[2] measure. This measure uses codes 1137F and 1138F to identify the denominator population and does not allow for exclusions. As a result, the reporting instructions included with this measure note that modifiers 1P, 2P, and 3P may not be used with any of the codes included with this measure. The reporting instructions also direct users to use either code 1137F or 1138F for each patient, and to use either code 4240F or 4242F to identify compliance with the measure.

Codes 4245F and 4248F are used as part of separate measures: Advice for Normal Activities for Back Pain Patients[2] and Advice Against Bed Rest for Back Pain Patients,[2] respectively. They both utilize the same codes to identify the denominator population—codes 0525F and 0526F—which separate back pain patients into initial visit patients (identified by code 0525F, which includes the target population) and subsequent visit patients (code 0526F). Neither of these measures allows for exclusions, as is noted in the reporting instructions. The instructions listed for the Advice for Normal Activities for Back Pain Patients[2] measure, however, provides additional advice for "normal" activities to further clarify the measure's intent, as this measure is intended to identify whether the patient was counseled regarding maintaining or resuming normal activities. This note clarifies what is considered "normal" by issuing a warning against "normal" activities that would be detrimental to the healing process.

●**4250F** Active warming used intraoperatively for the purpose of maintaining normothermia, OR at least one body temperature equal to or greater than 36 degrees Centigrade (or 96.8 degrees Fahrenheit) recorded within the 30 minutes immediately before or the 30 minutes immediately after anesthesia end time (CRIT)[1]

Rationale

Code 4250F is used to report whether the patient, regardless of age, undergoing a surgical or therapeutic procedure under general or neuraxial anesthesia of 60 minutes' duration or longer had *either* active warming used intraoperatively for the purpose of maintaining normothermia, *or* at least one body temperature equal to or greater than 36 degrees Centigrade (or 96.8 degrees Fahrenheit) recorded within the 30 minutes immediately before or the 30 minutes immediately after anesthesia end time. It is included as part of the Anesthesiology/Critical Care (CRIT) Perioperative Temperature Management for Surgical Procedures Under General Anesthesia[1] measure and is the only code used to identify the appropriate patient population and compliance with the measure. A definition has been included with this measure to note modalities that are included for active warming. Only medical exclusions exist for this measure, and therefore, only modifier 1P may be appended to this code to identify medical exclusions.

●**5020F** Treatment summary report communicated to physician(s) managing continuing care within 1 month of completing treatment (ONC)[1]

Rationale

Code 5020F is used to report performance measurement for the Treatment Summary Communication—Radiation Oncology[1] measure, which notes whether the patient with a diagnosis of cancer who has undergone radiation therapy has a treatment summary report in the chart that was communicated to the physician(s) providing continuing care within 1 month of completing treatment. To help to clarify the intent of the measure and use of the codes for users, a definition for treatment summary has been included with the numerator listing, noting that the treatment summary is a report that includes mention of (1) dose delivered; (2) relevant assessment of tolerance to and progress toward the treatment goals; and (3) subsequent care plans. The reporting instructions note that (1) the measure is reported once at the conclusion of each course of treatment (informing users of how often the service code should be reported) and (2) modifiers 2P and 3P may be used to identify patient and system exclusions for this measure.

Timely, accurate, and effective communications are critical to quality and value in contemporary medical practices. As both a consultant oncologist and the provider of radiation oncology services, the radiation oncologist has a dual role. Radiation therapy incorporates the science of complex, integrated treatment delivery and the art of individual cancer management. Through written focused reports and direct communications, the contribution of radiation oncologists concerning patient care, responsible utilization, and quality are provided, especially to primary care physicians, other oncologists and specialists, and allied health care providers (nurses, tumor registrars, quality assurance personnel, third-party reviewers, etc).

●**5050F** Treatment plan communicated to provider(s) managing continuing care within 1 month of diagnosis (ML)[5]

 Rationale

Code 5050F is used to report the communication of a treatment plan communicated to the provider managing continuing care within 1 month of the diagnosis of the disease. It is included within the Melanoma clinical topic as part of the Melanoma Coordination of Care[5] measure. Codes 1127F and 1128F are used as denominator codes for this measure, separating the target population (patients who are being treated for a new episode of the condition; code 1127F) from patients who are not a part of the target population (those with a subsequent episode of the condition; code 1128F). Patients being treated for a subsequent episode of the condition are not included as part of the target population, as the intent of this measure is to enable the primary care provider to support, facilitate, and coordinate the care of the patient. This is important due to the perception of a lack of follow-up with primary care providers for these patients (provision of a subsequent episode of care denotes follow-up with the patient, and therefore, patients for whom a subsequent visit is provided are inherently excluded from measurement). An explanation has been included in the numerator statement to educate users regarding the elements included for a treatment plan, which comprises the diagnosis, tumor thickness, and plan for surgery or alternate care. Patient and system exclusions exist for this measure; therefore, modifiers 2P and 3P may be used to identify the allowed exclusions for this measure.

●**5060F** Findings from diagnostic mammogram communicated to practice managing patient's on-going care within 3 business days of exam interpretation (RAD)[5]

●**5062F** Findings from diagnostic mammogram communicated to the patient within 5 business days of exam interpretation (RAD)[5]

Rationale

Codes 5060F and 5062F are used in separate measures: Communication of Suspicious Findings From the Diagnostic Mammogram to the Practice Managing Ongoing Care[5] and Communication of Suspicious Findings From the Diagnostic Mammogram to the Patient,[5] respectively. They are both used to indicate compliance with the respective measure in which they are listed. For more information regarding use of these codes, see the Rationale included for codes 3040F-3050F.

●**6030F** All elements of maximal sterile barrier technique including: cap AND mask AND sterile gown AND sterile gloves AND a large sterile sheet AND hand hygiene AND 2% chlorhexidine for cutaneous antisepsis, followed (CRIT)[1]

✍ Rationale

Code 6030F is used to report whether all elements of maximal sterile barrier technique were followed, including use of a cap, mask, sterile gown, sterile gloves, a large sterile sheet, adherence to hand hygiene, and 2% chlorhexidine for cutaneous antisepsis. Only code 6030F is listed for this measure, and therefore this code is used to identify compliance with the measure specifications. To exemplify this, all of the previously noted components are included as part of the code descriptor, alerting users to the importance of including all of these elements. To ensure that the appropriate population is included for this measure, a note has been incorporated into the denominator language directing users to the measure specifications on the developer's Web site for information regarding the central venous catheters that are appropriate for identifying the denominator population.

Catheter-related bloodstream infection is a costly complication of central venous catheter insertion. This condition may be avoided with routine use of aseptic technique during catheter insertion.

●**6040F** Use of appropriate radiation dose reduction devices OR manual techniques for appropriate moderation of exposure, documented (RAD)[5]

●**6045F** Radiation exposure or exposure time in final report for procedure using fluoroscopy, documented (RAD)[5]

✍ Rationale

Codes 6040F and 6045F are used to report compliance for different measures within the Radiology measure set. They are both used to help measure regulation of radiation dosage or exposure but include different descriptors to accomplish this. Code 6040F is included as part of the CT Radiation Dose Reduction[5] measure and determines whether there is documentation of use of appropriate radiation dose reduction devices for the radiation treatment or whether appropriate documentation exists identifying the use of manual techniques for appropriate moderation of exposure to radiation during treatment. Both elements are included as part of this code, and therefore, this code may be used to identify compliance if documentation for either element is provided. Code 6045F is used to identify documentation of radiation exposure or exposure time in the final report for procedures using fluoroscopy as part of the Exposure Time Reported for Procedures Using Fluoroscopy[5] measure. Neither procedure allows for exclusions as part of the measure. As a result, the reporting instructions note that modifiers 1P, 2P, and 3P may not be used to identify exclusions for these measures.

While the use of computed tomography (CT) in adults and children has increased nearly seven-fold in the past 10 years, data suggest that the lifetime risk of cancer can be increased, albeit by a small amount, with frequent or repeated exposure to ionizing radiation. The National Cancer Institute has noted "adjustments are not frequently made in the exposure parameters that determine the amount of radiation children receive from CT, resulting in a greater radiation dose than necessary." In order to monitor these long term effects, the exposure time or radiation dose that a patient receives as a result of the procedure should be measured and recorded in the patient's record.

▶Structural Measures◀

▶Structural measures codes are used to identify measures that address the setting or system of the delivered care. These codes also address aspects of the capabilities of the organization or health care professional providing the care.◀

- ●7010F   Patient information entered into a recall system with the target date for the next exam specified (ML)[5]

- ●7020F   Mammogram assessment category (eg, Mammography Quality Standards Act (MQSA), Breast Imaging Reporting and Data System (BI-RADS®), or FDA approved equivalent categories) entered into an internal database to allow for analysis of abnormal interpretation (recall) rate (RAD)[5]

- ●7025F   Patient information entered into a reminder system with a target due date for the next mammogram (RAD)[5]

Rationale

A new section was developed for the Category II Code section. The Structural Measures section was developed to capture measures that address the setting (location such as the ambulatory surgical center or the skilled nursing facility) or system (such as the computer record) of the delivery of care. As noted in the guideline, these codes also address aspects of the capabilities of the organization or health care professional providing the care.

With the addition of the new section to the Category II code set comes the addition of new codes, which include codes 7010F, 7025F, and the recently revised code 7020F. These codes are included as part of two different measures sets (Melanoma and Radiology) but are utilized to denote similar information within these measures.

Code 7010F is used to identify the inclusion of patient information into a recall system. As is noted in the guidelines, this code measures the capability of the organization via use of a recall system that allows recall of a target date for the next examination for the condition. The single measure in which this code is used (Melanoma Continuity of Care[5]) identifies whether the patient with a current diagnosis of melanoma or a history of melanoma had information entered into a recall system with the target date for the next complete physical skin examination specified, at least once within the 12-month reporting period. As is noted in the measure statement, the measure specifically targets the organization's ability to capture and schedule a future date for follow-up services with the patient for the specific condition. The measure notes that the follow-up is scheduled, but because the actual follow-up is also dependent upon patient compliance with the instructions, the measure allows for system exclusions for use of this measure, noting that the modifier 3P may be appended to this code when appropriate system exclusions exist. In addition, supplemental information has been included within the numerator listing to notify users regarding specific elements that should be available within the recall system abilities.

Codes 7020F and 7025F are used as part of separate measures within the Radiology clinical topic. Code 7020F is included within the Mammography Assessment Category Data Collection[5] measure. The title for this measure previously read "Breast Imaging-Reporting and Data System (BI-RADS) Data Collection[5]" on the American Medical Association Web site, but because this title included proprietary language, the phrase "Breast Imaging-Reporting and Data System (BI-RADS®)" was replaced by "Mammography Assessment Category." This language will allow use of other mammogram assessment systems. The proprietary language has been similarly removed from other parts of the Appendix H measure listing, including the code descriptor. In addition, examples have been incorporated into the code descriptor to cite the previous method of categorization as an example. The measure with which this code is listed does not allow for exclusions. As a result, modifiers 1P, 2P, and 3P should not be used with this code. Code 7025F is used to identify patient information entered into a reminder system with a target due date for the next mammogram as part of the Reminder System for Mammograms[5] measure. Special numerator instructions for this measure note that the reminder system should be linked to a process for notifying patients when their next mammogram is due and should include the following elements at a minimum: patient identifier, patient contact information, dates(s) of prior screening mammogram(s) (if known), and the target due date for the next screening mammogram. Since there are no exclusions for use of this code, modifiers 1P, 2P, and 3P may not be reported for this measure.

Recent studies have shown that while radiologists surpass recommendations for most mammography services, the recall rate for almost half of radiologists is higher than recommended. Collecting the data elements required to allow for internal calculation of recall rate is a first step in encouraging quality improvement activities

Although screening mammograms can reduce breast cancer mortality by 20-35% in women aged 40 years and older, recent evidence has suggested a decreasing trend in screening rates and a need for intervention. The use of patient reminders is associated with an increase in screening mammography. Encouraging the implementation of a reminder system could therefore help to reverse the trend and lead to an increase in mammography.

FOOTNOTES

1. Physician Consortium for Performance Improvement® (PCPI), www.physicianconsortium.org
2. National Committee on Quality Assurance (NCQA), Health Employer Data Information Set (HEDIS®), www.ncqa.org
3. Joint Commission on Accreditation of Healthcare Organizations (JCAHO), ORYX Initiative Performance Measures, www.jcaho.org/pms
4. National Diabetes Quality Improvement Alliance (NDQIA), www.nationaldiabetesalliance.org
5. Joint measure from the Physician Consortium for Performance Improvement, www.physicianconsortium.org and National Committee on Quality Assurance (NCQA), www.ncqa.org
6. The Society of Thoracic Surgeons, www.sts.org, National Quality Forum, www.qualityforum.org

Category III Codes

Revisions to this section include the addition of 13 new codes and the deletion of 22 codes, demonstrating the dynamic and transitional nature of this code category. Of the code deletions, seven codes have been converted to Category I codes, including the codes for reporting programming and analysis of gastric neurostimulators, template guided saturation prostate biopsies, cervical artificial disc arthroplasty, and actigraphy testing. The remaining 15 deleted Category III codes have been archived, without meeting the criteria for conversion to Category I codes.

Category III Codes

The following section contains a set of temporary codes . . .

The inclusion of a service or procedure in this section . . .

Services/procedures described in this section make use of alphanumeric characters. These codes have an alpha character as the 5th character in the string, preceded by four digits. The digits are not intended to reflect the placement of the code in the Category I section of CPT nomenclature. Codes in this section may or may not eventually receive a Category I CPT code. In either case, a given Category III code will be archived five years from its date of publication or revision in the CPT codebook unless it is demonstrated that a temporary code is still needed. ▶Services/procedures described by Category III codes which have been archived after five years, without conversion, may be reported using the Category I unlisted code.◀ New codes in this section are released semi-annually via the AMA/CPT Web site, to expedite dissemination for reporting. The full set of temporary codes for emerging technology, services, and procedures published annually in the CPT codebook. Go to www.ama-assn.org/go/cpt for the most current listing.

▶(0024T has been deleted)◀

▶(For non-surgical septal reduction therapy, use 93799)◀

▶(0026T has been deleted)◀

▶(For lipoprotein, direct measurement, intermediate density lipoproteins [IDL] [remnant lipoprotein], use 84999)◀

▶(0027T has been deleted)◀

▶(For endoscopic lysis of epidural adhesions with direct visualization using mechanical means or solution injection [eg, normal saline], use 64999)◀

▶(0028T has been deleted)◀

▶(For dual energy x-ray absorptiometry [DEXA] body composition study, use 76499)◀

▶(0029T has been deleted)◀

▶(For pulsed magnetic neuromodulation incontinence treatment, use 53899)◀

0030T Antiprothrombin (phospholipid cofactor) antibody, each 1g class

▶(0031T, 0032T have been deleted)◀

▶(For speculoscopy, including sampling, use 58999)◀

▶(0041T has been deleted)◀

▶(For urinalysis infectious agent detection, semi-quantitative analysis of volatile compounds, use 81099)◀

0042T Cerebral perfusion analysis using computed tomography with contrast administration, including post-processing of parametric maps with determination of cerebral blood flow, cerebral blood volume, and mean transit time

▶(0043T has been deleted)◀

▶(For carbon monoxide, expired gas analysis [eg, ETCO c/hemolysis breath test], use 84999)◀

▶(0046T, 0047T have been deleted)◀

▶(For mammary duct[s] catheter lavage, use 19499)◀

0048T Implantation of a ventricular assist device, extracorporeal, percutaneous transseptal access, single or dual cannulation

▶(0049T has been deleted)◀

▶(For prolonged extracorporeal percutaneous transseptal ventricular assist device, use 33999)◀

Rationale

The introductory guidelines of the Category III Codes subsection have been revised to include a statement to instruct that Category III codes archived after 5 years, without conversion, may be reported using Category I unlisted procedure codes. Previously, when a Category III code was deleted, according to provisions of the Category III code set guidelines, no reference was provided to direct the user to the appropriate code for the procedure. For CPT® 2009, a parenthetical note directing the user to the appropriate Category I unlisted code is now included in the Category III subsection.

Codes 0024T, 0026T, 0027T, 0028T, 0029T, 0031T, 0032T, 0041T, 0043T, 0046T, 0047T, 0049T and related cross-references have been deleted, according to the provisions of the Category III code set guidelines. To support the deletion of the Category III codes, cross-references have been established to instruct the use of the appropriate unlisted Category I code for each service as described as follows.

Code 0024T, which previously described non-surgical septal reduction therapy, should be reported with unlisted code 93799.

Code 0026T, which previously described lipoprotein, direct measurement, intermediate density lipoproteins (IDL) (remnant lipoproteins), should be reported with unlisted code 84999.

Code 0027T, which previously described endoscopic lysis of epidural adhesions with direct visualization using mechanical means or solution injection, should be reported with unlisted code 64999.

Code 0028T, which previously described dual energy X ray absorptiometry (DeXA) body composition study, should be reported with unlisted code 76499.

Code 0029T, which previously described treatment(s) for incontinence, pulsed magnetic neuromodulation, should be reported with unlisted code 53899.

Codes 0031T and 0032T, which previously described speculoscopy, with directed sampling, should be reported with unlisted code 58999.

Code 0041T, which previously described urinalysis infectious agent detection, semi-quantitative analysis of volatile compounds, should be reported with unlisted code 81099.

Code 0043T, which previously described carbon monoxide, expired gas analysis, should be reported with unlisted code 84999.

Codes 0046T and 0047T, which previously described catheter lavage of a mammary duct(s) for collection of cytology specimen(s), in high risk individuals, should be reported with unlisted code 19499.

Code 0049T, which previously described prolonged extracorporeal percutaneous transseptal ventricular assist device, greater than 24 hours, each subsequent 24-hour period, should be reported with unlisted code 33999.

+O 0054T   Computer-assisted musculoskeletal surgical navigational orthopedic procedure, with image-guidance based on fluoroscopic images (List separately in addition to code for primary procedure)

+O 0055T   Computer-assisted musculoskeletal surgical navigational orthopedic procedure, with image-guidance based on CT/MRI images (List separately in addition to code for primary procedure)

►(When CT and MRI are both performed, report 0055T only once)◄

►(0056T has been deleted. To report, use 20985)◄

Rationale

Codes 0054T and 0055T and the parenthetical instruction originally associated with code 0055T have been reinstated for reporting computer-assisted musculoskeletal surgical navigational procedures. Computer-assisted musculoskeletal surgical navigational preoperative and intraoperative imaging will now be reported with codes 0054T and 0055T and differentiated solely by the type of imaging (fluoroscopic [0054T], CT/MRI [0055T]) rather than the timing of the imaging (pre-operative, intraoperative). These codes were originally established for the CPT 2004 codebook. For 2008, three new Category I codes 20985-20987 were added to report these services. Only code 20985 has demonstrated the necessary frequency of performance for retention of this Category I code. Codes 0054T and 0055T will continue as Category III codes pending the availability of further information to demonstrate that the necessary criteria for Category I code status has been met. A new symbol has been added with the reinstatement of these codes to assist the user in identification of the source for these codes. This symbol will be included in the CPT codebook to identify recycled or reinstated codes.

►(0058T, 0059T have been deleted)◄

►(For cryopreservation, ovarian reproductive tissue, oocytes, use 89240)◄

►(0060T has been deleted)◄

►(For electrical impedance breast scan, use 76499)◄

►(0061T has been deleted)◄

►(For destruction/reduction of malignant breast tumor, microwave phased array thermotherapy, use 19499)◄

Rationale

Category III codes 0058T, 0059T, 0060T, 0061T and related cross-references have been deleted, according to the provisions of the Category III code set guidelines.

Codes 0058T and 0059T, which previously described cryopreservation of reproductive tissue, ovarian, oocytes(s), should be reported with unlisted code 89240.

Code 0060T, which previously described electrical impedance scan of the breast, should be reported with unlisted code 76499.

Code 0061T, which previously described destruction/reduction of malignant breast tumor including breast carcinoma cells in the margins, microwave phased array thermotherapy, disposable catheter with combined temperature monitoring probe and microwave sensor, should be reported with unlisted code 19499.

▶(0088T has been deleted. To report, use 41530)◀

Rationale

Category III code 0088T, which previously described radiofrequency tissue volume reduction of the tongue base, has been deleted. This procedure is now performed frequently enough to warrant Category I status. As such, Category I code 41530 has been established to report radiofrequency tissue volume reduction of the tongue base. A parenthetical note has been placed in the Category III section to direct users to code 41530.

▶(0089T has been deleted. For actigraphy testing, use 95803)◀

Rationale

In tandem with the establishment of code 95803 to report actigraphy sleep assessment, Category III code 0089T has been deleted. A cross-reference has been added to direct users to 95803 for this service.

▶(0090T has been deleted. To report total disc cervical arthroplasty, use 22856)◀

+ ▲ 0092T   Total disc arthroplasty (artificial disc), anterior approach, including discectomy with end plate preparation (includes osteophytectomy for nerve root or spinal cord decompression and microdissection), each additional interspace, cervical (List separately in addition to code for primary procedure)

(Use 0092T in conjunction with ▶22856◀)

▶(Do not report 0092T in conjunction with 22851 when performed at the same level)◀

▶(0093T has been deleted. To report removal of total disc cervical arthroplasty, use 22864)◀

+ ▲ 0095T   Removal of total disc arthroplasty (artificial disc), anterior approach, each additional interspace, cervical (List separately in addition to code for primary procedure)

(Use 0095T in conjunction with ▶22864◀)

▶(0096T has been deleted. To report revision of total disc cervical arthroplasty, use 22861)◀

+▲ 0098T   Revision including replacement of total disc arthroplasty (artificial disc), anterior approach, each additional interspace, cervical (List separately in addition to code for primary procedure)

(Use 0098T in conjunction with ▶22861◀)

(Do not report 0098T in conjunction with ▶0095T◀)

▶(Do not report 0098T in conjunction with 22851 when performed at the same level)◀

Rationale

In order to accommodate the addition of codes 22856, 22861, and 22864, codes 0092T, 0095T, and 0098T have been revised to specify the use of these codes for reporting performance of a total cervical disc arthroplasty, arthroplasty revision, and arthroplasty removal in an additional interspace. In addition to the revision of these codes, codes 0090T, 0093T, and 0096T have been deleted to support the addition of the new Category I codes 22856, 22861, and 22864. Exclusionary parenthetical instructions have been added following codes 0092T and 0098T to indicate that intervertebral biomechanical device application (22851) is inherent and, therefore, not separately reported with these codes.

▲ 0124T   Conjunctival incision with posterior extrascleral placement of pharmacological agent (does not include supply of medication)

▶(For suprachoroidal delivery of pharmacologic agent, use 0186T)◀

Rationale

Code 0124T was revised to list the more accurate anatomic site of delivery by deleting the term "juxtascleral" and replacing it with the term "extrascleral." A parenthetical note was added after code 0124T to direct users to code 0186T for suprachoroidal delivery of a pharmacologic agent.

Clinical Example (0124T)

A 67-year-old male presents with decreased visual acuity and metaphorphopsia secondary to subfoveal choroidal neovascularization. A posterior extrascleral injection of an anti-angiogenic pharmacologic agent is performed.

Description of Procedure (0124T)

After reclining the patient in an examination chair, topical anesthetic is administered and a lid and conjunctival preparation with 5% povidone iodine solution is administered. A lid speculum is positioned and topical 4% lidocaine applied to the incision site. A 2- to 3-mm conjunctival and Tenon's capsule incision is made in the superior temporal quadrant, 8 mm from the limbus and Tenon's space is entered. The injection cannula is passed into Tenon's space and follows the globe posteriorly to the macula where 0.5 cc is injected. An assistant provides pressure over the injection site to prevent reflux. The speculum is removed and a semi-pressure patch is applied.

▶(0137T has been deleted. For transperineal stereotactic template guided saturation prostate biopsies, use 55706)◀

🔍 Rationale

Code 0137T has been deleted. In its place, a parenthetical note has been included to direct users to the correct code to use to report transperineal stereotactic template guided saturation prostate biopsy (55706). For more information regarding use of code 55706 and other information regarding reporting for this procedure, see the Rationale included in the Surgery section for this code.

▶(0162T has been deleted. To report, see 95980–95982)◀

+▲ **0163T** Total disc arthroplasty (artificial disc), anterior approach, including discectomy to prepare interspace (other than for decompression), each additional interspace, lumbar (List separately in addition to code for primary procedure)

(Use 0163T in conjunction with 22857)

+▲ **0164T** Removal of total disc arthroplasty, (artificial disc), anterior approach, each additional interspace, lumbar (List separately in addition to code for primary procedure)

(Use 0164T in conjunction with 22865)

+▲ **0165T** Revision including replacement of total disc arthroplasty (artificial disc), anterior approach, each additional interspace, lumbar (List separately in addition to code for primary procedure)

(Use 0165T in conjunction with 22862)

(Do not report 0163T-0165T in conjunction with 22851, 49010, when performed at the same level)

(For decompression, see 63001-63048)

🔍 Rationale

Category III code 0162T, which previously described electronic analysis and programming of gastric neurostimulator pulse generator has been deleted. These physician services are adequately and appropriately described in codes 95980, 95981 and 95982 as indicated in the new cross-reference.

In support of revisions made to the cervical arthroplasty codes 0092T, 0095T, and 0098T, codes 0163T, 0164T, and 0165T have been revised to clarify the intent of each of these codes for total artificial disc arthroplasty and to standardize the descriptor nomenclature for consistency with other add-on codes and with the cervical arthroplasty codes.

●**0184T** Excision of rectal tumor, transanal endoscopic microsurgical approach (ie, TEMS)

▶(For non-endoscopic excision of rectal tumor, see 45160, 45170)◀

▶(Do not report 0184T in conjunction with 45300-45327, 69990)◀

Rationale

Category III code 0184T has been added to report transanal endoscopic microsurgical (TEMS) excision of rectal tumors. It is one of a number of procedures currently included in the CPT codebook for removing rectal tumors. The procedure was developed in the early 1980s and requires specially designed equipment. It also requires a surgeon who possesses advanced skills with use of the device and the instrumentation. The procedure involves manipulation of the instrument in the confined space of the operating scope (the procedure is performed inside a small diameter cylinder). The procedure described in code 0184T differs from other rectal resection procedures identified in the CPT codebook because it describes a minimally invasive endoscopic technique with magnification and insufflation for more proximal rectosigmoid tumors. Other procedures included in the codebook are suitable for transanal resection (45170) or sacral rectal resections (45160) and do not identify this additional effort. This procedure describes extensive dissection of the neoplasm, more proximal dissection, and reconstruction of the rectal wall. To direct users to the appropriate codes to report TEMS versus other rectal resections, parenthetical notes have been included in both the Surgery section and after the listing of code 0184T. Because many of the endoscopically performed services included in the 45300 series of codes and microsurgical technique are included as part of the TEMS procedures, a parenthetical note has been added to notify users of the restriction for reporting these codes in conjunction with code 0184T.

Clinical Example (0184T)

A 74-year-old male presents with a rectal mass 9-cm proximal to the dentate line that is biopsy-proven adenocarcinoma in-situ. No suspicious lymph nodes were seen on endorectal ultrasound. He undergoes transanal endoscopic microsurgery for full-thickness excision of the rectal mass and adjacent mesorectum.

Description of Procedure (0184T)

The patient is placed in the perinolithotomy or prone position (depending on the location and level of the tumor) such that the majority of the tumor will be in the 6:00 position through the microscope. Proctoscopy with the TEMs muffler is used to ensure the location of the tumor. Under anesthesia, the anal sphincter is dilated by means of a wide rectoscope with an outside diameter of 40 mm. A TEMs set is connected to the operating table via a grasping device and an arm support system, with insufflation, irrigation, light source, and magnification attached. Epinephrine is injected beneath the tumor for hemostasis. Scoring of the rectal mucosa is performed around the tumor. A full rectal wall thickness excision of the lesion and the adjacent mesorectum is performed. The specimen is removed and oriented for pathology, and the mesorectum identified for accurate staging of depth of invasion and nodal involvement. The rectal wall is reconstructed by transverse running 3–0 braided absorbable sutures under endoscopic guidance to avoiding postoperative rectal stenosis. Hemostasis is obtained. Proctoscopy is performed to assure there is no narrowing of the canal.

●**0185T** Multivariate analysis of patient-specific findings with quantifiable computer probability assessment, including report

▶(Do not report 0185T in conjunction with 99090)◀

Rationale

Code 0185T was established to report pretest probability assessment.

Quantitative pretest probability assessment is a procedure that enables the provider to estimate the numeric (ie, discrete) probability of disease, based upon information immediately available at the bedside. This assessment aids the provider in making the decision to perform certain diagnostic tests. A parenthetical note instructing users not to report code 0185T in conjunction with code 99090 was placed following code 0185T.

Clinical Example (0185T)

A 41-year-old male presents to the emergency department with a 2-day history of sporadic chest pain that lasts 5 minutes at most and which he rates the pain as 6 on a 10-point scale. He has had no diaphoresis, radiation, or nausea. He is free of pain now. His only cardiac risk factor is that his uncle died at the age of 51 from a heart attack. A chest X ray performed in the emergency department shows no abnormality. He has normal vital signs and his electrocardiogram shows nonspecific ST-segment changes but is otherwise normal. Physical examination is normal. The physician proceeds to order a troponin and CPK-MB for the evaluation of acute coronary syndrome. These results come back within normal limits, but now the physician must decide whether the patient should be admitted and evaluated with another set of enzymes, monitoring, and/or a cardiac imaging study (stress electrocardiogram, stress or dobutamine echocardiogram, nuclear cardiac imaging, multidetector coronary angiogram, formal cardiac catheterization, etc). The physician decides to perform a pretest probability test using the method of attribute matching to help provide a documentable, standardized pretest probability point estimate.

Description of Procedure (0185T)

The provider enters eight pieces of information about the patient that he gathered from the history and physical examination. The handheld or mobile manager, handheld computer, etc, which uses software, provides outputs of a probability of acute coronary syndrome, which is equal to 1.0%, with a diagram of risk to show to the patient. The physician then evaluates the precision and reliability of the result.

●**0186T** Suprachoroidal delivery of pharmacologic agent (does not include supply of medication)

Rationale

Code 0186T was established to report suprachoroidal drug delivery. Code 0124T was revised to list the more accurate anatomic site of delivery by deleting the term "juxtascleral" and replacing it with the term "extrascleral." A parenthetical note was added following code 0124T to direct users to code 0186T for suprachoroidal delivery of a pharmacologic agent. Suprachoroidal drug delivery is intended to treat choroidal neovascularization (CNV) associated with age-related macular degeneration (AMD), which is the leading cause of blindness in the United States. This procedure is performed using a microcatheter, which allows agents to be delivered directly to the choroids, versus traditional methodology (ie, injections of pharmacologic agents into the vitreous cavity). In general, pharmacologic agents injected into the vitreous for age-related macular degeneration must diffuse from the vitreous through the retina and Bruch's membrane in order to contact and affect the CNV. Each intravitreal injection raises risks associated with infection, retinal detachment, glaucoma, or cataract formation. Also, because of the difficulty in achieving adequate drug concentrations at the level of the choroid, injections must be repeated frequently. Suprachoroidal drug delivery eliminates the need for the drug to penetrate the retina and subretinal tissues, thus enabling site-specific delivery of drugs directly to the anatomic site of the pathology, the choroid. Additionally, suprachoroidal delivery no longer relies on the vitreous humor to be the carrier for sustained drug delivery.

Clinical Example (0186T)

A 65-year-old woman presents to the ophthalmologist with a recent history of sudden vision loss resulting from wet age-related macular degeneration in the right eye. She recently received conventional pharmacologic therapy, and her vision in the right eye has continued to deteriorate or she has a prior medical history of vitrectomy, which limits her ability to have a successful outcome with intravitreal injections. Visual acuity in the right eye is counting fingers at 3 feet. On fundus examination, there is subfoveal blood in the right eye and drusen in the left eye. Fluorescein angiography confirms that the patient has classic choroidal neovascularization (CNV) with submacular bleeding in the right eye and drusen in the left eye. The patient requires further treatment for the CNV in the right eye.

Description of Procedure (0186T)

Standard preparation (draping and anesthesia) of the patient for ocular surgery is performed. A limbal conjunctival peritomy is performed and the conjunctiva is retracted to expose the sclera. A 2-3 mm radial incision is made at the pars plana, through the sclera and exposing the choroid. The microcatheter is prepared and primed with the agent to be delivered. The microcatheter is attached to fiberoptic illuminator to provide illumination at the distal tip for surgical location guidance. The microcatheter distal tip is then placed into the incision, into the suprachoroidal space, and advanced posteriorly for approximately 15mm. The globe is rotated so as to be able to view the posterior surface through the pupillary aperture. The illuminated microcatheter distal tip is located visually, and the microcatheter is then advanced to the appropriate target site (usually at or near the macula). The agent is delivered to the site and the microcatheter is withdrawn. The radial incision is closed with 1 or 2 sutures, the conjunctiva is closed per usual procedures, and standard post-operative medications are administered.

●0187T   Scanning computerized ophthalmic diagnostic imaging, anterior segment, with interpretation and report, unilateral

🖉 Rationale

Code 0187T has been established to report anterior segment imaging with optical coherence tomography. Anterior segment imaging with optical coherence tomography is a non-contact, high-resolution tomographic and biomicroscopic procedure for imaging of anterior segment ocular structures for patients with selected macular abnormalities and glaucoma. The operation of anterior segment imaging with optical coherence tomography is analogous to ultrasound B-mode imaging, reflected in code 76513, except that light is used rather than acoustic waves. In support of this addition, the descriptor for code 92135 was revised in CPT 2008 to clarify the intent of this code for posterior segment imaging to distinguish it from code 0187T, which was released on the AMA's CPT Web site on July 1, 2007, and implemented January 1, 2008.

🩺 Clinical Example (0187T)

An 82-year-old male presents with a history of pterygium excision X6 with growth into the central pupillary axis with significant visual loss. An anterior segment scan using optical coherence tomography is undertaken to evaluate the extent (depth) of the pterygium and determine whether an additional excision could be performed safely with or without the need for a patch graft to avoid corneal perforation.

Description of Procedure (0187T)

Clinical staff performs the acquisition-related tasks of anterior segment imaging with optical coherence tomography. These tasks include entering patient data into the device database, aligning the patient, instructing the patient on how to fixate the target within the system, aligning and centering the scan, freezing the scan, reviewing and accepting the scan result, and acquiring all scans within a given scan protocol. The physician reviews the multiple image results within the system's planning and analysis software component, and he or she identifies key landmarks in each image to assist diagnosis and planning. After landmark identification, the physician performs caliper measurements as needed for diagnostic decisions and for surgical planning.

▶Remote Real-Time Interactive Videoconferenced Critical Care Services◀

▶Remote real-time interactive videoconferenced critical care is the direct delivery by a physician(s) of medical care for a critically ill or critically injured patient from an offsite location. Remote real-time interactive videoconferenced critical care is intended to supplement onsite critical care services at times when a critically ill or injured patient requires additional critical care resources than are available onsite. (For definitions of critical illness or injury and critical care services, see **Critical Care Services** section.)

In order to report remote real-time interactive video-conferenced critical care, the physician(s) in the remote location must have real-time access to the patient's medical record including progress notes, nursing notes, current medications, vital signs, clinical laboratory test results, other diagnostic test results, and radiographic images. The physician must have real-time capability to enter electronic orders; document the remote care services provided in the hospital medical record; videoconference with the on-site health care team in the patient room; assess patients in their individual rooms, using high fidelity audio and video capabilities, including clear observation of the patient, monitors, ventilators, and infusion pumps; and speak to patients and family members.

The review and/or interpretation of all diagnostic information is included in reporting remote real-time interactive video-conferenced critical care when performed during the critical period by the physician(s) providing remote real-time interactive video-conferenced critical care and should not be reported separately.

The remote real-time interactive video-conferenced critical care codes 0188T and 0189T are used to report the total duration of time spent by a physician providing remote real-time interactive video-conferenced critical care services to a critically ill or critically injured patient, even if the time spent by the physician on that date is not continuous. For any given period of time spent providing remote real-time interactive video-conferenced critical care services, the physician must devote his or her full attention to the patient and, therefore, cannot provide services to any other patient during the same period of time.

Time spent with the individual patient should be recorded in the patient's record. The time that can be reported as remote real-time interactive video-conferenced critical care is the time spent engaged in work directly related to the individual patient's care. For example, time spent reviewing test results or imaging studies, discussing the critically ill patient's care with other medical staff or documenting remote real-time interactive video-conferenced critical care services in the medical record would be reported as remote real-time interactive video-conferenced critical care, even though it does not occur at the bedside. Also, when the patient is unable or lacks capacity to participate in discussions, time spent from the remote site with family members or surrogate decision makers obtaining a medical history, reviewing the patient's condition or prognosis, or discussing treatment or limitation(s) of treatment may be reported as remote real-time interactive video-conferenced critical care, provided that the conversation bears directly on the management of the patient.

Time spent in activities that occur away from the bedside when the physician does not have the real-time capabilities described above may not be reported as remote real-time interactive video-conferenced critical care because the physician is not immediately available to the patient. Time spent in activities that do not directly contribute to the treatment of the patient may not be reported as remote real-time interactive video-conferenced critical care, even if they are performed in the remote site (eg, participation in administrative meetings or telephone calls to discuss other patients). Only one physician may report either Critical Care Services (99291, 99292) or remote real-time interactive video-conferenced Critical Care for the same period of time. Do not report remote real-time interactive video-conferenced critical care if another physician reports Pediatric or Neonatal Critical Care or Intensive Care services (99468-99476).

Code 0188T is used to report the first 30 to 74 minutes of remote real-time interactive video-conferenced, critical care on a given date. It should be used only once per date even if the time spent by the physician is not continuous on that date. Remote real-time interactive video-conferenced, critical care of less than 30 minutes total duration on a given date should not be reported.

Code 0189T is used to report additional block(s) of time, of up to 30 minutes each, beyond the first 74 minutes (see table below).

The following examples illustrate the correct reporting of remote critical care services:

Total Duration of Critical Care	Code(s)
Less than 30 minutes (less than 1/2 hour)	Do not report
30-74 minutes (1/2 hr. -1 hr. 14 min.)	0188T X 1
75-104 minutes (1 hr. 15 min. - 1 hr. 44 min.)	0188T X 1 AND 0189T X 1
105-134 minutes (1 hr. 45 min. - 2 hr. 14 min	0188T X 1 AND 0189T X 2

●0188T Remote real-time interactive video-conferenced critical care, evaluation and management of the critically ill or critically injured patient; first 30-74 minutes

+●0189T each additional 30 minutes (List separately in addition to code for primary service)

▶(Use 0189T in conjunction with 0188T)◀

Rationale

Over the past 10 years, critical care Evaluation and Management (E/M) services provided by means of remote real-time interactive videoconference technology have become more prevalent. Remote real-time interactive videoconferenced critical care is intended to supplement available onsite critical care services and is provided at the request of the patient's attending physician. The existing critical care E/M codes (99291 and 99292) describe critical care services provided at the immediate bedside or elsewhere on the floor or unit. Codes 99291 and 99292 are not appropriate for reporting remote real-time interactive videoconferenced critical care. To reflect this new mode of providing critical care E/M services, Category III codes 0188T and 0189T, as well as new guidelines to report remote real-time interactive videoconferenced critical care services, have been established for 2009.

It is important to note that a physician may not report code 0188T or 0189T during the same period of time for which a physician reports Critical Care services (99291, 99292) or Pediatric or Neonatal Critical Care or Intensive Care services (99468-99480). For example, if a physician provides onsite critical care services from 10 a.m. to 12 p.m., another physician cannot report remote real-time interactive videoconferenced critical care services during the same period of time.

Code 0188T is used to report the first 30-74 minutes of services. Code 0189T is an add-on code and is used to report each additional 30 minutes of services. A parenthetical note was added following code 0189T instructing users to report this code in conjunction with code 0188T.

Clinical Example (0188T)

A 66-year-old woman with suspected community-acquired pneumonia is intubated in the emergency department (ED) of a rural hospital. The patient is admitted to the intensive care unit and is initially evaluated by her family practitioner who contacts the offsite remote physician. They agree on a care plan that includes mechanical ventilation and empiric intravenous antibiotic therapy (to be adjusted based upon culture results) administered via subclavian catheter placed in the ED. During the night, the patient develops septic shock and acute respiratory distress syndrome. The offsite remote physician spends 50 minutes managing these problems.

Clinical Example (0189T)

A 66-year-old woman with suspected community-acquired pneumonia is intubated in the emergency department (ED) of a rural hospital. The patient is admitted to the intensive care unit and is initially evaluated by her family practitioner who contacts the offsite remote physician. They agree on a care plan that includes mechanical ventilation and empiric intravenous antibiotic therapy (to be adjusted based upon culture results) administered via subclavian catheter placed in the ED. During the night, the patient develops septic shock and acute respiratory distress syndrome. The offsite remote physician spends 90 minutes managing these problems.

Description of Procedure (0188T, 0189T)

After admission, a computer-based alert notifies the remote physician that the patient is hypotensive. The remote physician contacts the patient's nurse, electronically writes and signs an order that is transmitted to the intensive care unit (ICU) and the patient is given additional fluid boluses and placed on intravenous norepinephrine to maintain an adequate blood pressure. In addition, the remote physician is in constant communication with the respiratory therapist and nurse increasing the positive end-expiratory pressure (PEEP) to 15 while having to maintain the FiO2 at 100%. The chest X ray, visualized by the remote physician, now is compatible with adult respiratory distress syndrome (ARDS). The remote physician repeatedly reviews the patient's data screens throughout the night to assess for clinical changes. The patients mottling, as seen by the remote physician, has slowly improved in response to the 3 liters of saline ordered by the remote physician throughout the night. At 2 AM, six hours following the patient's admission to the ICU, the laboratory reports microbiology for the patient's sputum sample which shows gram negative bacilli. The remote physician enters an electronic order to change antibiotic therapy based on the laboratory results, local antibiotic sensitivity patterns and the established care plan with the attending physician.

At 6 AM the remote physician identifies that the patient's blood pressure is improving; after a review of the laboratory data, ventilator settings and direct visual assessment of the patient, the remote physician notes that the patient is adequately sedated, well perfused, and clearing the metabolic acidosis.

+●0190T   Placement of intraocular radiation source applicator (List separately in addition to primary procedure)

▶(Use 0190T in conjunction with 67036)◀

▶(For application of the source by radiation oncologist, see Clinical Brachytherapy section)◀

Rationale

Code 0190T was established as an add-on code to allow ophthalmologists to report placement of intraocular radiation source applicator for epiretinal radiation therapy to be used in conjunction with vitrectomy code 67036. This procedure is a new type of treatment for neovascular age-related macular degeneration. A vitrectomy (67036) is performed to allow the insertion of an applicator containing a high-intensity radioactive source. Once the applicator is in position, the radioactive source is advanced out of the applicator's protected storage compartment to a closed-chamber cannula tip where the radiation is delivered. In a separate procedure, the radiation oncologist applies the radioelement while the applicator is held in place by the surgeon, in light contact with the retina, for no more than 5 minutes. After completion of the radioelement application, the applicator is removed from the eye and the eye is closed by the surgeon.

A cross-reference was added to direct users to the Clinical Brachytherapy section for application of the radioelement by a radiation oncologist. As part of the separate radiation brachytherapy procedure, the radiation oncologist performs a radiation survey of the patient and the apparatus based on standard radiation safety protocol. The patient will return to the surgeon's office based on standard surgical postoperative protocol.

Clinical Example (0190T)

A 70-year-old man presents to the physician with rapid, progressive loss of his central vision due to the onset of neovascular, subfoveal age-related macular degeneration.

Description of Procedure (0190T)

A core vitrectomy is performed to gain access to the patient's vitreous cavity. An applicator containing a strontium-90 beta radiation source is inserted into the patient's vitreous cavity and positioned over the patient's subfoveal choroidal neovascular lesion. Once in place, the radioactive source is advanced out of the applicator's protected storage compartment to a closed-chamber cannula tip where the radiation is delivered. The applicator is held in place, in light contact with the retina, for no more than 5 minutes.

The radioactive source is retracted back into the applicator's protected storage compartment, the applicator is removed from the eye, and the eye is properly closed following current medical protocol. The patient will return to the surgeon's office based on standard surgical postoperative protocol.

●**0191T** Insertion of anterior segment aqueous drainage device, without extraocular reservoir; internal approach

●**0192T** external approach

Rationale
Codes 0191T and 0192T were established to report the insertion of an anterior segment drainage device utilizing either an internal or external approach. The internal approach technique involves the insertion of a microstent into the anterior chamber of the eye (ab interno) through a small self-sealing, clear corneal incision under gonioscopy (or other visualization enhancement technique). The external approach technique requires a conjunctival incision and creation of a partial-thickness scleral flap in which to secure the aqueous drainage device beneath.

The services described by code 66180, Aqueous shunt to extraocular reservoir, generally involve the cutting of conjuctiva and sclera; fixation of an aqueous shunt device (approximately 5 mm in diameter) to the outside of the eye (ab externo); the creation of a sclerostomy from the outside of the eye into the anterior chamber; placement of a drainage tube (attached to the aqueous shunt device) through the sclerostomy into the anterior chamber, and the fixation of the tube to avoid movement within the sclerostomy and underneath the conjunctival tissue.

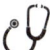
Clinical Example (0191T)
A 67-year-old man presents with a 5-year history of progressive open-angle glaucoma. The patient is receiving 2 topical ophthalmic anti-glaucoma medications (eg, prostaglandin, beta-blocker). His intraocular pressure is not controlled.

Description of Procedure (0191T)
A small clear cornea incision is created. A viscoelastic agent is used to deepen the anterior chamber. Under gonioscopy, the applicator is introduced into the anterior chamber of the eye through the incision, and the aqueous drainage device is inserted into the anterior chamber angle opposite the location of the clear cornea incision.

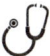
Clinical Example (0192T)
A 65-year-old man presents with a history of chronic open-angle glaucoma and intraocular pressures uncontrolled in the right eye by maximum medical therapy and laser trabeculoplasty. Visual field testing of the right eye reveals progressive loss of visual field.

Description of Procedure (0192T)
A limbal- or fornix-based conjunctival incision is prepared. Next, a partial-thickness scleral flap is formed with a base at the limbus. Aqueous flow from the anterior chamber is produced by an incision into the anterior chamber beneath the scleral flap or by excising the inner wall of Schlemm's canal. The aqueous drainage device is implanted under the scleral flap in order to maintain the aqueous flow out of the eye. The scleral flap is secured with sutures, and the conjunctiva is repositioned over the wound site and closed with sutures to create a watertight seal.

●**0193T** Transurethral, radiofrequency micro-remodeling of the female bladder neck and proximal urethra for stress urinary incontinence

▶(Do not report 0193T in conjunction with 51701)◀

Rationale
Code 0193T was established to report transurethral radiofrequency micro-remodeling of the female bladder neck and proximal urethra. This radiofrequency procedure is a non-surgical alternative for women with stress urinary incontinence (SUI) who have failed conservative non-surgical alternatives or who are not viable candidates for surgery. Transurethral radiofrequency micro-remodeling increases the compliance of the bladder neck and proximal urethra for SUI under local anesthesia.

Insertion of a non-indwelling catheter is included in code 0193T. Therefore, a parenthetical note was added following code 0193T, instructing users not to report this code in conjunction with code 51701.

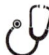
Clinical Example (0193T)
A 43-year-old markedly obese (BMI 35) woman presents with P3G2 with Type II diabetes and a 5-year history of stress urinary incontinence of more than two episodes a day requiring pad changes and not sufficiently treated with biofeedback and pelvic floor strengthening, despite more than 18 months of therapy. She is not a good candidate for surgical treatment due to her desire for more children, her obesity, and her diabetes.

Description of Procedure (0193T)
The patient undergoes an in-office non-surgical transurethral radiofrequency treatment to increase the compliance of the bladder neck and proximal urethra for stress urinary incontinence under local anesthesia. The procedure is performed by the urologist/urogynecologist under a peri-urethral local anesthetic block. The patient is placed in the dorsal lithotomy position, the angle of the urethra is determined and the local anesthetic is injected. Once the local anesthesia has taken effect, the bladder is drained with a catheter and the device is placed transurethrally without image guidance and the balloon inflated. The proper position of the device is determined prior to treatment through palpation of the balloon at the bladder neck and verifying on visual markings at the urethral meatus. Nine treatment cycles are performed at varying positions to complete the treatment.

●**0194T** Procalcitonin (PCT)

Rationale
Category III code 0194T was established to report procalcitonin (PCT) testing for detection and monitoring of bacterial infections and sepsis.

PCT is a marker for the early detection and therapeutic monitoring of bacterial infections and sepsis. PCT levels are specifically elevated in bacterial infections compared to inflammation or viral infection. PCT concentrations are also sensitive to severity of infection and can help in the monitoring and diagnosis of more serious conditions.

PCT measurements may be used in the intensive care unit as well as in the hospital emergency department in the differential diagnosis of bacterial versus non-bacterial disorders; the diagnosis of severe sepsis and septic shock; for the early detection of infectious complications; and risk assessment of patients with suspected bacterial infection. Physicians may also refer samples to independent reference labs for managing patients on an outpatient basis.

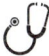

Clinical Example (0194T)
Example 1:
A 23-year-old male patient with multiple trauma and open fracture of the lower leg presents with septic symptoms after admission, obviously due to soft tissue infection.

Description of Procedure (0194T–Example 1)
During the subsequent course, elevated procalcitonin (PCT) levels indicated a systemic bacterial infection. Following amputation of the lower leg the patient's condition improved and PCT decreased back to normal levels.

Procalcitonin measurements are made using a "sandwich" type luminescence immunoassay. The assay uses two monoclonal antibodies that are directed against the C-terminal and mid-regional catacalcin sequences. The anti-catacalcin antibody is immobilized on the surface of the coated tube, and the anti-calcitonin antibody is labelled using a luminescent acridine derivative. The immunoassay method includes pipetting, incubation washing and measuring steps.

Example 2:
A 57-year-old male patient undergoes coronary artery bypass graft surgery with an uncomplicated course. On day 7 after surgery the patient presents with mild hypotension, a pale skin, sweating, mild hypothermia, and loss of appetite.

Description of Procedure (0194T–Example 2)
Because of hypotension the patient is transferred to the intensive care unit. Chest X ray and echocardiography reveal normal findings: no pericardial effusion, no impaired ejection function, no pneumonia or pleural effusion. The next day, the PCT value is 2.5 ng/mL. Volume resuscitation improves hypotension and the patient is scheduled to return to the normal ward. Due to the increased PCT value, which is inappropriately high for this patient, a CT-scan is performed, and shows a sternum osteomyelitis. The diagnosis is confirmed during a surgical procedure. A local drainage is performed and the patient recovered within 10 days.

The laboratory analysis involves sophisticated technology including immunoassay procedures with two antigen-specific monoclonal antibodies that bind PCT at two different binding sites. One of these antibodies is luminescence labeled and the other is fixed to the inner walls of the tube.

During the course of incubation, both antibodies react with PCT molecules in the sample to form "sandwich complexes."

The amount of PCT in serum or plasma is quantified by measuring the luminescence signal using a suitable Luminescence Instrument. The intensity of the luminescence signal (Relative Light Units) is directly proportional to the PCT concentration in the sample. After a standard curve has been established using standards with known antigen concentrations (calibrated against recombinant intact human PCT), the unknown PCT concentrations can then be quantified by comparison of test values with the curve. The results are reported as procalcitonin levels in ng/ml. The assay is aided by sophisticated software and instrumentation support.

●0195T Arthrodesis, pre-sacral interbody technique, including instrumentation, imaging (when performed), and discectomy to prepare interspace, lumbar; single interspace

+●0196T each additional interspace (List separately in addition to code for primary procedure)

▶(Use 0196T in conjunction with 0195T)◀

▶(Do not report 0195T, 0196T in conjunction with 22558, 22845, 22851, 76000, 76380, 76496, 76497)◀

Rationale

Two Category III codes, 0195T, 0196T, were established to report percutaneous lumbar discectomy and preparation of the interspace for fusion.

This procedure represents a new technique that involves both a unique approach and surgical technique for lumbar fusion and for the treatment of lumbar degenerative disc, annular tear, low back pain, and spondylolisthesis.

The instructional parenthetical note included in the code descriptor indicates that any imaging guidance required for this service is included and not reported separately. Code 0195T should be reported in addition to code 0196T for each additional level. An exclusionary parenthetical note was also added to instruct that it would not be appropriate to report codes 0195T and 0196T in conjunction with 22558, 22845, 22851, 76000, 76380, 76496, 76497 because these services are considered an inclusive component of the percutaneous lumbar discectomy Category III codes 0195T and 0196T.

Clinical Example (0195T)

A 40-year-old male presents with a history of low back pain unresponsive to non-operative management for more than 1 year. Work-up and evaluation show a degenerative disc and/or annular tear at L5/S1. The patient continues to have limitations to his activities both at home and at work despite adequate physical therapy and other non-operative interventions. Examination of the patient is consistent with lumbar annular tear with increased pain with forward bending and or lifting. The patient is a candidate for lumbar fusion and desires to proceed with surgery.

Description of Procedure (0195T)

The patient undergoes an anterior L5/S1 lumbar discectomy and fusion via a pre-sacral approach. Bone grafting is performed and an anterior screw is inserted into

S1, across the L5/S1 interspace and into the L5 vertebral body. Posterior supplemental instrumentation and/or fusion is performed through a separate incision.

Clinical Example (0196T)

A 45-year-old male presents with a history of low back pain unresponsive to non-operative management for more than 1 year. Work-up and evaluation show a degenerative disc and/or annular tear at L4/L5 and L5/S1. The patient continues to have limitations to his activities both at home and at work despite adequate physical therapy and other non-operative interventions. Examination of the patient is consistent with lumbar annular tear with increased pain with forward bending and or lifting. The patient is a candidate for a level 2 lumbar fusion and desires to proceed with surgery. At the completion of the first level, the second level procedure is performed.

Description of procedure (0196T)

After a L5-S1 anterior, pre-sacral discectomy and interbody arthrodesis has been performed, the surgeon performs a L4-5 discectomy and arthrodesis through the same anterior, pre-sacral approach. Bone grafting is performed and the screw across L5-S1 is advanced across the L4-5 disc space. Posterior supplemental instrumentation and/or fusion is performed through a separate incision.

Appendices

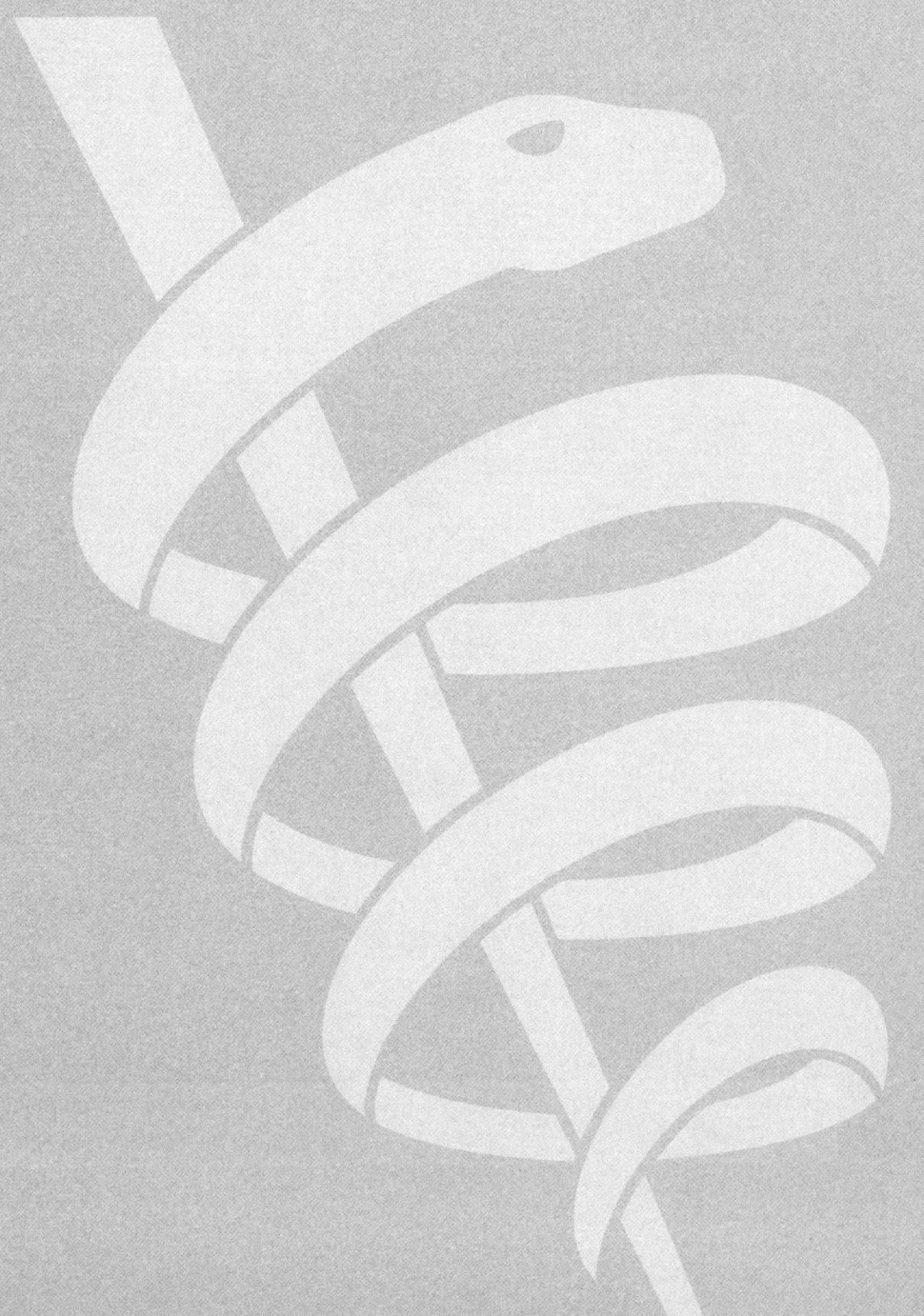

Appendix A

Modifiers

This list includes all of the modifiers applicable to CPT 2009 codes.

▶(Modifier 21 has been deleted. To report prolonged physician services, see 99354-99357)◀

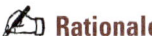 **Rationale**

Modifier 21 for reporting a prolonged evaluation and management service has been deleted. This modifier provided a duplicate mechanism for the same concept that is reported with the prolonged Evaluation and Management Services codes 99354-99359, violating the CPT® concept of unique methods of concept reporting.

Appendix H

Alphabetic Index of Performance Measures by Clinical Condition or Topic

As has been true in the past few years, the Appendix H document has many revisions, including new codes, clinical conditions/topics, and revisions to existing topics, measures, and codes. The following listing includes an itemization of the added and revised topics and measures included in the Appendix H document:

New/Added Clinical Topics/Conditions (12)

Acute Bronchitis (A-BRONCH)
    Avoidance of (Inappropriate) Antibiotic Treatment in Adults with Acute Bronchitis[2] (New measure)

Acute Otitis Externa/Otitis Media with Effusion (AOE/OME)
    Acute Otitis Externa: Topical Therapy[1] (New measure)
    Acute Otitis Externa: Pain Assessment[1] (New measure)
    Systemic Antimicrobial Therapy: Avoidance of Inappropriate Use[1] (New measure)
    Diagnostic Evaluation: Assessment of Tympanic Membrane Mobility[1] (New measure)
    Otitis Media with Effusion: Hearing Testing[1] (New measure)
    Otitis Media with Effusion Antihistamines or Decongestants: Avoidance of Inappropriate Use[1] (New measure)
    Systemic Antimicrobials: Avoidance of Inappropriate Use[1] (New measure)
    Otitis Media with Effusion Systemic Steroids: Avoidance of Inappropriate Use[1] (New measure)

Anesthesiology/Critical Care (CRIT)
    Prevention of Ventilator-Associated Pneumonia: Head Elevation[1] (New measure)
    Prevention of Catheter-Related Bloodstream Infections (CRBSI)–Central Venous Catheter Insertion Protocol[1] (New measure)
    Anesthesiology/Critical Care (CRIT) Perioperative Temperature Management for Surgical Procedures Under General Anesthesia[1] (New measure)

Annual Monitoring (AM)
    Annual monitoring for patients on angiotensin converting enzyme (ACE) inhibitors or angiotensin receptor blockers (ARB)[2] (New measure)

Back Pain (BkP)
    Initial Visit for Back Pain[2] (New measure)
    Physical Exam after Back Pain Onset[2] (New measure)
    Mental Health Assessment after Back Pain Onset[2] (New measure)
    Appropriate Imaging for Acute Back Pain[2] (New measure)
    Advice for Normal Activities for Back Pain Patients[2] (New measure)
    Advice Against Bed Rest for Back Pain Patients[2] (New measure)
    Recommendation for Exercise for Back Pain Patients[2] (New measure)

---

[1] Physician Consortium for Performance Improvement, www.physicianconsortium.org
[2] National Committee on Quality Assurance (NCQA), Health Employer Data Information Set (HEDIS®), www.ncqa.org
[3] Joint Commission on Accreditation of Healthcare Organizations (JCAHO), ORYX Initiative Performance Measures, www.jcaho.org/pms
[4] National Diabetes Quality Improvement Alliance (NDQIA), www.nationaldiabetesalliance.org
[5] Joint measure from the Physician Consortium for Performance Improvement, www.physicianconsortium.org and National Committee on Quality Assurance (NCQA), www.ncqa.org
[6] The Society of Thoracic Surgeons, www.sts.org, National Quality Forum, www.qualityforum.org

Chronic Kidney Disease (CKD)
  Blood Pressure Management[1] (New measure)
  ACE Inhibitor (ACE) or Angiotensin Receptor Blocker (ARB) Therapy[1] (New measure)
  Laboratory Testing (Calcium, Phosphorus, and Intact Parathyroid Hormone [PTH], and Lipid Profile)[1] (New measure)
  Plan of Care: Elevated Hemoglobin for Patients Receiving Erythropoiesis-Stimulating Agents (ESA)[1] (New measure)
  Influenza Immunization[1] (New measure)
  Referral for AV Fistula[1] (New measure)

Hematology (HEM)
  Myelodysplastic Syndrome (MDS) and Acute Leukemias-Baseline Cytogenetic Testing Performed on Bone Marrow[1] (New measure)
  Myelodysplastic Syndrome (MDS)-Documentation of Iron Stores in Patients Receiving Erythropoietin Therapy[1] (New measure)
  Multiple Myeloma: Treatment with Bisphosphonates[1] (New measure)
  Chronic Lymphocytic Leukemia (CLL)-Baseline Flow Cytometry[1] (New measure)

Pathology (PATH)
  Breast Cancer Resection Pathology Reporting-pT Category (Primary Tumor) and pN (Regional Lymph Nodes) with Histologic Grade[1] (New measure)
  Colorectal Cancer Resection Pathology Reporting-pT Category (Primary Tumor) and pN Category (Regional Lymph Node) with Histologic Grade[1] (New measure)

Prenatal Care (PRENATAL)
  Anti-D Immune Globulin[1] (New measure)
  Screening for Human Immunodeficiency Virus (HIV)[1] (New measure)

Prostate Cancer (PRCA)
  Initial Evaluation[1]
  Overuse Measure—Bone Scan for Staging Low-Risk Patients[1] (New measure)
  Treatment Options for Patients with Clinically Localized Disease[1] (New measure)
  Adjuvant Hormonal Therapy for High-Risk Patients[1] (New measure)
  Three-Dimensional Radiotherapy[1] (New measure)

Radiology (RAD)
  Stenosis Measurement in Carotid Imaging Reports[5] (New measure)
  Mammography Assessment Category Data Collection[5] (New measure)
  Inappropriate Use of "Probably Benign" Assessment Category in Mammography Screening[5] (New measure)
  Communication of Suspicious Findings From the Diagnostic Mammogram to the Practice Managing Ongoing Care[5] (New measure)
  Communication of Suspicious Findings From the Diagnostic Mammogram to the Patient[5] (New measure)
  Reminder system for mammograms[5] (New measure)
  CT Radiation Dose Reduction[5] (New measure)
  Exposure Time Reported for Procedures Using Fluoroscopy[5] (New measure)

Rheumatoid Arthritis (RA)
  Disease Modifying Anti-Rheumatic Drug Therapy in Rheumatoid Arthritis (New measure)

---

[1] Physician Consortium for Performance Improvement, www.physicianconsortium.org
[2] National Committee on Quality Assurance (NCQA), Health Employer Data Information Set (HEDIS®), www.ncqa.org
[3] Joint Commission on Accreditation of Healthcare Organizations (JCAHO), ORYX Initiative Performance Measures, www.jcaho.org/pms
[4] National Diabetes Quality Improvement Alliance (NDQIA), www.nationaldiabetesalliance.org
[5] Joint measure from the Physician Consortium for Performance Improvement, www.physicianconsortium.org and National Committee on Quality Assurance (NCQA), www.ncqa.org
[6] The Society of Thoracic Surgeons, www.sts.org, National Quality Forum, www.qualityforum.org

Revised Clinical Topics/Conditions (14 Revised)

Chronic Obstructive Pulmonary Disease (COPD)
    Recommendation of Influenza Immunization[1] (New measure)
    Influenza Immunization Administered[1] (New measure)
    Assessment of Pneumococcus Immunization Status[1] (New measure)
    Pneumococcus Immunization Administered[1] (New measure)

Community-Acquired Bacterial Pneumonia (CAP)
    Assessment of Influenza Immunization Status[1,2] (New measure)
    Assessment of Pneumococcus Immunization Status[1,2] (New measure)

Diabetes
    Urine Protein Screening (Medical Attention for Nephropathy)[2,4] (New measure)
    Blood Pressure Management[2] (Revised)
    Appropriate Eye Exam for People with Diabetes[2] (New measure)

Emergency Medicine (EM)
    Assessment of Oxygen Saturation for Community-Acquired Bacterial Pneumonia[5] (Revised)

End Stage Renal Disease (ESRD)
    Plan of Care for Inadequate Hemodialysis[1] (New measure)
    Plan of Care for Inadequate Peritoneal Dialysis[1] (New measure)
    Influenza Immunization[1] (New measure)
    Vascular Access-Patients Receiving Hemodialysis[1] (New measure)
    Vascular Access-Patients Receiving Hemodialysis with a Permanent Catheter[1] (New measure)
    Plan of Care for Anemia[1] (New measure)

Eye Care (EC)
    Primary Open-Angle Glaucoma: Reduction of Intraocular Pressure (IOP) by 15% OR Documentation of a Plan of Care[5] (New measure)
    Primary Open-Angle Glaucoma: Counseling on Glaucoma[5] (New measure)
    Cataracts: 20/40 or Better Visual Acuity within 90 Days Following Cataract Surgery[5] (New measure)
    Cataracts: Comprehensive Pre-operative Assessment for Cataract Surgery with Intraocular Lens (IOL) Placement[5] (New measure)
    Age-Related Macular Degeneration (AMD): Counseling on Antioxidant Supplement[5] (New measure)

Gastroesophageal Reflux Disease (GERD)
    Continuous Medication Therapy - Assessment of GERD Symptoms[5] (New measure)

Geriatrics (GER)
    Advance Care Plan[5] (New measure)
    Risk Assessment for Falls[5] (New measure)
    Plan of Care for Falls[5] (New measure)

Hepatitis C (HEP C)
    Testing for Chronic Hepatitis C: Confirmation of Hepatitis C Viremia (HCV)[1] (New measure)
    Hepatitis C Ribonucleic Acid (RNA) Testing Before Initiating Therapy[1] (New measure)

---

[1] Physician Consortium for Performance Improvement, www.physicianconsortium.org
[2] National Committee on Quality Assurance (NCQA), Health Employer Data Information Set (HEDIS®), www.ncqa.org
[3] Joint Commission on Accreditation of Healthcare Organizations (JCAHO), ORYX Initiative Performance Measures, www.jcaho.org/pms
[4] National Diabetes Quality Improvement Alliance (NDQIA), www.nationaldiabetesalliance.org
[5] Joint measure from the Physician Consortium for Performance Improvement, www.physicianconsortium.org and National Committee on Quality Assurance (NCQA), www.ncqa.org
[6] The Society of Thoracic Surgeons, www.sts.org, National Quality Forum, www.qualityforum.org

HCV Genotype Testing Prior to Therapy[1] (New measure)
Consideration for Antiviral Therapy[1] (New measure)
Combination Antiviral Therapy[1] (New measure)
HCV Quantitative RNA Testing at Week 12 of Therapy[1] (New measure)
Hepatitis A Vaccination[1] (New measure)
Hepatitis B Vaccination[1] (New measure)
Education Regarding Risk of Alcohol Consumption[1] (New measure)
Counseling Regarding Use of Contraception Prior to Antiviral Therapy[1] (New measure)

Hypertension (HTN)
Plan of Care[1] (Revised)

Major Depressive Disorder (MDD)
Depression Screening and Assessment in High Risk Patients SUP[2] (New measure)
Major Depressive Disorder: Diagnostic Evaluation[1] (New measure)

Melanoma (ML)
Melanoma Follow Up Measures[5] (New measure)
Melanoma Continuity of Care[5] (New measure)
Melanoma Coordination of Care[5] (New measure)
Over Utilization of Imaging Studies in Stage 0-IA Melanoma[5] (New measure)

Oncology (ONC)
Cancer Stage Documented[1] (New measure)
Hormonal Therapy for Stage IC-IIIC, ER/PR Positive Breast Cancer[1] (New measure)
Adjuvant Chemotherapy for Stage IIIA Through Stage IIIC Colon Cancer Patients[1] (New measure)
Plan for Chemotherapy Documented Before Chemotherapy Administered[1] (New measure)
Treatment Summary Communication—Radiation Oncology[1] (New measure)
Normal Tissue Dose Constraints Specified[1] (New measure)
Pain Intensity Quantified-Medical Oncology and Radiation Oncology[1] (New measure)
Plan of Care for Pain—Medical Oncology and Radiation Oncology[1] (New measure)
Pathology Report—Medical Oncology and Radiation Oncology[1] (New measure)

Preventive Care & Screening (PV)
Adult Colorectal Cancer Screening[1,2] (Revised Measure)
Colorectal Cancer Screening[2] (New measure)
Breast Cancer Screening[2] (New measure)
Pneumococcal Vaccination for Patients 65 Years and Older[2] (New measure)
Advising Smokers to Quit[2] (New measure)

The rationales for each of the code changes can be found within the discussion for the Category II Code section of this book. This includes information regarding reporting instructions, intended use of codes, and other helpful information regarding the use of the codes. New clinical topics within Appendix H have been noted with bow ties (▶◀) to alert the user to the added topic. Revised Clinical Topics (whether through changes to existing measures or via addition of new measures to the existing topic) have been noted with bow ties as well.

[1] Physician Consortium for Performance Improvement, www.physicianconsortium.org
[2] National Committee on Quality Assurance (NCQA), Health Employer Data Information Set (HEDIS®), www.ncqa.org
[3] Joint Commission on Accreditation of Healthcare Organizations (JCAHO), ORYX Initiative Performance Measures, www.jcaho.org/pms
[4] National Diabetes Quality Improvement Alliance (NDQIA), www.nationaldiabetesalliance.org
[5] Joint measure from the Physician Consortium for Performance Improvement, www.physicianconsortium.org
and National Committee on Quality Assurance (NCQA), www.ncqa.org
[6] The Society of Thoracic Surgeons, www.sts.org, National Quality Forum, www.qualityforum.org

As has been noted in other sources of CPT educational materials, since the Category II section and Appendix H are intended to be complementary sections of the codebook, it is important to use both sections to identify important information regarding the use of these codes, complete code descriptor language, and location of measure information necessary for appropriate use. In addition, as a result of frequent updates to clinical practice and measure development, the Category II code section and Appendix H documents are both subject to changes that may supercede the ability of the printed publication of the CPT Codebook to sustain. As a result, it is important that users of this coding system use both the latest printed publication of the CPT codebook and the listing on the AMA coding Web site for these codes. It is both of these publications that comprise the entire current set of published codes. In most instances, the Web site will include the latest information regarding this code set (the exception being the Category II code listing as only updates are included in the Category II code section). The Appendix H document on the AMA Web site has been included with the complete listing of all Category II codes because all of the Category II codes have been listed within their specific clinical conditions, topics, or disease conditions.

The complete listing of the diseases, clinical condition, or clinical topic and the associated acronyms are included in alphabetical order in Appendix H. As is true using Category II codes, users are directed to review the complete measure associated with each code prior to use. This allows the user the ability to comply with the intent of the measure according to the developer's specifications. Specific measure information may be found on the measure developer's Web site or appropriate publication (Example: NCQA's HEDIS® Technical Specifications). The measure developer's Web addresses have been included in the footnotes located in both the Category II section and in Appendix H.

Tabular Review of the Changes

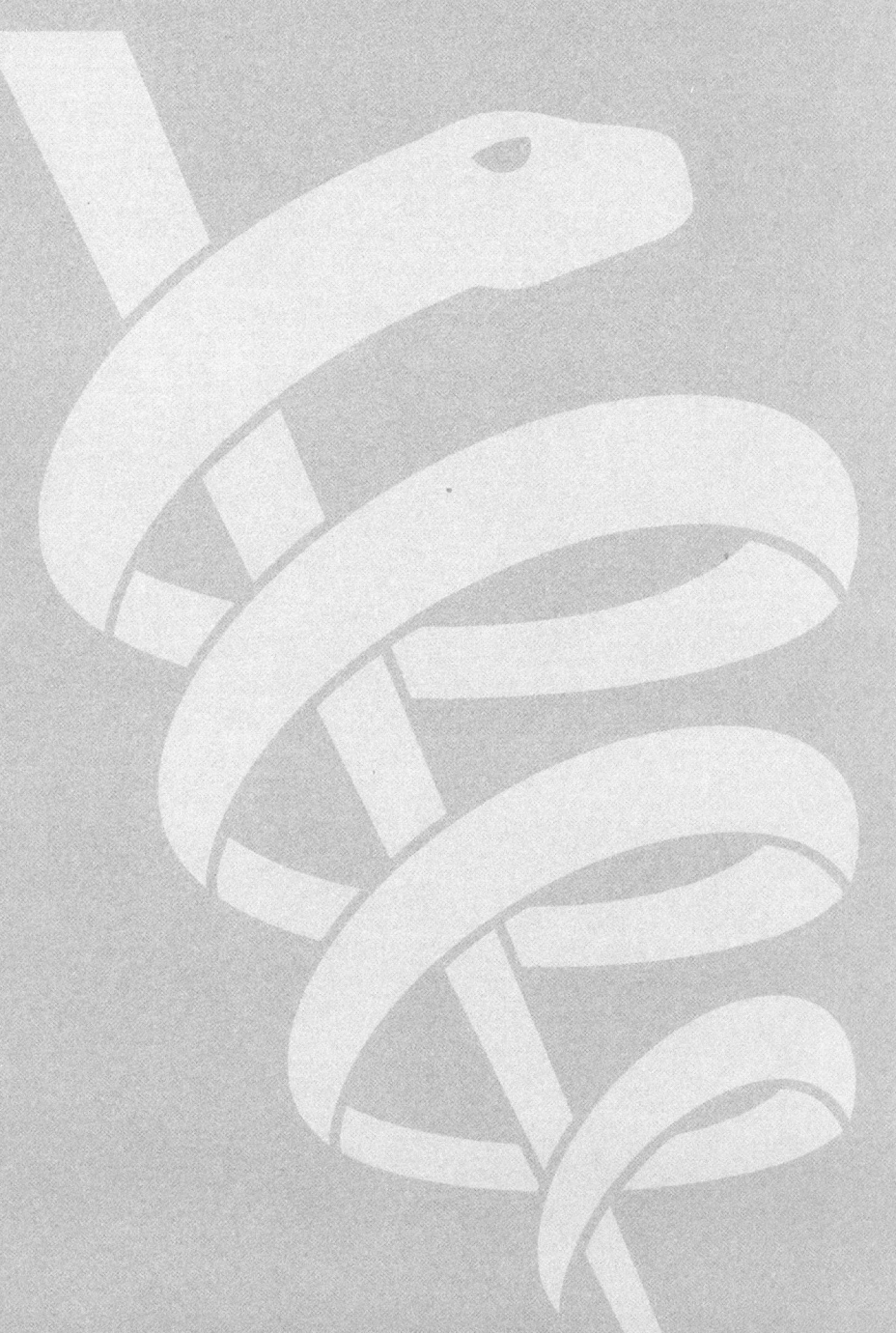

Section/Code	Added	Deleted	Revised	Grammatical Revision	Cross-reference

Evaluation and Management

Emergency Department Services

Other Emergency Services

New or Established Patient

Section/Code	Added	Deleted	Revised	Grammatical Revision	Cross-reference
99289		X			
99290		X			

Critical Care Services

Section/Code	Added	Deleted	Revised	Grammatical Revision	Cross-reference
99293		X			
99294		X			
99295		X			
99296		X			
99298		X			
99299		X			
99300		X			

Prolonged Services

Prolonged Physician Service With Direct (Face-To-Face) Patient Contact

Section/Code	Added	Deleted	Revised	Grammatical Revision	Cross-reference
99354			X		X
99355			X		
99356			X		X
99357			X		

Preventive Medicine Services

New Patient

Section/Code	Added	Deleted	Revised	Grammatical Revision	Cross-reference
99381			X		
99382			X		
99383			X		
99384			X		
99385			X		
99386			X		
99387			X		

Section/Code	Added	Deleted	Revised	Grammatical Revision	Cross-reference
Established Patient					
99391			X		
99392			X		
99393			X		
99394			X		
99395			X		
99396			X		
99397			X		
Counseling Risk Factor Reduction and Behavior Change Intervention					
Other Preventive Medicine Services					
99431		X			
99432		X			
99433		X			
99435		X			
99436		X			
99440		X			
Newborn Care Services					
99460	X				
99461	X				
99462	X				
99463	X				X
Delivery/Birthing Room Attendance and Resuscitation Services					
99464	X				X
99465	X				X
Inpatient Neonatal Intensive Care Services and Pediatric and Neonatal Critical Care Services					
Pediatric Critical Care Patient Transport					
99466	X				
99467	X				X

Section/Code	Added	Deleted	Revised	Grammatical Revision	Cross-reference
Inpatient Neonatal and Pediatric Critical Care					
99468	X				
99469	X				
99471	X				
99472	X				
99475	X				
99476	X				
Initial and Continuing Intensive Care Services					
99478	X				
99479	X				
99480	X				

Anesthesia

Head

00211	X				

Intrathoracic

00561				X	
00562			X		
00566			X		
00567	X				

Surgery

Integumentary System

Skin, Subcutaneous and Accessory Structures					
Excision - Debridement					
11001			X		
Removal of Skin Tags					
11201			X		
Nails					
11720				X	

Section/Code	Added	Deleted	Revised	Grammatical Revision	Cross-reference
11721				X	
Introduction					
11922			X		
Repair (Closure)					
Repair - Intermediate					
12031			X		
12032			X		
12034			X		
12035			X		
12036			X		
12037			X		
12041			X		
12042			X		
12044			X		
12045			X		
12046			X		
12047			X		
12051			X		
12052			X		
12053			X		
12054			X		
12055			X		
12056			X		
12057			X		
Skin Replacement Surgery and Skin Substitutes					
15003			X		
15005			X		
15201			X		
15221			X		
15241			X		

Section/Code	Added	Deleted	Revised	Grammatical Revision	Cross-reference
15261			X		
15341			X		
Breast					
Introduction					
19296			X		
19297			X		
Musculoskeletal System					
General					
Introduction or Removal					
20552				X	
20553				X	
20693				X	
20696	X				X
20697	X				X
Other Procedures					
20985			X		
20986		X			
20987		X			
Head					
Repair, Revision, and/or Reconstruction					
21122				X	
21142				X	
21143				X	
21146				X	
21147				X	
Spine (Vertebral Column)					
Spinal Instrumentation					
22856	X				X
22857			X		

▲=Revised Code   ●=New Code   ▶◀=New or Revised Text   ○=Reinstated Code

Section/Code	Added	Deleted	Revised	Grammatical Revision	Cross-reference
22861	X				X
22862			X		
22864	X				X
22865			X		X

Shoulder

Fracture and/or Dislocation

Section/Code	Added	Deleted	Revised	Grammatical Revision	Cross-reference
23585			X		

Forearm and Wrist

Fracture and/or Dislocation

Section/Code	Added	Deleted	Revised	Grammatical Revision	Cross-reference
25630				X	
25645				X	

Hand and Fingers

Repair, Revision, and/or Reconstruction

Section/Code	Added	Deleted	Revised	Grammatical Revision	Cross-reference
26517				X	
26518				X	

Pelvis and Hip Joint

Incision

Section/Code	Added	Deleted	Revised	Grammatical Revision	Cross-reference
27027	X				X

Excision

Section/Code	Added	Deleted	Revised	Grammatical Revision	Cross-reference
27057	X				X

Fracture and/or Dislocation

Section/Code	Added	Deleted	Revised	Grammatical Revision	Cross-reference
27215			X		X
27216			X		X
27217			X		X
27218			X		X

Femur (Thigh Region) and Knee Joint

Repair, Revision, and/or Reconstruction

Section/Code	Added	Deleted	Revised	Grammatical Revision	Cross-reference
27396			X		
27397			X		
27455				X	

Section/Code	Added	Deleted	Revised	Grammatical Revision	Cross-reference
Respiratory System					
Trachea and Bronchi					
Endoscopy					
31620				X	
Cardiovascular System					
Arteries and Veins					
Endovascular Repair of Abdominal Aortic Aneurysm					
34806			X		
Bypass Graft					
35535	X				X
35570	X				X
35632	X				X
35633	X				X
35634	X				X
Digestive System					
Tongue and Floor of Mouth					
Other Procedures					
41512	X				X
41530	X				
Esophagus					
Endoscopy					
43273	X				X
Laparoscopy					
43279	X				X
Manipulation					
43460			X		
Anus					
Destruction					
46930	X				X

▲=Revised Code ●=New Code ▶◀=New or Revised Text O=Reinstated Code

Section/Code	Added	Deleted	Revised	Grammatical Revision	Cross-reference
46934		X			
46935		X			
46936		X			

Liver

Liver Transplantation

47144				X	

Abdomen, Peritoneum, and Omentum

Repair

49568			X		

Laparoscopy

49652	X				X
49653	X				X
49654	X				X
49655	X				X
49656	X				X
49657	X				X

Urinary System

Bladder

Vesical Neck and Prostate

52606		X			
52612		X			
52614		X			
52620		X			
52630			X		X

Urethra

Repair

53410				X	
53415				X	
53420				X	

Section/Code	Added	Deleted	Revised	Grammatical Revision	Cross-reference
Other Procedures					
53853		X			

Male Genital System

Prostate

Section/Code	Added	Deleted	Revised	Grammatical Revision	Cross-reference
Incision					
55706	X				X

Female Genital System

Vagina

Section/Code	Added	Deleted	Revised	Grammatical Revision	Cross-reference
Manipulation					
57400			X		
57410			X		
57415			X		

Nervous System

Skull, Meninges, and Brain

Section/Code	Added	Deleted	Revised	Grammatical Revision	Cross-reference
Stereotaxis					
61793		X			
Stereotactic Radiosurgery (Cranial)					
61796	X				X
61797	X				X
61798	X				X
61799	X				X
61800	X				X

Spine and Spinal Cord

Section/Code	Added	Deleted	Revised	Grammatical Revision	Cross-reference
Injection, Drainage, or Aspiration					
62267	X				X
62287			X		X
Posterior Extradural Laminotomy or Laminectomy for Exploration/ Decompression of Neural Elements or Excision of Herniated Intervertebral Discs					
63020			X		

▲=Revised Code   ●=New Code   ▶◀=New or Revised Text   O=Reinstated Code

Section/Code	Added	Deleted	Revised	Grammatical Revision	Cross-reference
63030			X		
63035			X		
Incision					
63180				X	
63182				X	
63185				X	
63190				X	
63194				X	
63196				X	
63198				X	
Stereotactic Radiosurgery (Spinal)					
63620	X				X
63621	X				X

Extracranial Nerves, Peripheral Nerves, and Autonomic Nervous System

Section/Code	Added	Deleted	Revised	Grammatical Revision	Cross-reference
Introduction/Injection of Anesthetic Agent (Nerve Block), Diagnostic or Therapeutic					
64416			X		
64446			X		
64448			X		
64449			X		
64455	X				X
Destruction by Neurolytic Agent (eg, Chemical, Thermal, Electrical or Radiofrequency)					
64632	X				X
Neuroplasty (Exploration, Neurolysis or Nerve Decompression)					
64702				X	
Excision					
64776				X	
Neurorrhaphy					
64831				X	

Section/Code	Added	Deleted	Revised	Grammatical Revision	Cross-reference
Eye and Ocular Adnexa					
Anterior Segment					
Cornea					
65710			X		
65730			X		
65756	X				
65757	X				X
Anterior Chamber					
65855				X	
Iris, Ciliary Body					
66761				X	
66762				X	
Lens					
66821				X	
66840				X	
Intraocular Lens Procedures					
66983				X	
66984				X	
Posterior Segment					
Vitreous					
67031				X	
Retina or Choroid					
67101				X	
67141				X	
67208				X	
67220				X	
67227				X	
67228				X	

▲=Revised Code ●=New Code ▶◀=New or Revised Text O=Reinstated Code

Section/Code	Added	Deleted	Revised	Grammatical Revision	Cross-reference
Ocular Adnexa					
Extraocular Muscles					
67311				X	
67312				X	
67314				X	
67316				X	
Eyelids					
67971				X	
67973				X	
67974				X	
Auditory System					
External Ear					
Removal					
69210				X	
Middle Ear					
Repair					
69633				X	
69637				X	

Radiology

Section/Code	Added	Deleted	Revised	Grammatical Revision	Cross-reference
Diagnostic Radiology (Diagnostic Imaging)					
Head and Neck					
70100				X	
70110				X	
70120				X	
70130				X	
70140				X	
70150				X	
70200				X	
70210				X	

Section/Code	Added	Deleted	Revised	Grammatical Revision	Cross-reference
70220				X	
70250				X	
70260				X	
Chest					
71020				X	
71030				X	
71100				X	
71101				X	
71110				X	
71111				X	
71120				X	
71130				X	
Spine and Pelvis					
72040				X	
72050				X	
72070				X	
72072				X	
72074				X	
72080				X	
72100				X	
72110				X	
72120				X	
72170				X	
72190				X	
72200				X	
72202				X	
72220				X	
72270				X	
Upper Extremities					
73020				X	

▲=Revised Code ●=New Code ►◄=New or Revised Text ○=Reinstated Code

Section/Code	Added	Deleted	Revised	Grammatical Revision	Cross-reference
73030				X	
73060				X	
73070				X	
73080				X	
73090				X	
73092				X	
73100				X	
73110				X	
73120				X	
73130				X	
73140				X	
Lower Extremities					
73500				X	
73510				X	
73520				X	
73540				X	
73550				X	
73560				X	
73562				X	
73564				X	
73590				X	
73592				X	
73600				X	
73610				X	
73620				X	
73630				X	
73650				X	
73660				X	
Gastrointestinal Tract					
74270			X		

Section/Code	Added	Deleted	Revised	Grammatical Revision	Cross-reference
Diagnostic Ultrasound					
Pelvis					
Obstetrical					
76815				X	
Radiation Oncology					
Medical Radiation Physics, Dosimetry, Treatment Devices, and Special Services					
77305				X	
77310				X	
77326				X	
Radiation Treatment Delivery					
77407				X	
77412				X	
Radiation Treatment Management					
77427				X	
77431				X	
77432				X	X
77435				X	X
Clinical Brachytherapy					
77750				X	
77781		X			
77782		X			
77783		X			
77784		X			
77785	X				
77786	X				
77787	X				

Section/Code	Added	Deleted	Revised	Grammatical Revision	Cross-reference
Nuclear Medicine					
Diagnostic					
Musculoskeletal System					
78315				X	
78350				X	
78351				X	
Respiratory System					
78588				X	
Other Procedures					
78804				X	
78808	X				X
78890		X			
78891		X			

Pathology and Laboratory

Organ or Disease-Oriented Panels

Section/Code	Added	Deleted	Revised	Grammatical Revision	Cross-reference
80048			X		
80053			X		
80069			X		

Evocative/Suppression Testing

Section/Code	Added	Deleted	Revised	Grammatical Revision	Cross-reference
80438				X	
80439				X	

Urinalysis

Section/Code	Added	Deleted	Revised	Grammatical Revision	Cross-reference
81020				X	

Chemistry

Section/Code	Added	Deleted	Revised	Grammatical Revision	Cross-reference
82040			X		
82375			X		
82376			X		X
82652				X	

Section/Code	Added	Deleted	Revised	Grammatical Revision	Cross-reference
83876	X				
83890			X		
83891			X		
83892			X		
83893			X		
83894			X		
83897			X		
83900				X	
83903				X	
83907			X		
83909			X		
83914				X	
83925			X		
83950			X		
83951	X				
84132			X		
84155			X		
84295			X		

Hematology and Coagulation

85046				X	
85397	X				

Microbiology

87186				X	
87810			X		
87901				X	
87905	X				X

Cytopathology

88155				X	

▲=Revised Code ●=New Code ▶◀=New or Revised Text ○=Reinstated Code

Section/Code	Added	Deleted	Revised	Grammatical Revision	Cross-reference
Surgical Pathology					
88400		X			
In Vivo (eg, Transcutaneous) Laboratory Procedures					
88720	X				X
88740	X				X
88741	X				X
Other Procedures					
89135				X	

Medicine

Section/Code	Added	Deleted	Revised	Grammatical Revision	Cross-reference
Vaccines, Toxoids					
90650	X				
90681	X				
90696	X				
90698			X		
90738	X				
90760		X			
90761		X			
90765		X			
90766		X			
90767		X			
90768		X			
90769		X			
90770		X			
90771		X			
90772		X			
90773		X			
90774		X			
90775		X			

Section/Code	Added	Deleted	Revised	Grammatical Revision	Cross-reference
90776		X			
90779		X			

Dialysis

Section/Code	Added	Deleted	Revised	Grammatical Revision	Cross-reference
90918		X			
90919		X			
90920		X			
90921		X			
90922		X			
90923		X			
90924		X			
90925		X			

End-Stage Renal Disease Services

Section/Code	Added	Deleted	Revised	Grammatical Revision	Cross-reference
90951	X				
90952	X				
90953	X				
90954	X				
90955	X				
90956	X				
90957	X				
90958	X				
90959	X				
90960	X				
90961	X				
90962	X				
90963	X				
90964	X				
90965	X				
90966	X				
90967	X				

▲=Revised Code ●=New Code ►◄=New or Revised Text ○=Reinstated Code

Section/Code	Added	Deleted	Revised	Grammatical Revision	Cross-reference
90968	X				
90969	X				
90970	X				

Gastroenterology

Section/Code	Added	Deleted	Revised	Grammatical Revision	Cross-reference
91100		X			

Ophthalmology

General Ophthalmological Services

New Patient

Section/Code	Added	Deleted	Revised	Grammatical Revision	Cross-reference
92004				X	

Established Patient

Section/Code	Added	Deleted	Revised	Grammatical Revision	Cross-reference
92014				X	

Special Ophthalmological Services

Other Specialized Services

Section/Code	Added	Deleted	Revised	Grammatical Revision	Cross-reference
92265				X	

Contact Lens Services

Section/Code	Added	Deleted	Revised	Grammatical Revision	Cross-reference
92311				X	
92315				X	

Cardiovascular

Cardiography

Section/Code	Added	Deleted	Revised	Grammatical Revision	Cross-reference
93040				X	
93224			X		
93225			X		
93226			X		
93227			X		
93228	X				X
93229	X				X
93230			X		
93231			X		
93232			X		

Section/Code	Added	Deleted	Revised	Grammatical Revision	Cross-reference
93233			X		
93235			X		
93236			X		
93237			X		X
93268			X		
93270			X		
93271			X		
93272			X		X
Cardiovascular Device Monitoring - Implantable and Wearable Devices					
93279	X				X
93280	X				X
93281	X				X
93282	X				X
93283	X				X
93284	X				X
93285	X				X
93286	X				X
93287	X				X
93288	X				X
93289	X				X
93290	X				X
93291	X				X
93292	X				X
93293	X				X
93294	X				X
93295	X				X
93296	X				X
93297	X				X
93298	X				X
93299	X				X

▲=Revised Code   ●=New Code   ▶◀=New or Revised Text   O=Reinstated Code

Section/Code	Added	Deleted	Revised	Grammatical Revision	Cross-reference
Echocardiography					
93306	X				X
93307			X		X
93308			X		
93312				X	
93350			X		X
93351	X				X
93352	X				X
Noninvasive Physiologic Studies and Procedures					
93727		X			
93731		X			
93732		X			
93733		X			
93734		X			
93735		X			
93736		X			
93741		X			
93742		X			
93743		X			
93744		X			
93760		X			
93762		X			

Allergy and Clinical Immunology

Allergy Testing					
95010			X		
95015			X		
Allergen Immunotherapy					
95117				X	
95125				X	

Section/Code	Added	Deleted	Revised	Grammatical Revision	Cross-reference
95131				X	
95132				X	
95133				X	
95134				X	
95146				X	
95147				X	
95148				X	
95149				X	
Endocrinology					
95250			X		X
95251			X		X
Neurology and Neuromuscular Procedures					
Sleep Testing					
95803	X				X
Routine Electroencephalography (EEG)					
95813				X	
Electromyography					
95861				X	
95863				X	
95864				X	
Autonomic Function Tests					
95922				X	
Other Procedures					
95992	X				X
Motion Analysis					
96000				X	

Section/Code	Added	Deleted	Revised	Grammatical Revision	Cross-reference
Hydration, Therapeutic, Prophylactic, Diagnostic Injections and Infusions, and Chemotherapy and Other Highly Complex Drug or Highly Complex Biologic Agent Administration					
Hydration					
96360	X				X
96361	X				X
Therapeutic, Prophylactic, and Diagnostic Injections and Infusions (Excludes Chemotherapy and Other Highly Complex Drug or Highly Complex Biologic Agent Administration)					
96365	X				
96366	X				X
96367	X				X
96368	X				X
96369	X				X
96370	X				X
96371	X				X
96372	X				X
96373	X				
96374	X				
96375	X				X
96376	X				X
96379	X				X
Chemotherapy and Other Highly Complex Drug or Highly Complex Biologic Agent Administration					
Intra-Arterial Chemotherapy and Other Highly Complex Drug or Highly Complex Biologic Agent Administration					
96422				X	
Physical Medicine and Rehabilitation					
Modalities					
Supervised					
97010				X	

Section/Code	Added	Deleted	Revised	Grammatical Revision	Cross-reference
Osteopathic Manipulative Treatment					
98925				X	
98926				X	
98927				X	
98928				X	
98929				X	
Chiropractic Manipulative Treatment					
98940				X	
98941				X	
98942				X	
98943				X	
Non-Face-to-Face Nonphysician Services					
Telephone Services					
98966				X	
Qualifying Circumstances for Anesthesia					
99100				X	

Category II Codes

Section/Code	Added	Deleted	Revised	Grammatical Revision	Cross-reference
Composite Codes					
0014F	X				
0015F	X				
Patient Management					
0513F	X				
0514F	X				
0516F	X				
0517F	X				
0518F	X				
0519F	X				
0520F	X				

Section/Code	Added	Deleted	Revised	Grammatical Revision	Cross-reference
0521F	X				
0525F	X				
0526F	X				

Patient History

Section/Code	Added	Deleted	Revised	Grammatical Revision	Cross-reference
1040F			X		
1080F		X			
1116F	X				
1118F	X				
1119F	X				
1121F	X				
1123F	X				
1124F	X				
1125F	X				
1126F	X				
1127F	X				
1128F	X				
1130F	X				
1134F	X				
1135F	X				
1136F	X				
1137F	X				

Physical Examination

Section/Code	Added	Deleted	Revised	Grammatical Revision	Cross-reference
2000F				X	
2010F				X	
2022F				X	
2024F				X	
2026F				X	
2028F				X	
2035F	X				

Section/Code	Added	Deleted	Revised	Grammatical Revision	Cross-reference
2040F	X				
2044F	X				

Diagnostic/Screening Processes or Results

Section/Code	Added	Deleted	Revised	Grammatical Revision	Cross-reference
3014F				X	
3017F			X		
3027F				X	
3035F				X	
3037F				X	
3042F				X	
3046F				X	
3060F				X	
3061F				X	
3062F				X	
3066F				X	
3072F				X	
3073F			X		
3075F				X	
3077F				X	
3079F				X	
3080F				X	
3082F				X	
3083F				X	
3084F				X	
3095F				X	
3096F				X	
3215F	X				
3216F	X				X
3218F	X				X
3220F	X				

Section/Code	Added	Deleted	Revised	Grammatical Revision	Cross-reference
3230F	X				
3260F	X				
3265F	X				
3266F	X				
3268F	X				
3269F	X				
3270F	X				
3271F	X				
3272F	X				
3273F	X				
3274F	X				
3278F	X				
3279F	X				
3280F	X				
3281F	X				
3284F	X				
3285F	X				
3288F	X				
3290F	X				
3291F	X				
3292F	X				
3300F	X				
3301F	X				
3302F	X				
3303F	X				
3304F	X				
3305F	X				
3306F	X				
3307F	X				
3308F	X				

Section/Code	Added	Deleted	Revised	Grammatical Revision	Cross-reference
3309F	X				
3310F	X				
3311F	X				
3312F	X				
3315F	X				
3316F	X				
3317F	X				
3318F	X				
3319F	X				
3320F	X				
3325F	X				
3330F	X				
3331F	X				
3340F	X				
3341F	X				
3342F	X				
3343F	X				
3344F	X				
3345F	X				
3350F	X				
3351F	X				
3352F	X				
3353F	X				
3354F	X				

Therapeutic, Preventive, or Other Interventions

4006F				X	
4007F		X			
4009F				X	
4012F				X	

Section/Code	Added	Deleted	Revised	Grammatical Revision	Cross-reference
4014F				X	
4040F			X		
4044F				X	
4047F				X	
4048F				X	
4052F				X	
4053F				X	
4058F				X	
4066F				X	
4070F				X	
4120F				X	
4124F				X	
4130F	X				
4131F	X				
4132F	X				
4133F	X				
4134F	X				
4135F	X				
4136F	X				
4150F	X				
4151F	X				
4152F	X				
4153F	X				
4154F	X				
4155F	X				
4156F	X				
4157F	X				
4158F	X				
4159F	X				
4163F	X				

Section/Code	Added	Deleted	Revised	Grammatical Revision	Cross-reference
4164F	X				
4165F	X				
4167F	X				
4168F	X				
4169F	X				
4171F	X				
4172F	X				
4174F	X				
4175F	X				
4176F	X				
4177F	X				
4178F	X				
4179F	X				
4180F	X				
4181F	X				
4182F	X				
4185F	X				
4186F	X				
4187F	X				
4188F	X				
4189F	X				
4190F	X				
4191F	X				
4200F	X				
4201F	X				
4210F	X				
4220F	X				
4221F	X				
4230F	X				
4240F	X				

▲=Revised Code ●=New Code ▶◀=New or Revised Text O=Reinstated Code

Section/Code	Added	Deleted	Revised	Grammatical Revision	Cross-reference
4242F	X				
4245F	X				
4248F	X				
4250F	X				
Follow-up or Other Outcomes					
5020F	X				
5050F	X				
5060F	X				
5062F	X				
Patient Safety					
6010F				X	
6015F				X	
6030F	X				
6040F	X				
6045F	X				
Structural Measures					
7010F	X				
7020F	X				
7025F	X				

Category III Codes

Section/Code	Added	Deleted	Revised	Grammatical Revision	Cross-reference
0026T		X			
0027T		X			
0028T		X			
0029T		X			
0031T		X			
0032T		X			
0041T		X			
0043T		X			

Section/Code	Added	Deleted	Revised	Grammatical Revision	Cross-reference
0046T		X			
0047T		X			
0049T		X			
0054T	X				
0055T	X				
0058T		X			
0059T		X			
0060T		X			
0061T		X			
0073T				X	
0078T				X	
0080T				X	
0088T		X			
0089T		X			
0090T		X			
0092T			X		X
0093T		X			
0095T			X		X
0096T		X			
0098T			X		X
0124T			X		X
0137T		X			
0162T		X			
0163T			X		
0164T			X		
0165T			X		
0184T	X				X
0185T	X				X
0186T	X				
0187T	X				

▲=Revised Code   ●=New Code   ▶◀=New or Revised Text   O=Reinstated Code

Section/Code	Added	Deleted	Revised	Grammatical Revision	Cross-reference
0188T	X				
0189T	X				X
0190T	X				X
0191T	X				
0192T	X				
0193T	X				X
0194T	X				
0195T	X				
0196T	X				X

Timesaving, money-saving and easy to use

Meet all your coding needs with *CodeManager® 2009 with Netter's Atlas of Human Anatomy for CPT® Coding*. Get access to 11 essential medical coding references plus links to 400 detailed, true-to-life Frank Netter illustrations. This combination provides a complete visual rending to help you better understand anatomic structures described within Current Procedural Terminology (CPT®) codes.

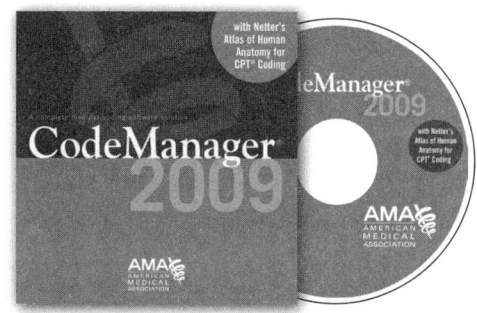

- **AMA exclusive! RBRVS Payment Calculator** lets you calculate the Medicare physician fee schedule payment amounts and RBRVS units for CPT codes for any region in the United States
- **AMA exclusive!** More than 1,700 CPT clinical examples
- **AMA exclusive!** Access the entire Dorland's Illustrated Medical Dictionary
- **New! Code report** allows you to gather all information related to a specific CPT code
- **New! Enhanced searching** enables you to search within the Surgery section for a CPT code by anatomy, method and/or device

Users	Order #	Price	AMA member price	ISBN
Single	OP135309DMZ	$546	**$464**	978-1-57947-962-6
Network 2-5	OP135409DMZ	$2,060	**$1,710**	978-1-57947-963-3
Network 6-10	OP135509DMZ	$3,840	**$3,190**	978-1-57947-964-0

CD-ROM, shipping included. Available December 2008!

For additional product and ordering information, visit *www.amabookstore.com* or call (800) 621-8335.

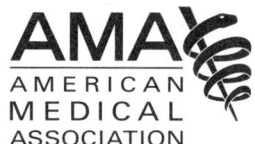

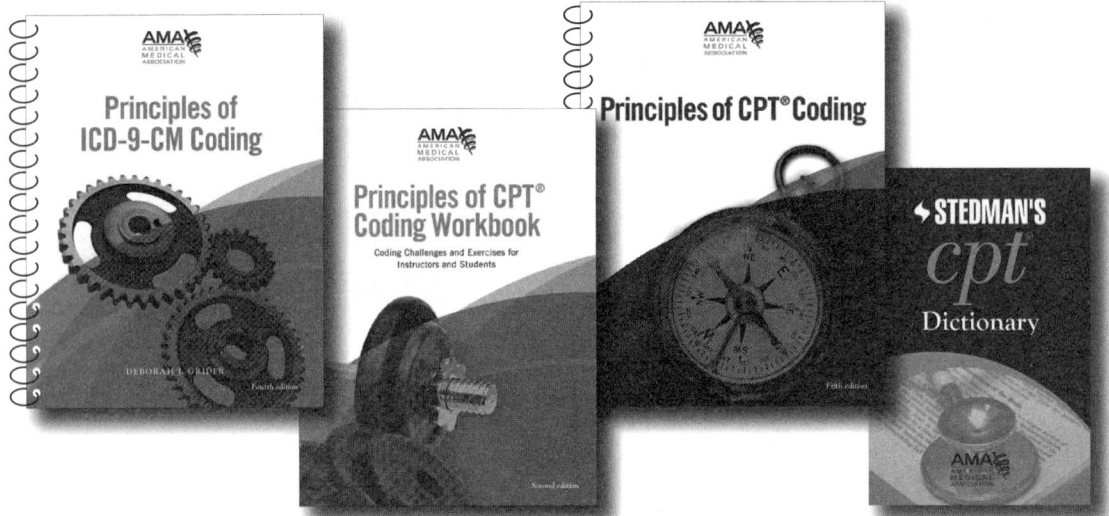

Principles of ICD-9-CM, fourth edition
This coding resource from the American Medical Association (AMA) provides helpful guidelines for identifying and locating the most appropriate codes for your practice and informative coding tips. Practical and educational, the fourth edition includes chapter learning objectives and checkpoint exercises, as well as a new timesaving CD-ROM teaching tool that lets instructors administer tests using AMA-developed questions and answers. New chapters cover symptoms, signs, ill-defined conditions, injury and poisoning, and an overview of ICD-9-CM, Volume 3, with a comparison to ICD-10-CM conventions.
Spiralbound, 8½" x 11", 356 pages, includes CD-ROM   ISBN: 978-1-57947-899-5

Principles of CPT® Coding Workbook, second edition
Newly revised and expanded, *Principles of CPT® Coding Workbook* provides in-depth instruction on key coding concepts, organized by Current Procedural Terminology (CPT®) code section. Extensive coding scenarios and operative procedure exercises accompany each chapter to test knowledge. The second edition features new chapters on Category II codes and appendixes found in the CPT codebook. This edition also contains new illustrations, decision-tree flowcharts and expanded chapters on E/M, medicine, surgery, anesthesiology and radiology.
Softbound, 8½" x 11", 300 pages   ISBN: 978-1-57947-883-4

Principles of CPT® Coding, fifth edition
Updated and revised by the AMA, this resource provides the most in-depth review available of the entire CPT codebook. Broad enough to educate the beginning coder while still offering relevant insight to those with more experience, the fifth edition explains the use of CPT codes and guidelines in a practical, easy-to-read style that addresses everyday coding challenges. Included are instructions on how to code from an operative report, and coding tips with hints on code assignments, bundling and payer policies.
Spiralbound, 8½" x 11", 580 pages   ISBN: 978-1-57947-967-1

Stedman's CPT® Dictionary
Understanding medical definitions can be one of the biggest struggles a coding or reimbursement professional faces. Developed by the AMA's CPT experts in conjunction with *Stedman's Medical Dictionary*, this resource makes coding easier by providing definitions of medical terms found within the CPT codebook descriptions.
Hardbound, 8" x 10", 425 pages   ISBN: 978-1-57947-882-7

For more information and to order online, visit *www.amabookstore.com* or call (800) 621-8335.

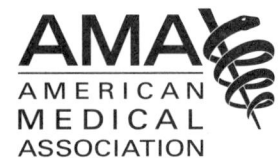

All the coding educational resources you need from the authors of CPT®

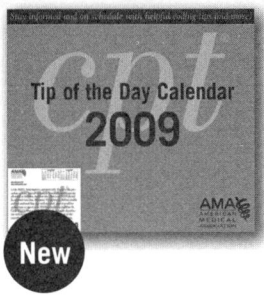

CPT® Calendar

Let the American Medical Association (AMA) help you keep track of appointments and important industry dates throughout the year. Featuring valuable coding tips from the source of Current Procedural Terminology (CPT®), the 2009 calendar is available in a convenient tear-off format perfect for the desktop.

Order #: OP060209
Price: $34.99
AMA member price: $24.99

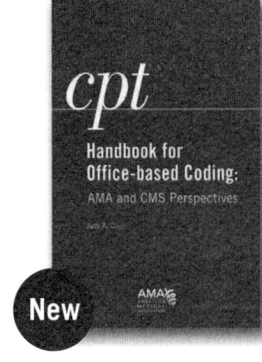

CPT® Handbook for Office-based Coding

Developed as an easy-to-navigate and timesaving handbook, this resource allows readers to quickly find coding and policy information needed to accurately report and reduce claim denials. Includes information for both national Medicare policy and CPT code information for the office-based physician.

Order #: OP057409
Price: $84.95
AMA member price: $63.95

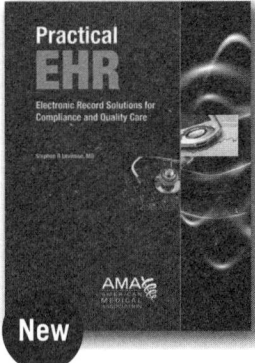

Practical EHR

An essential reference for physicians and their staff seeking to better understand critical components of electronic health records (EHRs) and their impact on physicians and patients at the point of care.

Order #: OP324408
Price: $84.95
AMA member price: $64.95

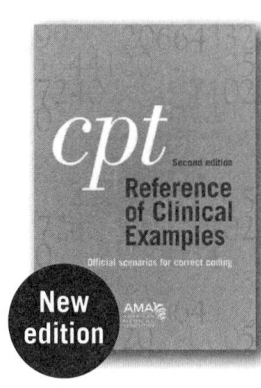

CPT® Reference of Clinical Examples, second edition

Straight from the AMA, the only reference organized by CPT codebook section that provides more than 1,000 clinical examples of the top-reported codes pulled from the proprietary CPT information database and Medicare claim data. New illustrations enhance this one-of-a-kind resource.

Order #: OP153907
Price: $99.95
AMA member price: $74.95

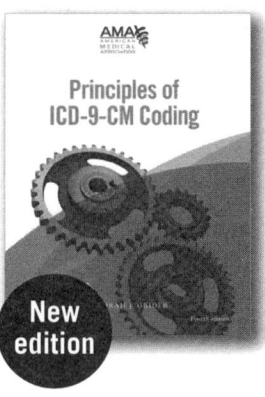

Principles of ICD-9-CM

This coding resource provides helpful guidelines for identifying and locating the most appropriate codes for your practice, as well as chapter learning objectives, checkpoint exercises and informative coding tips. Practical and educational, the fourth edition includes a new CD-ROM teaching tool so instructors can administer tests using questions and answers developed by the AMA; new chapters covering symptoms, signs, ill-defined conditions, injury and poisoning; an overview of ICD-9-CM, Volume 3 and a comparison between ICD-9-CM and ICD-10-CM conventions; and more.

Order #: OP065808
Price: $74.95
AMA member price: $59.95

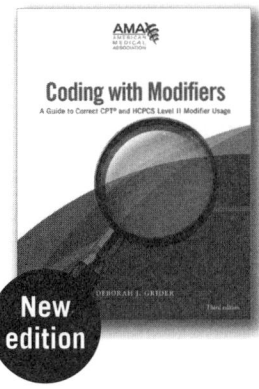

Coding with Modifiers: A Guide to Correct CPT® and HCPCS Level II Modifier Usage, third edition

Coding with Modifiers, third edition, is the definitive guide on modifier usage. This must-have resource is filled with the largest number of modifier changes since 2000, including revisions to modifiers 25, 32, 51, 58, 59, 76, 78 and new modifier 92. This new edition also contains updated CMS, third-party payer and AMA-modifier guidelines to assist in coding accurately.

Order #: OP322007
Price: $92.95
AMA member price: $69.95

To order today or to learn more, visit www.amabookstore.com or call (800) 621-8335.

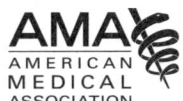

Online tool puts CPT® coding answers at your fingertips!

CPT® Network from the AMA provides expert answers and data fast—all from your desktop.

Brought to you by the American Medical Association (AMA), *CPT® Network* is a subscription-based online inquiry system that helps you find fast, accurate answers to all of your coding questions—straight from the professionals who developed the Current Procedural Terminology (CPT®) code system.

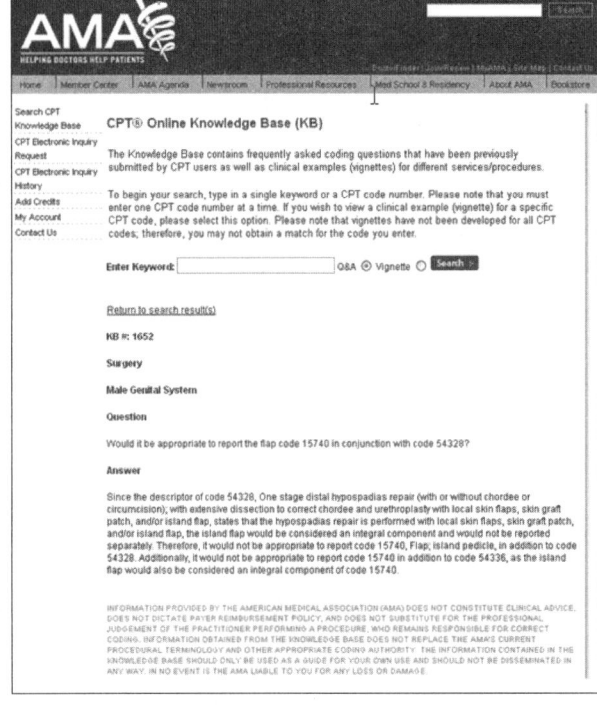

AMA member bonus: Six electronic inquiries and Knowledge Base access for one year free!

Quickly research the network's online Knowledge Base of commonly asked coding questions and clinical examples, as well as:

- Submit electronic inquiries directly to a CPT expert for timely, accurate results
- Track inquiry history
- Add credits to your account toward additional electronic inquiries (special pricing available)
- Easily update customer profile information

Subscribe today!

Call (800) 621-8335 to determine the subscription package that best meets your needs or visit **www.cptnetwork.com** for details.

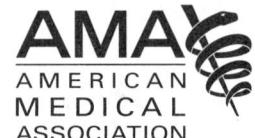

MAKING THE SWITCH
FROM PAPER TO DIGITAL?

Let the American Medical Association's many resources help you move from paper-based to electronic health records.

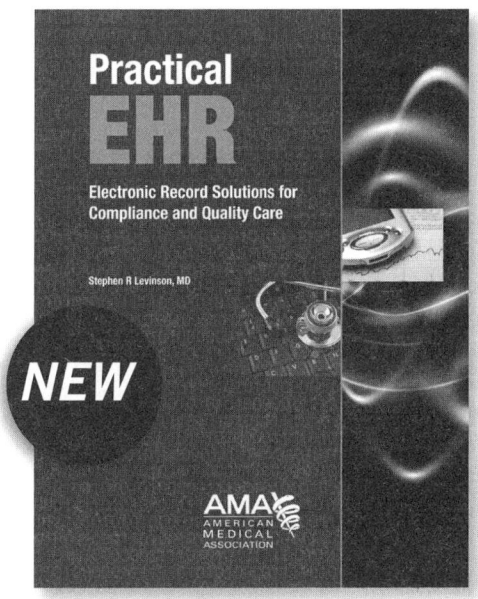

Practical EHR: Electronic Record Solutions for Compliance and Quality Care

Filled with practical information, this new resource is designed to help physicians and medical practices get the most from their current Electronic Health Record (EHR) system. In addition to delivering compliance and quality of care solutions, this book offers valuable insight on topics such as:

- EHR review at the point of care
- Medical records and E/M compliance
- Evaluation and design of the electronic history and physical
- Practice transition and health information transformation

NEW

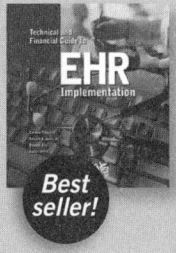

"If you don't have EHR Implementation: A Step by Step Guide for the Medical Practice, you have no business going into electronic health records. This is your guide. Follow it. I did."
—Stephen Z. Fadem,

Best seller!

Guides physicians and administrators through the evaluation, selection, negotiation and culture management transition [that often accompanies the move] to an electronic environment.

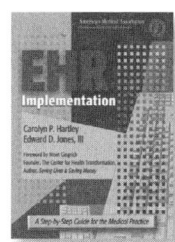

A must-have working guidebook that addresses security preparedness, measuring your EHR "ROI," remittance implementation, work flow analyses and more!

Order today! Visit www.amabookstore.com or call (800) 621-8335.

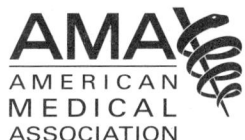

AMERICAN MEDICAL ASSOCIATION

Improve the health of your practice.

The AMA can show you how.

Helping doctors help patients begins with helping you build a stronger practice. That's why the American Medical Association (AMA) offers proven resources to help you better manage the business side of medicine.

Practice management resources that improve reimbursement
Access AMA resources on topics ranging from claims management and fee scheduling to model managed care contracts, performing internal billing audits and protecting your practice from unfair payment practices.

Discounts of up to 25 percent on AMA books and products
Enjoy members-only discounts on AMA books and products, as well as programs and services from partners such as Henry Schein medical supplies and equipment, First National credit card processing, Chase and Hertz.

Award-winning publications
Stay up to date with print or online subscriptions to *AMNews*, *JAMA*, *Archives* journals and *AMA Morning Rounds* — free for AMA members.

Powerful advocacy that's shaping the future
Stand united with AMA members nationwide on professional and public health issues, from ensuring access to medical care to pursuing fair Medicare payment.

The AMA helps its members save time, save money and build a better practice.

Join the AMA today.

Visit *www.ama-assn.org/go/join*
or call (800) 262-3211.

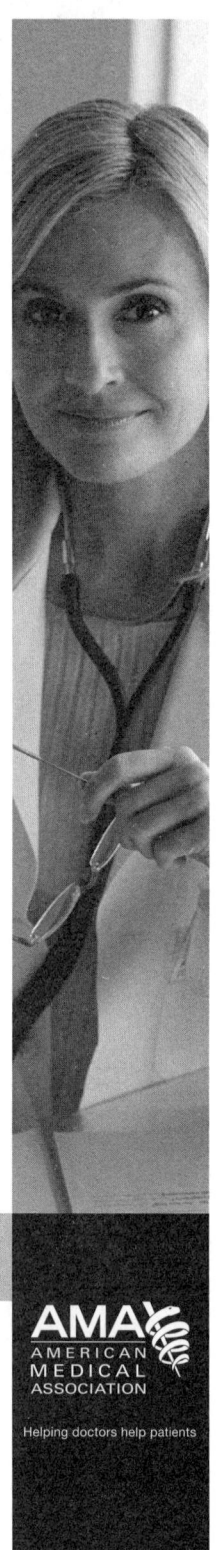

AMA
AMERICAN MEDICAL ASSOCIATION

Helping doctors help patients